Lippincott's Obstetrics
Case-Based Review

Lippincott's Obstetrics Case-Based Review

EDITORS

■■■ **MARIE H. BEALL, MD**

Professor of Obstetrics and Gynecology
David Geffen School of Medicine at UCLA
Los Angeles, California

■■■ **MICHAEL G. ROSS, MD, MPH**

Professor of Obstetrics and Gynecology
David Geffen School of Medicine at UCLA
Professor of Public Health
UCLA School of Public Health
Los Angeles, California

⊞. Wolters Kluwer | Lippincott Williams & Wilkins
Health

Philadelphia • Baltimore • New York • London
Buenos Aires • Hong Kong • Sydney • Tokyo

Acquisitions Editor: Sonya Seigafuse
Product Manager: Nicole Walz
Vendor Manager: Bridgett Dougherty
Senior Manufacturing Manager: Benjamin Rivera
Marketing Manager: Kimberly Schonberger
Design Coordinator: Terry Mallon
Production Service: Aptara, Inc.

© 2011 by LIPPINCOTT WILLIAMS & WILKINS, a WOLTERS KLUWER business
Two Commerce Square
2001 Market Street
Philadelphia, PA 19103 USA
LWW.com

Printed in China

Library of Congress Cataloging-in-Publication Data

Lippincott's obstetrics case-based review / [edited by] Marie H. Beall, Michael G. Ross.
    p. ; cm.
  Obstetrics case-based review
  Includes bibliographical references and index.
  ISBN 978-0-7817-9849-5 (pbk. : alk. paper)
1. Pregnancy—Complications—Case studies.   I. Beall, Marie H.
II. Ross, Michael G.   III. Title: Obstetrics case-based review.
  [DNLM: 1. Pregnancy Complications.   2. Case Reports. WQ 240]
  RG571.L545 2011
  618.2—dc22

                       2011004403

To purchase additional copies of this book, call our customer service department at (800) 638-3030 or fax orders to (301) 223-2320. International customers should call (301) 223-2300.

Visit Lippincott Williams & Wilkins on the Internet: at LWW.com. Lippincott Williams & Wilkins customer service representatives are available from 8:30 am to 6:00 pm, EST.

10 9 8 7 6 5 4 3 2 1

RRS1105

For Antonia, Bonnie, and Ursula.

Contributors

DAVID E. ABEL, MD
Attending Physician
Maternal-Fetal Medicine
Deaconess Medical Center
Spokane, Washington

CAROL L. ARCHIE, MD, FACOG
Associate Clinical Professor
Department of Obstetrics and Gynecology
David Geffen School of Medicine at UCLA
Los Angeles, California;
Maternal-Fetal Medicine Division
Department of Obstetrics and Gynecology
Harbor-UCLA Medical Center
Torrance, California

MARIE H. BEALL, MD
Professor of Obstetrics and Gynecology
David Geffen School of Medicine at UCLA
Los Angeles, California

JENNIFER BENEDICT, MD
Department of Obstetrics and Gynecology
Harbor-UCLA Medical Center
Torrance, California

HELENE B. BERNSTEIN, MD, PhD
Associate Professor of Reproductive Biology
Molecular Biology and Microbiology
Case Western Reserve University School of Medicine
Cleveland, Ohio

JULIE BOLES, MD
Fellow Maternal-Fetal Medicine
Department of Obstetrics and Gynecology
Harbor-UCLA Medical Center
Torrance, California

ELENA BRONSHTEIN, MD
Clinical Instructor
Department of Obstetrics and Gynecology
New York College of Osteopathic Medicine of New York
    Institute of Technology
New York, New York
Attending Physician
Department of Obstetrics and Gynecology
Newark Beth Israel Medical Center
Newark, New Jersey

RICHARD BURWICK, MD
Department of Obstetrics and Gynecology
Harbor-UCLA Medical Center
Torrance, California

ROBERT EDEN, MD
Assistant Professor
Department of Obstetrics and Gynecology
David Geffen School of Medicine at UCLA
Los Angeles, California;
Department of Obstetrics and Gynecology
Harbor-UCLA Medical Center
Torrance, California

RACINE N. EDWARDS-SILVA, MD, FACOG
Visiting Assistant Professor
Department of Obstetrics and Gynecology
David Geffen School of Medicine at UCLA
Los Angeles, California;
Division of Maternal-Fetal Medicine
Department of Obstetrics and Gynecology
Olive View-UCLA Medical Center
Sylmar, California

RAMY ESKANDER, MD
Department of Obstetrics and Gynecology
Harbor-UCLA Medical Center
Torrance, California

RIZWANA FAREEDUDDIN, MD, FACOG
Attending Physician
Division of Maternal Fetal Medicine
St. John Providence Hospital & Medical Centers
Southfield, Michigan

LAUREN FERRARA, MD
Assistant Professor
Obstetrics, Gynecology and Reproductive Science
Mount Sinai School of Medicine
Mount Sinai Medical Center
New York, New York

MARTIN L. GIMOVSKY, MD
Clinical Professor
Obstetrics, Gynecology and Reproductive Medicine
Mount Sinai School of Medicine
New York, New York;
Vice Chair and Program Director
Obstetrics and Gynecology
Newark Beth Israel Medical Center
Newark, New Jersey

JEOTSNA GROVER, MD, FACOG
Associate Clinical Professor
Obstetrics & Gynecology
David Geffen School of Medicine at UCLA
Los Angeles, California;
Director Maternal-Fetal Medicine
Obstetrics & Gynecology
Olive View UCLA Medical Center
Sylmar, California

TASMIA Q. HENRY, MD
Fellow, Maternal-Fetal Medicine
Department of Obstetrics and Gynecology
Harbor-UCLA Medical Center
Torrance, California

SAMUEL S. IM, MD
Assistant Professor
Department of Obstetrics and Gynecology
David Geffen School of Medicine at UCLA
Los Angeles, California;
Chief, Division of Gynecologic Oncology
Department of Obstetrics and Gynecology
Harbor UCLA Medical Center
Torrance, California

SHERRI JACKSON, MD, MPH
Fellow, Maternal Fetal Medicine
Department of Obstetrics and Gynecology
Cedars-Sinai Medical Center
8635 West Third Street, Suite 160 West
Los Angeles, California

MARQUIS JESSIE, MD
Fellow Maternal-Fetal Medicine
Department of Obstetrics and Gynecology
Harbor-UCLA Medical Center
Torrance, California

MATTHEW KIM, MD
Assistant Clinical Professor
Obstetrics and Gynecology
David Geffen School of Medicine at UCLA
Los Angeles, California;
Department of Obstetrics and Gynecology
Cedars-Sinai Medical Center
Los Angeles, California

STEVEN A. LAIFER, MD
Assistant Clinical Professor
Obstetrics, Gynecology and Reproductive Sciences
Yale University School of Medicine
New Haven, Connecticut;
Chief of Obstetrics
Obstetrics and Gynecology
Bridgeport Hospital
Bridgeport, Connecticut

MEN-JEAN LEE, MD
Associate Professor
Department of Obstetrics and Gynecology
Indiana University School of Medicine
Indianapolis, Indiana

RICHARD H. LEE, MD
Assistant Professor of Clinical Obstetrics and Gynecology
Keck School of Medicine
University of Southern California
Los Angeles, California

ROY Z. MANSANO, MD
Fellow Maternal-Fetal Medicine
Department of Obstetrics and Gynecology
Harbor-UCLA Medical Center
Torrance, California

AISLING MURPHY, MD
Department of Obstetrics and Gynecology
David Geffen School of Medicine at UCLA
Los Angeles, California

DOTUN OGUNYEMI, MD
Vice Associate Professor
Obstetrics & Gynecology
David Geffen School of Medicine at UCLA;
Los Angeles, California;
Vice Chair of Education
Obstetrics & Gynecology
Cedars Sinai Medical Center
Los Angeles, California

LAWRENCE D. PLATT, MD
Professor of Obstetrics and Gynecology
David Geffen School of Medicine at UCLA;
Director, Center for Fetal Medicine and Woman's Ultrasound
Los Angeles, California

JOHN D. RICHARD, MD
Fellow Maternal-Fetal Medicine
Department of Obstetrics and Gynecology
Harbor-UCLA Medical Center
Torrance, California

MICHAEL G. ROSS, MD, MPH
Professor of Obstetrics and Gynecology
David Geffen School of Medicine at UCLA
Professor of Public Health
UCLA School of Public Health
Los Angeles, California

SIEGFRIED ROTMENSCH, MD
Professor, Clinical Health Sciences
Obstetrics and Gynecology
David Geffen School of Medicine at UCLA
Director, Obstetrics and Maternal-Fetal Medicine
Obstetrics and Gynecology
Cedars-Sinai Medical Center
Los Angeles, California

NEIL SILVERMAN, MD
Clinical Professor
Department of Obstetrics and Gynecology
David Geffen School of Medicine at UCLA
Los Angeles, California

LISA VASQUEZ, MD
Department of Obstetrics and Gynecology
Harbor-UCLA Medical Center
Torrance, California

DIANA S. WOLFE, MD
Fellow Maternal-Fetal Medicine
Department of Obstetrics and Gynecology
Harbor-UCLA Medical Center
Torrance, California

SARAH YAMAGUCHI, MD
Department of Obstetrics and Gynecology
Harbor-UCLA Medical Center
Torrance, California

NOELIA ZORK, MD
Department of Obstetrics and Gynecology
Harbor-UCLA Medical Center
Torrance, California

Preface

Teaching rounds are a traditional part of the education of medical students and house officers. A patient is presented to the faculty attending, who formulates a plan for the patient at hand, but who also provides a brief overview of the topic. This overview may take the form of a brief lecture, though many faculties employ a Socratic dialog, a technique known to the house staff as "pimping." Although being questioned in front of friends and colleagues is seldom a pleasant experience, it does provide a powerful incentive to learn the material, if only to avoid future embarrassment. The dialog also allows the faculty member to determine the level of knowledge of the trainee. Add to this the practical application of the material to a real patient, and patient rounds remain one of our most effective means of teaching. Unfortunately, there remain some defects in the teaching rounds paradigm. The topics discussed are determined by the patients available and may not cover the full range of the specialty. The faculty member is usually speaking "off the cuff" and may not present a full discussion, or provide the trainee with references for further reading. Finally, the trainee has no ability to revisit the information in a less-stressful setting to solidify the lessons learned. This book represents our effort to remedy these defects, while hopefully retaining some of the flavor of morning rounds.

Taken as a whole, the book covers a wide range of medical, obstetrical, and fetal complications. Each chapter in the book concerns a single patient with a problem in clinical obstetrics. Some of the authors based their chapters on actual patients, although names and medical details were altered; others described a patient who was a composite. Each chapter begins with a description of the patient at presentation and concludes with delivery of the infant. The student is asked a number of multiple-choice questions, usually concerning management of the patient, and the correct answer is then explained. In addition, each chapter has didactic sections covering areas such as pathophysiology, not amenable to a multiple-choice format. The patient care described in these chapters is based on current evidence and recommendations, and thus represents our optimum faculty input. We chose not to reference each statement, but each chapter concludes with a list of references for additional reading. The old saying is that "good judgment comes from experience." We hope that you, the trainee, will use this book to get practical experience with patients, some of whom you may never have met, and some of whom may seem all too familiar.

Acknowledgments

We would like to acknowledge the efforts of Dr. Robert Eden, who initially proposed this book, and Dr. Roy Mansano, who was instrumental in the early recruitment of chapter authors. Drs. Susan Ballagh and David Abel assisted with editing. Our authors generously contributed time, effort, and expertise, and we thank them. Jenny Koleth attempted to keep us on schedule and on track. Our residents keep us in touch with what they need to learn.

Finally, we would like to thank our patients, who are the reason for morning rounds.

Contents

Contributors vi
Preface ix
Acknowledgments x

1   Cardiac Disease in Pregnancy 1
    Marie H. Beall

2   Pulmonary Disease in Pregnancy 7
    Marie H. Beall and Jeotsna Grover

3   Pyelonephritis in Pregnancy 12
    David E. Abel

4   Preeclampsia 17
    Rizwana Fareeduddin

5   Chronic Hypertension and Pregnancy 23
    Lisa Vasquez and Marquis Jessie

6   HELLP Syndrome 28
    Richard Burwick

7   Gestational Diabetes 32
    Jeotsna Grover

8   Diabetes in Pregnancy 36
    Dotun Ogunyemi

9   RBC Alloimmunization 41
    Steven A. Laifer

10 Pelvic Mass in Pregnancy 48
    Samuel S. Im

11 Venous Thromboembolism 53
    Steven A. Laifer

12 Trauma in Pregnancy 60
    Martin L. Gimovsky and Elena Bronshtein

13 Sexually Transmitted Diseases in Pregnancy 67
    Neil Silverman

14 Thyroid Disease in Pregnancy 74
    David E. Abel

15 HIV in Pregnancy 80
    Lauren Ferrara, Men-Jean Lee, and Helene B. Bernstein

16 Acute Abdominal Pain in Pregnancy 87
    Ramy Eskander

17 Ultrasound Diagnosis of a Congenital Anomaly 92
    Aisling Murphy and Lawrence D. Platt

18 Fetal Chromosomal Anomaly 97
    Marie H. Beall

19 Multiple Gestation 103
    Julie Boles

20 Intrauterine Growth Restriction 109
    Michael G. Ross

21 Macrosomia 114
    Marquis Jessie

22 Oligohydramnios 119
    Michael G. Ross and Marie H. Beall

23 Polyhydramnios 125
    Marie H. Beall and Michael G. Ross

24 Teratogens in Pregnancy 130
    Noelia Zork

25 Cervical Incompetence 137
    Sarah Yamaguchi

26 Preterm Labor 142
    Roy Z. Mansano

27 Uterine Anomalies 149
    Tasmia Q. Henry

28 Premature Rupture of Membranes and
    Chorioamnionitis 154
    Carol L. Archie

29 Breech Presentation 160
    Tasmia Q. Henry

30 Placenta Accreta 165
    Richard H. Lee and Jeotsna Grover

31 Placenta Previa 170
    Racine N. Edwards-Silva

32 Placental Abruption 176
    Matthew Kim

33 Postdated Pregnancy 182
    Robert Eden

34 Abnormal Labor 188
    Robert Eden

35 **Shoulder Dystocia** 195
    Sherri Jackson and Siegfried Rotmensch

36 **Postpartum Hemorrhage** 202
    Diana S. Wolfe

37 **Uterine Rupture** 208
    John D. Richard

38 **Amniotic Fluid Embolism** 213
    Robert Eden

39 **Operative Delivery** 219
    John Richard

40 **Breastfeeding** 225
    Jennifer Benedict

Index 231

Cardiac Disease in Pregnancy

Marie H. Beall

 CASE PRESENTATION

Your first patient on Monday morning is Ms. Forsythe, a 27-year-old G2 P0 Caucasian female who is at 15 and 2/7 weeks of gestation by her last menstrual period. At her initial examination 4 weeks ago, she gave a history of heart disease, and so the nurse practitioner requested her medical records and scheduled her second visit with the physician.

Ms. Forsythe reports feeling well and specifically denies any exercise limitation, shortness of breath, or palpitations. She does not yet feel fetal movement and denies any bleeding, cramping, or loss of fluid. She was born in another country and reports that 5 years ago she came to the United States to attend graduate school. She subsequently married one of her classmates and is now a U.S. citizen. Since adolescence she has had moderate exercise intolerance. After coming to the United States she was told that she had a problem with her heart. She denies other significant medical problems, or medication use; she has a history of one pregnancy termination 2 years ago.

On physical examination, she is a slender woman in no apparent distress. Her blood pressure is 110/55 mm Hg and her pulse is 95 bpm. Her physical examination is unremarkable except for a grade III/VI holosystolic murmur, heard best in the lower left sternal border. The oxygen saturation in her right index finger is 98%.

Review of medical records reveals that Ms. Forsythe had an echocardiogram 3 years ago that revealed a ventricular septal defect (VSD) with left-to-right flow. She was scheduled for a cardiac catheterization, but this was never performed.

 Decision 1: Evaluation

Which of the following suggests worsening cardiac status in a pregnant patient?

- A. Mild shortness of breath
- B. Dependent edema
- C. Increased pulse rate
- D. Rales on lung examination

The correct answer is D: Rales on lung examination. Rales are not heard in the examination of a normal pregnant woman. By contrast, shortness of breath (Answer A), dependent edema (Answer B), and an increase in pulse rate (Answer C) may be seen in normal pregnant patients.

 NEED TO KNOW

Cardiac Physiology in Pregnancy

The diagnosis of cardiac disease in pregnancy may be complicated by the normal physiologic changes occurring in pregnant women. In pregnancy, the diaphragm elevates by about 4 cm, causing the heart to assume a more horizontal position in the chest. This results in lateral deviation of the cardiac apex, with a larger cardiac silhouette on chest x-ray and a shift in the electrical axis. In addition to the changes in position, the heart increases in size by about 12%. Cardiac output increases by 30% to 50%, with most of the increase occurring in the first trimester. The increase in cardiac output is the consequence of an increase in both the heart rate and the stroke volume: In a pregnant woman, the heart rate increases by about 17%, with the maximum reached by the middle of the third trimester (32 weeks). The stroke volume increases by 32%, with the maximum reached by midgestation. Although the cardiac output generally increases, in late pregnancy the cardiac output may decrease significantly (25%–30%) when the patient lies in the supine position (as compared with the left lateral position) because of compression of the inferior vena cava by the pregnant uterus, with resultant decreased venous return.

The distribution of blood flow is altered in pregnancy: At term, 17% of the cardiac output is directed to the uterus and its contents, and an additional 2% goes to the breasts. The skin and kidneys receive additional blood flow when compared with the nonpregnant state, and blood flow to the brain and liver may increase. Perfusion of other organs such as the skeletal muscle and gut remains unchanged.

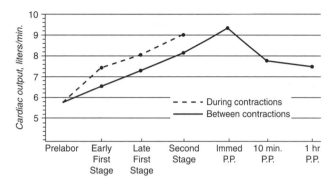

Figure 1.1 Hemodynamics during parturition. Cardiac output during the various phases of labor between and during contractions. Note the progressive increase between the contractions and a further 15% to 20% increase during contractions.
(Adapted from Bonica JJ. *Obstetric Analgesia and Anesthesia.* 2nd ed. Amsterdam: World of Societies of Anesthesiologists; 1980:6, with permission.)

Vascular resistance, both systemic and pulmonary, decreases during pregnancy. A concomitant decrease in systemic blood pressure reaches its nadir at about 24 weeks of gestation. Blood pressure then rises gradually until term but generally does not exceed nonpregnant levels. Mean arterial pressure, pulmonary capillary wedge pressure, central venous pressure, and left ventricular stroke work index remain unchanged, whereas colloid osmotic pressure is decreased.

Labor and delivery are associated with additional cardiac stress. Cardiac output may increase by as much as 40% in patients not receiving pain relief, although those with adequate anesthesia experience much smaller rises. The rise in cardiac output increases with progressive stages of labor, and there is a further rise of approximately 15% during each uterine contraction resulting from the expression of 300 to 500 mL of blood from the uterus back into the mother's circulation (Fig. 1.1). Delivery is associated with as much as a 59% increase in cardiac output, presumably a result of autotransfusion of blood contained in the uterus. This increase may be blunted by the blood loss at delivery.

 CASE CONTINUES

An ultrasound reveals a normally grown fetus; the fetal anatomy appears to be normal, consistent with a 15-week gestation. A serum screen is obtained.

You question Ms. Forsythe about her exercise tolerance. She reports that she can usually walk 5 to 6 blocks without shortness of breath and that she regularly does household chores. However, she states that lately (for about 6 months) she has had increased shortness of

breath with exercise, so much so that she has stopped dancing with her husband. You refer her to the cardiologist for an echocardiogram and consultation.

 Decision 2: Risk assessment

What information is most important to obtain from a maternal echocardiogram in this patient?

   A. Pulmonic valve area
   B. Left ventricular ejection fraction
   C. Amount and direction of flow across the VSD
   D. Left ventricular wall thickness

The correct answer is C: Amount and direction of flow across the VSD. With a large VSD, blood will flow from the left ventricle to the lower-pressure right heart and the lungs. Over time, this volume overload leads to damage to the pulmonary vasculature and pulmonary hypertension (Eisenmenger's syndrome). Eventually, the pulmonary pressure may exceed that in the systemic circulation, with reversal of the shunt, resulting in right-to-left flow. This may be more severe during exercise, when systemic pressure drops. Eisenmenger's syndrome has been associated with a 50% maternal mortality, and it represents one of the highest-risk cardiac lesions in pregnancy.

 NEED TO KNOW

Counseling the Patient with Heart Disease About Pregnancy

Given the dramatic increase in demand on the heart in pregnancy, patients with cardiac disease may be at increased risk for morbidity and mortality with pregnancy. Patients with symptomatic heart disease are the most at risk. The New York Heart Association Functional Classification of heart disease (Table 1.1) is often used to describe the patient's functional status, and it has been shown to correlate with maternal morbidity. Certain cardiac lesions carry a much higher risk of maternal morbidity; left ventricular dysfunction and pulmonary hypertension carry especially poor prognoses. A matrix for maternal risk in pregnancy depending on the cardiac lesion is presented in Table 1.2. Notably, the causes of maternal heart disease are evolving; in the past the most common cardiac finding in young women was valvular stenosis as a consequence of rheumatic fever. Improvements in antibiotics and in the care of children with congenital heart disease mean that in developed countries, the majority of gravidas with cardiac complications are survivors of congenital heart disease.

TABLE 1.1

NEW YORK HEART ASSOCIATION (NYHA) FUNCTIONAL CLASSES OF HEART DISEASE

NYHA Class	Symptoms
I	No symptoms and no limitation in ordinary physical activity, e.g., shortness of breath when walking or climbing stairs
II	Mild symptoms (mild shortness of breath and/or angina) and slight limitation during ordinary activity
III	Marked limitation in activity due to symptoms, even during less-than-ordinary activity, e.g., walking short distances (20–100 m) Comfortable only at rest
IV	Severe limitations. Experiences symptoms even while at rest. Mostly bedbound patients

Reprinted with permission. www.heart.org. Copyright 2011, American Heart Association, Inc.

Postrheumatic changes are now responsible for about 20% of cases. The number of pregnant women with ischemic or atherosclerotic heart disease is very small.

Prior to pregnancy, a woman with heart disease should be aware of the special risks associated with her diagnosis. In terms of counseling the cardiac patient regarding pregnancy, several issues must be addressed:

■ The risk of death or disability related to pregnancy to the patient. (In a recent report, it was found that there was a 20% risk of death or serious cardiac event in a mixed population of pregnant cardiac patients.)
■ The life expectancy of the patient and her likely ability to raise the child.

■ The possibility of effect of the maternal heart disease (see below) on the fetus or pregnancy.
■ The teratogenicity of any medications, and what alternatives are available.
■ The need to optimize maternal functional status prior to pregnancy. This may involve a change in medication, or it may mean performing cardiac surgery (e.g., to repair a stenotic valve) prior to initiating pregnancy.

In addition to the cardiac risk to the mother, the presence of maternal cardiac disease poses a substantial risk of poor perinatal outcome (Table 1.3). The highest rate of pregnancy complications occurs in patients with cyanotic congenital heart disease. In one report, the live birth rate was only 43% in mothers with cyanotic congenital heart disease, and up to 50% of the surviving newborns may be premature or growth restricted, or both.

Many patients, especially those with mechanical heart valves and other foreign bodies in their vascular system, will require lifelong anticoagulation. Of note, warfarin is teratogenic and should be avoided in pregnancy if possible, particularly in the first trimester. Unfortunately, heparin is not as well studied in the context of the patient with an artificial valve, and the patient may have to make a choice between potential harm to the fetus and the potential of a valve thrombosis.

The best management of the patient with cardiac disease would include a preconception visit with an obstetrician or cardiologist experienced in the management of such complications. The patient could then be provided with her risks and recommendations and could elect to become pregnant with appropriate knowledge.

TABLE 1.2

EXPECTED MATERNAL MORTALITY IN PREGNANCY FROM VARIOUS MATERNAL CARDIAC ABNORMALITIES

Groups	Underlying Cardiac Disease	Mortality
Group 1	Atrial septal defect, uncomplicated ventricular septal defect, patent ductus arteriosus in the absence of pulmonary hypertension, pulmonic and tricuspid disease, repaired tetralogy of Fallot, bioprosthetic valve, and mitral stenosis (functional class I and II)	<1%
Group 2	Mitral stenosis with atrial fibrillation, mechanical valve prostheses, mitral stenosis (functional class >II), aortic stenosis, uncomplicated coarctation of the aorta, unrepaired tetralogy of Fallot, previous myocardial infarction with preserved left ventricular function, and Marfan syndrome with aortic dimension <40 mm.	5%–15%
Group 3	Pulmonary hypertension, complicated coarctation of the aorta, and Marfan syndrome with aortic dimension ≥40 mm	25%–50%

From Abbas AE, Lester SJ, Connolly H. Pregnancy and the cardiovascular system. Int J Cardiol. 2005;98(2): 179–89, with permission.

TABLE 1.3

ADVERSE OBSTETRIC EVENTS, 74 PREGNANCIES AMONG 69 WOMEN

Maternal Lesion	Number of Pregnancies With Events/ Category	Total Number of Obstetric Events	Preterm Birth	Preeclampsia	Small for Gestational Age (Less Than 10th Percentile)	NICU Admission
Overall	34/74 (45.9)	44	13 (17.7)	7 (9.5)	16 (21.6)	8 (10.8)
Right obstructive	2/3 (66.7)	2	0	0	2	0
Left obstructive[a]	3/14 (21.4)	4	1	0	2	1
Right regurgitant	1/4 (25.0)	1	1	0	0	0
Left regurgitant	4/6 (66.7)	4	1	1	1	1
Shunts[a]	14/19 (73.7)	20	9	3	4	4
Conotruncal[a]	9/19 (47.4)	12	2	1	7	2
Miscellaneous	1/4 (25.0)	1	0	1	0	0

Note: Data are n/N (%). As in other studies, the highest rate of complications occurred in patients with cyanotic congenital heart disease (those with shunts and conotruncal abnormalities). There were no cases of stillbirth.
[a]Ten pregnancies experienced two adverse obstetric events, including six shunts, three conotruncal defects, and one left obstructive defect.
NICU, neonatal intensive care unit.
From Ford AA, Wylie BJ, Waksmonski CA, Simpson LL. Maternal congenital cardiac disease: outcomes of pregnancy in a single tertiary care center. Obstet Gynecol. 2008;112(4):828–33, with permission.

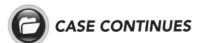 **CASE CONTINUES**

The echocardiogram, performed at rest, demonstrates left-to-right flow across the VSD. The pulmonary artery systolic pressure is estimated to be 35 mm Hg, which is above normal, but which does not predict pulmonary hypertension. The cardiologist suggests that the patient consider pregnancy termination because of the risk of death with pregnancy.

You discuss the issue with Ms. Forsythe, and she is adamant about continuing the pregnancy. You agree to care for her during the pregnancy. Her maternal serum screen (quadruple screen) is negative. You send her to the perinatologist for consultation regarding her and her fetus' risk. The perinatologist points out that she is at increased risk for fetal cardiac malformations and recommends a fetal echocardiogram.

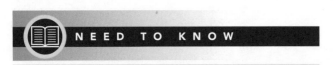 **N E E D   T O   K N O W**

Inheritance of Heart Disease

In the United States, 70% to 80% cases of cardiac disease seen in pregnancy are the result of congenital cardiac malformations. The presence of a congenital lesion raises the question of the risk of genetically

mediated heart disease in the fetus of the affected mother.

Some congenital heart disease is associated with other malformations. Examples would be Down Syndrome or the VATERR (vertebral defects, anal atresia, tracheoesophageal fistula, radial and renal defects) association. In nonsyndromic congenital heart disease, some families exhibit Mendelian inheritance, with identifiable gene defects, while others show apparent multifactorial inheritance, with recurrence risks of 1% to 5% with one affected child (Table 1.4). The risk of recurrence increases to 10% if there are two affected persons in a family. Older work suggests that the recurrence risk of congenital heart disease with multifactorial inheritance is higher with affected parents than with affected siblings and that it is the highest of all with an affected mother. Small series have suggested that the recurrence risk of congenital heart disease when the mother has a VSD may be as high as 16%, although these studies may have included families with a dominantly inherited form of VSD. In recurrent heart defects due to multifactorial inheritance, the defects belong to the same general group about 50% of the time, but there may be a wide variation in the severity and specific type of defect.

In the pregnancy at risk for congenital cardiac defects, prenatal diagnosis may be offered with fetal echocardiography. Recent reviews suggest that experienced centers will detect up to 85% of significant anomalies when performing the examination in the late first or early second trimester.

TABLE 1.4
RECURRENCE RISK FOR NONSYNDROMIC CONGENITAL HEART DISEASE

Congenital Heart Defect	Mode of Inheritance	Recurrence Risk (One Affected First-Degree Relative)
Atrioventricular canal defect	Multifactorial Autosomal dominant	3%–4% 50% (affected parent only)
Tetralogy of Fallot	Multifactorial Autosomal dominant Autosomal recessive	2.5%–3% 50% (affected parent only) 25% (affected sibling only)
Transposition of the great arteries	Multifactorial Autosomal dominant	2.5%–3% 50% (affected parent only)
Congenitally corrected transposition of the great arteries	Multifactorial	5.8%
Left-sided obstructions	Multifactorial Autosomal dominant Autosomal recessive	3% 50% (affected parent only) 25% (affected sibling only)
Atrial septal defect	Multifactorial Autosomal dominant	3% 50% (affected parent only)

[a]Adapted from Calcagni G, Digilio MC, Sarkozy A, Dallapiccola B, Marino B. Familial recurrence of congenital heart disease: an overview and review of the literature. Eur J Pediatr. 2007;166(2):111–6.

 CASE CONTINUES

Ms. Forsythe undergoes fetal echocardiography at 20 weeks of gestation, with no fetal abnormalities found. At 28 and at 32 weeks of gestation she has a fetal evaluation by ultrasound for growth, and fetal growth proceeds at the 30th percentile. She continues to function at New York Heart Association Class I to II, with minimal symptoms of shortness of breath with exercise. At 35 weeks of gestation, she comes for a fetal evaluation and is found to have decreased amniotic fluid, with an amniotic fluid index (AFI) of 5 cm. She is admitted to the hospital, and an amniocentesis reveals fetal lung maturity.

 Decision 3: Delivery

What is the optimum delivery plan?

A. Ample intravenous (IV) fluid, antibiotics for endocarditis prophylaxis
B. Ample IV fluid, no antibiotics for endocarditis prophylaxis
C. Limit IV fluid, antibiotics for endocarditis prophylaxis
D. Limit IV fluid, no antibiotics for endocarditis prophylaxis

The correct answer is B: Ample IV fluid, no antibiotics for endocarditis prophylaxis. With a connection between the right and left circulations, a drop in the systemic vascular resistance may precipitate right-to-left shunting and systemic hypoxia. In general, such a patient is managed with an ample amount of IV fluid so as to reduce the risk of hypotension with delivery. In terms of antibiotic prophylaxis, the American Heart Association currently recommends antibiotic prophylaxis for vaginal delivery only for patients with prosthetic valves or those with unrepaired or palliated cyanotic heart disease.

 CASE CONCLUSION

Ms. Forsythe is admitted to the hospital. She undergoes labor induction with oxytocin, and delivers a 2200-g female infant with Apgar score of 7/9 at 1 and 5 minutes. The mother and the baby subsequently do well, and she is discharged home, with planned follow-up with the cardiologist.

SUGGESTED READINGS

Abbas AE, Lester SJ, Connolly H. Pregnancy and the cardiovascular system. Int J Cardiol. 2005;98(2):179–89.
Calcagni G, Digilio MC, Sarkozy A, Dallapiccola B, Marino B. Familial recurrence of congenital heart disease: an overview and review of the literature. Eur J Pediatr. 2007;166(2):111–6. Epub 2006 Nov 8.

Clapp JF III, Capeless E. Cardiovascular function before, during, and after the first and subsequent pregnancies. Am J Cardiol. 1997; 80(11):1469–73.

Duvekot JJ, Peeters LL. Maternal cardiovascular hemodynamic adaptation to pregnancy. Obstet Gynecol Surv. 1994;49(12, suppl): S1–14.

Ford AA, Wylie BJ, Waksmonski CA, Simpson LL. Maternal congenital cardiac disease: outcomes of pregnancy in a single tertiary care center. Obstet Gynecol. 2008;112(4):828–33.

Kovacs AH, Harrison JL, Colman JM, Sermer M, Siu SC, Silversides CK. Pregnancy and contraception in congenital heart disease: what women are not told. J Am Coll Cardiol. 2008;52(7):577–8.

Mabie WC, DiSessa TG, Crocker LG, Sibai BM, Arheart KL. A longitudinal study of cardiac output in normal human pregnancy. Am J Obstet Gynecol. 1994;170(3):849–56.

Pierpont ME, Basson CT, Benson DW Jr, et al. Genetic basis for congenital heart defects: current knowledge: a scientific statement from the American Heart Association Congenital Cardiac Defects Committee, Council on Cardiovascular Disease in the Young: endorsed by the American Academy of Pediatrics. Circulation. 2007;115(23):3015–38.

Sermer M, Colman J, Siu S. Pregnancy complicated by heart disease: a review of Canadian experience. J Obstet Gynaecol. 2003;23(5): 540–4.

Silversides CK, Colman JM, Sermer M, Siu SC. Cardiac risk in pregnant women with rheumatic mitral stenosis. Am J Cardiol. 2003; 91(11): 1382–5.

Siu SC, Colman JM. Heart disease and pregnancy. Heart. 2001;85(6): 710–5.

Warnes CA, Williams RG, Bashore TM, et al. ACC/AHA 2008 Guidelines for the Management of Adults with Congenital Heart Disease: Executive Summary: a report of the American College of Cardiology/American Heart Association Task Force on Practice Guidelines. Circulation. 2008;8(23):2395–451.

Pulmonary Disease in Pregnancy

Marie H. Beall   Jeotsna Grover

CASE PRESENTATION

You are called by the nurse on labor and delivery. Ms. June, a patient of the hospital clinic, has presented in labor and delivery for respiratory distress. She is 21 years old, G2 P0, with an intrauterine pregnancy at 30 weeks of gestation by last menstrual period, confirmed by a 14-week ultrasound. She has had no prior problems in this pregnancy. Prenatal labs are unremarkable. Her prior pregnancy ended at 10 weeks with an elective termination. Her past medical history is significant for a history of asthma, currently not requiring medication. She is allergic to seafood and reports asthma exacerbations with exercise. She uses an inhaler before running, but she has not done this since 18 weeks of pregnancy. The nurse reports that the patient is wheezing.

You see the patient in the triage room where she reports feeling short of breath. She has obvious wheezes in all lung fields. Her oxygen saturation is 97%. She is breathing 18 times per minute. Pulmonary function testing reveals a forced expiratory volume in 1 second (FEV_1) that is 80% of normal for this patient her. Fetal heart tones are 135 bpm with normal variability.

NEED TO KNOW

Respiratory Physiology in Pregnancy

During pregnancy, the respiratory system undergoes both anatomic and functional changes. Anatomically, the thoracic cavity becomes wider and shorter. The subcostal angle increases from about 68 degrees to about 103 degrees, with a concomitant increase in the transthoracic diameter. The resting level of the diaphragm is 4 cm higher at term than in the nongravid state. Many authors state that this elevation is a result of pressure from the expanding uterus. However, diaphragmatic excursions are increased by 1 to 2 cm over nonpregnant values, suggesting that uterine pressure is not the sole cause of the elevation.

Several aspects of pulmonary function change during pregnancy (Fig. 2.1). Vital capacity (the total amount of air that can be forcibly inspired or expired) is unchanged. However, during pregnancy, expiratory reserve volume decreases by about 200 mL and inspiratory reserve volume increases by about 300 mL. The net result of these changes is that both the tidal volume (normal breath volume) and the inspiratory capacity (the maximal inspiration from rest) increase, while the total lung volume decreases.

Total body oxygen uptake at rest increases by about 30 to 40 mL/min in pregnancy, or about 12% to 20%. Most of the oxygen is needed to meet maternal metabolic alterations. The increased oxygen need is met by increased tidal volume alone, as the pulmonary diffusing capacity appears to be decreased in pregnancy and the respiratory rate does not significantly increase. There is a total increase in minute ventilation of 48% at term, which exceeds the need for increased oxygen delivery. This "hyperventilation of pregnancy" appears to be hormonally mediated and results in a decrease in $Paco_2$ to approximately 30 mm Hg in normal women. Maternal pH does not change because there is a reciprocal decline in bicarbonate concentration. The net result of these acid–base alterations is facilitation of fetal–maternal CO_2 exchange.

? Decision 1: Treatment

What is the most appropriate initial treatment?

- **A.** Theophylline PO
- **B.** Inhaled steroids
- **C.** Cromolyn sodium
- **D.** Inhaled albuterol

The correct answer is D: Inhaled albuterol. Although inhaled steroids may be very useful in the treatment of the pregnant asthmatic, their onset of action is slow, making them a poor choice for an acute event. Theophylline and cromolyn sodium have also been used safely in pregnancy,

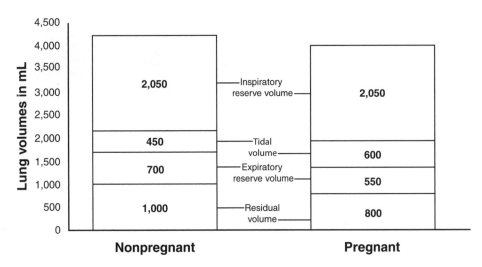

Figure 2.1 Changes in pulmonary function during pregnancy. The residual volume is the air left in the lung after maximal expiration. Tidal volume is the usual breath volume, while inspiratory and expiratory reserve volumes are the additional volumes that can be voluntarily inhaled or exhaled by the patient. Total lung capacity is the sum of all measurements (4,200 mL for nonpregnant and 4,000 mL for pregnant patients), and vital capacity is total lung capacity minus the residual volume. (Adapted from Creasy RK, Resnik R, Iams JD, et al. eds. Creasy and Resnik's Maternal Fetal Medicine Principles and Practice, 6th edition. Elsevier, 2009, p. 1299.)

although less common than albuterol and inhaled steroids. Their onset of action is also too slow to treat an acute exacerbation.

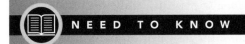

Management of Asthma in Pregnancy

The clinical course of asthma in pregnancy is unpredictable. Patients' condition may worsen, improve, or remain the same in approximately equal numbers. The reason for worsening asthma is unclear in most patients. In managing asthma, the first priority is to have the patient avoid asthma triggers. These vary with the patient, but may include allergens, exercise, or even cold (Table 2.1). When medication is needed, asthma is man-

TABLE 2.1
COMMON ASTHMA TRIGGERS

Category of Trigger	Examples
Allergens	Dust, molds, pollen, animal dander, dust mites, bugs
Irritants	Air pollution, cigarette smoke, wood burning stoves
Medical complications	Infections, sinusitis, esophageal reflux
Medications	Aspirin, nonsteroidal anti-inflammatory drugs, β-blockers, contrast media
Psychological stress	Stress, excessive laughter or crying, menses
Others	Food, exercise, changes in weather

From Curran CA. The effects of rhinitis, asthma, and acute respiratory distress syndrome as acute or chronic pulmonary conditions during pregnancy. J Perinat Neonatal Nurs. 2006 Apr-Jun;20(2):147–54. (Table 2).

aged using "step therapy," with the dose and number of medications increasing as the patient's asthma worsens (Tables 2.2 and 2.3). Most often, inhaled albuterol is used for acute asthma, with inhaled steroids for maintenance therapy. None of the medications commonly used to treat asthma is contraindicated in pregnancy. Although some medications, such as leukotriene modulators, have not been well studied in pregnancy, the possibility of fetal harm from the medication must be balanced with the likelihood of fetal harm if the mother has an asthma exacerbation due to inadequate treatment.

In order to guide management, it is important to query the patient on the presence of symptoms suggestive of exacerbation at each office visit. The clinical signs suggestive of a serious exacerbation include use of accessory muscles of respiration and tachypnea. In addition, centers specialized in treating asthma use an objective measure of lung function to track the patient's progress. Although the FEV_1 (forced expiratory volume in 1 second) is the gold standard for lung function, this test requires formal pulmonary function testing. The peak expiratory flow rate (PEFR or "peak flow") can be obtained using a peak flow meter, an inexpensive portable device. Patients with mild asthma might have their peak flow measured once or twice a month in the clinic, but patients with severe or worsening asthma may benefit from more frequent testing. In many cases, these patients are given a meter to take home and are asked to test frequently, often daily.

To effectively use the peak flow meter, the patient must know her usual PEFR. Expected peak flow rates in pregnancy are 380 to 550 L/min; however, this is a wide range. When the patient's usual peak flow has been established, she can be given a chart with cutoffs for action. In general, it is desirable to have a PEFR at

TABLE 2.2

DEFINITION OF ASTHMA STAGES. ASTHMA STAGE IS USED TO GUIDE MEDICAL THERAPY

	Disease Features Before Treatment		
	Symptoms in Daytime	Symptoms at Night	Peak Flow (% of Personal Best)
Mild intermittent	≤2 days per week	≤2 nights per month	≥80%
Mild persistent	>2 days per week, but less than daily	>2 nights per month	≥80%
Moderate persistent	Daily	>1 night per week	60–80%
Severe persistent	Continual	Frequent	≤60%

Adapted from National Heart, Lung and Blood Institute; National Asthma Education and Prevention Program Asthma and Pregnancy Working Group. NAEPP expert panel report. Managing asthma during pregnancy: recommendations for pharmacologic treatment-2004 update. J Allergy Clin Immunol. 2005;115(1):34–46.

least 80% of usual. When the patient experiences symptoms, a peak flow of 50% to 80% indicates an incomplete response to treatment, while a peak flow of <50% indicates a need for acute management and possible hospitalization (Fig. 2.2).

CASE CONTINUES

The patient is treated on labor and delivery with inhaled albuterol, oxygen, and hydration. Her white blood cell count is 8.4 × 10³/mL, and she is afebrile. She reports no recent exposures to her known triggers. She has resolution of her acute symptoms but continues to have daily episodes of wheezing requiring albuterol use. You decide to begin inhaled corticosteroids, and give the patient a peak flow meter with instructions to use it daily and whenever she experiences symptoms. She is discharged from the hospital.

Decision 2: Follow Up

What factors are assessed regularly in prenatal care in a pregnant asthmatic?

A. Maternal O_2 saturation
B. Fetal growth
C. Placental grade
D. Maternal weight

The correct answer is B: Fetal growth. Moderate and severe asthma, as well as poorly controlled asthma, have been associated with an increased risk of fetal growth restriction. Especially in a patient with worsening asthma or frequent exacerbations, the fetus may benefit from a regular program of fetal testing both for growth and fetal well-being. In addition to monitoring fetal growth, consideration could be given to serial testing by modified biophysical profile after 32 weeks of gestation, and to Doppler interrogation of the umbilical vessels.

TABLE 2.3

STEP THERAPY OF ASTHMA IN PREGNANCY

	Management	
Type	Preferred	Alternative
Mild intermittent asthma	No daily medications; albuterol as needed	
Mild persistent asthma	Low-dose inhaled corticosteroid	Cromolyn, leukotriene receptor antagonist, or theophylline (serum level 5–12 μg/mL
Moderate persistent asthma	Low-dose inhaled corticosteroid and salmeterol or medium-dose inhaled corticosteroid or (if needed) medium-dose inhaled corticosteroid and salmeterol	Low-dose or (if needed) medium-dose inhaled corticosteroid and either leukotriene receptor antagonist or theophylline (serum level 5–12 μg/mL)
Severe persistent asthma	High-dose inhaled corticosteroid and salmeterol and (if needed) oral corticosteroid	High-dose inhaled corticosteroid and theophylline (serum level 5–12 μg/mL) and oral corticosteroid if needed

From Dombrowski MP. Asthma and pregnancy. Obstet Gynecol. 2006;108(3 Pt 1):667–81 used with permission.

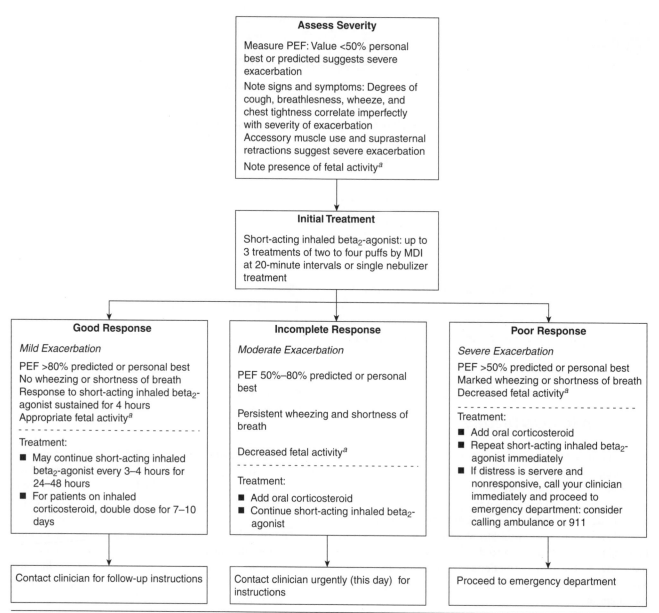

MDI, metered-dose inhaler; PEF, peak expiratory flow.
[a]Fetal activity is monitored by observing whether fetal kick counts decrease over time.

Figure 2.2 Outpatient management algorithm for the pregnant asthmatic (from NAEPP expert panel report National Heart, Lung and Blood Institute; National Asthma Education and Prevention Program Asthma and Pregnancy Working Group. NAEPP expert panel report. Managing asthma during pregnancy: recommendations for pharmacologic treatment-2004 update. J Allergy Clin Immunol. 2005;115(1):34–46.(Figure 4)). Management is guided by the response to treatment, as measured by the PEF (peak expiratory flow). To utilize this algorithm, the patient must have access to a peak flow meter and must know her expected peak flow.

Maternal O_2 saturation is not a sensitive indicator of maternal oxygenation. Placental grade may be accelerated in the hypoxic gestation, but it is not the most sensitive indicator of fetal harm. Although maternal obesity may increase the incidence of asthma, enhanced monitoring of maternal weight is not useful in the management of the asthmatic patient.

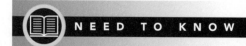

Prognosis of Asthma in Pregnancy

Asthma is a common complication of pregnancy, affecting about 8% of pregnant women. The incidence of asthma is increasing worldwide. The cause for the increase is uncertain, but increasing air pollution and obesity have both been implicated. Asthma in pregnancy, especially severe asthma (Table 2.2), may be associated with increased perinatal morbidity. In several trials, moderate or severe asthma has been associated with preterm delivery (<37 weeks), fetal growth restriction, preeclampsia, gestational diabetes, and cesarean delivery. Abnormal outcomes are more common in patients with poor lung function, indicating the importance of optimal asthma treatment in pregnancy. Most authors agree that active management of asthma in pregnancy will improve pregnancy outcomes, and there is observational data that the risk of low birth weight is significantly increased only in those asthmatic mothers not treated optimally.

In addition to effects during pregnancy, maternal asthma is a risk factor for asthma in the child. The mechanism is unknown, but it may be due to inflammatory mediators being transferred from mother to fetus, rather than a genetic cause.

 ## CASE CONTINUES

Ms. June continues in prenatal care. She receives influenza vaccine. She experiences gradually worsening asthma, with daily wheezing despite the use of inhaled steroids and albuterol. You elect to monitor her with ultrasounds every 4 weeks for fetal growth and modified biophysical profiles weekly after 32 weeks. At 37 weeks of gestation, a scheduled ultrasound reveals that the fetal abdominal circumference is lagging 2 weeks behind the other measurements. The estimated fetal weight is 2,400 g (less than the 10th percentile), the amniotic fluid index is 6.6 cm, and the placenta appears to be grade 2. You decide to admit Ms. June and induce her labor for fetal growth restriction at term.

 ### Decision 3: Management

What should be a part of the delivery plan due to the asthma?

- A. Prophylactic antibiotics
- B. Avoid pushing
- C. Avoid carboprost use
- D. Avoid oxygen use

The answer is C: Avoid carboprost use. Carboprost tromethamine (Hemabate) is $PGF_{2\alpha}$, a prostaglandin that

acts as a bronchoconstrictor. It should be used with caution in a patient with asthma. Methylergonovine may also cause bronchospasm, so the treatment of postpartum bleeding in a severely asthmatic patient should be very closely monitored no matter the treatment being used. In this case, the patient's allergy to seafood may also indicate a sensitivity to iodine, and the use of iodine-containing solutions on her skin may cause a reaction.

In labor, the asthmatic mother should be kept hydrated. Good pain control may help to reduce her oxygen consumption. There is no contraindication to pushing and vaginal delivery. Oxygen is not typically necessary, but is not contraindicated. There is no indication for prophylactic antibiotics due to asthma, although those on systemic steroids may benefit from a stress dose of steroids during labor.

 ## CASE CONCLUSION

Ms. June is admitted to the hospital. She undergoes mechanical cervical ripening with a balloon catheter, after which her Bishop score is 7. She undergoes labor induction with oxytocin, and during labor she receives 125 mL/hr of lactated Ringer's solution and 4 L of oxygen by nasal cannula. At 4 cm of cervical dilation, she asks for, and receives, a labor epidural. After a total of 15 hours, she delivers a 2,570-g male infant with Apgar score of 8 and 9 at 1 and 5 minutes. The infant is initially taken to the special care nursery for observation but is with his mother by 6 hours of age. On postpartum day 2 the mother and baby are discharged home. Ms. June continues her inhaled steroid but has noticed a decrease in her need for albuterol. You plan to attempt to wean her medications after several months. She is advised to get influenza vaccine annually.

SUGGESTED READINGS

Bakhireva LN, Schatz M, Chambers CD. Effect of maternal asthma and gestational asthma therapy on fetal growth. J Asthma. 2007;44(2): 71–6.

Barrett EG. Maternal influence in the transmission of asthma susceptibility. Pulm Pharmacol Ther. 2008;21(3):474–84. Epub 2007 Jul 12.

Dombrowski MP. Asthma and pregnancy. Obstet Gynecol. 2006;108 (3 Pt 1):667–81.

Dombrowski MP. Outcomes of pregnancy in asthmatic women. Immunol Allergy Clin North Am. 2006;26(1):81–92.

Murphy VE, Gibson PG, Smith R, Clifton VL. Asthma during pregnancy: mechanisms and treatment implications. Eur Respir J. 2005;25(4):731–50.

National Heart, Lung and Blood Institute; National Asthma Education and Prevention Program Asthma and Pregnancy Working Group. NAEPP expert panel report. Managing asthma during pregnancy: recommendations for pharmacologic treatment-2004 update. J Allergy Clin Immunol. 2005;115(1):34–46.

Pyelonephritis in Pregnancy

David E. Abel

3

CASE PRESENTATION

You are called by your patient Ms. Montoya, a primigravida at 29 weeks of gestation. She has experienced some retropubic discomfort over the past few days. Currently, she complains of a fever of 38.3°C (101°F), shaking chills, nausea, and flank pain. Her pregnancy has thus far been uncomplicated, and she has no significant past medical or surgical history. Her prenatal labs are unremarkable, including a baseline urine culture.

Ms. Montoya is instructed to come to your office for an assessment. She appears ill. Her vital signs include a temperature of 38.6°C (101.5°F) and a pulse of 108 bpm. Her blood pressure is 110/72 mm Hg, and her respiratory rate is normal. On examination, cardiac and respiratory assessment is unremarkable. Her abdominal examination reveals a gravid uterus without fundal tenderness. There is mild suprapubic tenderness, and significant right costovertebral angle tenderness is elicited.

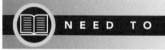

NEED TO KNOW

Physiologic Changes in the Urinary Tract During Pregnancy

Renal plasma flow (RPF) increases significantly during pregnancy (60%–80% above nonpregnant values), peaking in the first trimester. At term, it remains higher than that in the nonpregnant state. The glomerular filtration rate (GFR) increases as well, and by the end of the first trimester, it peaks with a value of 50% greater than that seen in the nonpregnant individual. It remains increased for the rest of the pregnancy. As the percentage increase in GFR is greater than the percentage increase for RPF, this leads to an elevation in the filtration fraction and a subsequent decrease in blood urea nitrogen (BUN) and serum creatinine values. The increase in the GFR during pregnancy leads to glucosuria and aminoaciduria that provide an excellent growth medium for bacteria.

In addition to changes in urine content, physiologic changes in the urinary tract in pregnancy promote urine stasis, predisposing the patient to both asymptomatic bacteriuria (ASB) and symptomatic infection. Both mechanical and hormonal factors are involved (Fig. 3.1). Hormonal changes include ureteral and calyceal dilation, presumably due to progesterone-induced relaxation of smooth muscle. The dilatation is significant, as the hydroureter may retain as much as 200 cc of urine. The urothelium is also affected, with an increase in vascularity and congestion due to hyperplasia. Similar changes occur in the bladder, including a decrease in vesical tone that leads to an increase in vesical capacity, and may contribute to vesicoureteral reflux in some patients. Mechanical alterations in the urinary tract in pregnancy include ureteral compression by the uterus at the pelvic brim that can lead to obstruction of urine flow. Hydroureter is more common on the right in pregnancy, presumably due to uterine dextrorotation that may in turn be due to the presence of the sigmoid colon on the left. Some physiologic changes in the urinary system are noted as early as 12 weeks of gestation and the urinary system may not return to normal until more than 6 weeks postpartum.

NEED TO KNOW

Definitions

ASB is defined as a urine culture yielding at least 100,000 colony-forming units of bacteria per milliliter in an asymptomatic patient. It occurs in 2% to 7% of pregnant patients. Untreated ASB will progress to pyelonephritis in up to 30% of patients, and there is also an association between ASB and preterm birth and low birth weight. For this reason, the American Congress of Obstetricians and Gynecologists recommends routine screening for ASB at the first prenatal visit.

Cystitis is an infection in the lower urinary tract (the bladder). The diagnosis of acute cystitis is based on

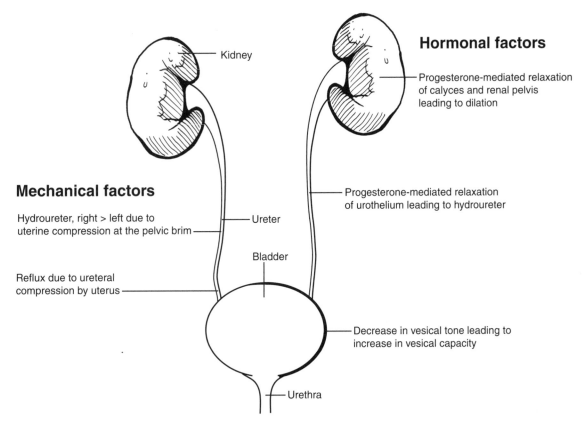

Figure 3.1 Hormonal/mechanical factors contributing to an increased risk of pyelonephritis during pregnancy.

clinical findings, with varying degrees of dysuria, frequency, and urgency, associated with evidence of urinary tract infection. A finding of either nitrite or leukocyte esterase on urine dipstick testing is a fast and convenient way to confirm the diagnosis.

Pyelonephritis is an infection of the renal parenchyma, pelvis, and calices, occurring in 1% to 2% of all pregnancies. It represents a systemic illness, characterized by flank pain, chills, and fever. It is the leading cause of nonobstetric hospital admissions in the antepartum period. Most cases (80%) occur in the antepartum period, particularly in the second and third trimester. In women with diabetes, pyelonephritis may be seen early in pregnancy. In more than 50% of cases, it is unilateral and right sided. In addition to diabetes, risk factors for pyelonephritis include obesity, sexual activity, substance abuse, low socioeconomic status, sickle cell trait, urolithiasis, congenital urinary tract anomalies, and conditions that warrant intermittent or indwelling catheterization. The effect of maternal age and parity are controversial; most reports find the incidence of pyelonephritis to be increased in younger mothers and nulliparas, while some find an increased incidence in multiparas and gravidas of advanced maternal age.

 Decision 1: Initial management

What is the most appropriate initial treatment?

A. A course of oral antibiotics
B. Obtain a clean catch urinalysis and culture and send the patient home
C. Admit the patient for intravenous antibiotics
D. Order a renal ultrasound

The correct answer is C: Admit the patient for intravenous antibiotics. Although there are some data that suggest that pyelonephritis may be effectively treated as an outpatient, most pregnant patients are admitted to the hospital for intravenous antibiotics and hydration. Laboratory assessment includes a complete blood cell count, chemistry panel, urinalysis, and urine culture. Approximately 15% to 20% of patients will be bacteremic, thus blood cultures may be reasonable, especially in the patient who appears septic or has a fever of >39°C (102.2°F). In some cases, electrolyte abnormalities and a decrease in creatinine clearance may occur. Cooling blankets and acetaminophen should be considered for fever, particularly in early pregnancy when hyperthermia may pose a teratogenic risk. Vital signs are monitored frequently, and an indwelling catheter may be needed. Intravenous antibiotic therapy is recommended until the patient is afebrile for 48 hours and demonstrates clinical improvement. Once discharged, oral antibiotics are prescribed to complete a 10- to 14-day course, followed by daily suppression therapy for the remainder of the pregnancy. Many recommend follow-up monthly surveillance urine cultures.

The pathogen most commonly seen in both ASB and pyelonephritis is *Escherichia coli*, noted in 75% to 80% of pregnant patients who are infected. Other pathogens include *Klebsiella*, *Proteus mirabilis*, *Enterobacter*, and *Enterococcus*. These organisms may be associated with nephrolithiasis or structural abnormalities. Group B streptococci are isolated more frequently in the urine of pregnant patients. The data on anaerobic bacteria and mycoplasma are limited.

Options for intravenous treatment of pyelonephritis during pregnancy commonly include ampicillin and gentamicin or a cephalosporin. Of note, the rates of *E. coli* resistance to ampicillin appear to be increasing (in one study, susceptibility testing demonstrated 46% resistance to ampicillin). Otherwise, there is no evidence that one regimen is superior to any other. A comparison of ampicillin and gentamicin versus cephalosporin revealed no difference in the rate of cure or recurrent infection. In addition, a comparison of a once-a-day (ceftriaxone) versus a multiple-dose (cefazolin) cephalosporin regimen showed no differences. Various intravenous treatment regimens are listed in Table 3.1.

Nitrofurantoin is often selected as the oral agent to complete the antibiotic course when the patient is discharged from the hospital. It is also the most commonly prescribed medication for lower urinary tract infections in pregnancy. At present, resistance to nitrofurantoin is not common. As 30% to 40% of patients develop recurrent bacteriuria after completion of therapy for pyelonephritis, suppression with nitrofurantoin for the remainder of therapy is used to reduce the risk of recurrent pyelonephritis.

TABLE 3.1

INTRAVENOUS ANTIBIOTIC REGIMENS FOR THE TREATMENT OF PYELONEPHRITIS

Ampicillin 2 g every 6 hours plus Gentamicin 2 mg/kg initially followed by 1.5 mg/kg every 8 hours (once daily dosing 3–5 mg/kg/d also an option)
Aztreonam 2 g every 8 hours
Cefazolin 1–2 mg every 8 hours
Ceftriaxone 1–2 g every 12–24 hours
Cefotetan 2 g every 12 hours
Cefotaxime 2 g every 8 hours

 CASE CONTINUES

Ms. Montoya is admitted to the hospital. On admission, her temperature is 38.3°C (101.0°F). Her serum creatinine is 0.7 mg/dL, her hemoglobin is 12 g/dL, and her white blood cell count is 18,000/mm³. A catheterized urine specimen is obtained, and aggressive intravenous hydration is initiated. Cefazolin is selected as the treatment regimen. After 48 hours, the patient remains febrile with a maximum temperature of 38.6°C (101.5°F) and continues to complain of significant flank pain. The costovertebral angle tenderness elicited on initial presentation has not improved.

 Decision 2: Management

What is the next step when the patient fails to respond to intravenous antibiotics?

A. Consider a renal ultrasound
B. Check antibiotic sensitivities
C. Order an intravenous urogram
D. A and B

The correct answer is D: A renal ultrasound and check antibiotic sensitivities. Most patients respond to therapy within 48 to 72 hours. For those who do not respond, one must consider renal obstruction due to nephrolithiasis or a resistant microorganism. A ureteral stent may be required to relieve an obstruction from a ureteral calculus. In addition to assessment of the collecting system, renal ultrasonography allows visualization of the renal parenchyma. Some patients may have a perinephric abscess requiring drainage, and usually the hospital course is prolonged in these patients. An intravenous urogram (answer C) may also be used to diagnose a renal obstruction but is seldom necessary with the use of ultrasound. In some cases, (approximately 10%) ultrasonography fails to identify obstructive nephrolithiasis, and a one-shot intravenous urogram at 20 to 30 minutes after contrast may be considered.

 CASE CONTINUES

You order a renal ultrasound, which is negative for calculi, obstruction, or parenchymal abnormalities. The urine culture result is now available and *E. coli* is identified. Susceptibility testing reveals resistance to cefazolin. The antibiotic regimen is adjusted accordingly, and the patient clinically improves. However, approximately 24 hours later, the patient develops dyspnea and tachypnea to 30 breaths/min, and her oxygen saturation is 91%. A chest x-ray suggests pulmonary edema. She is transferred to the intensive care unit, and the intensivist suggests intubation.

Decision 3: Maternal complications of pyelonephritis

Your patient's symptoms worsen, with increasing oxygen requirements leading to the need for intubation. What is the likely cause for this deterioration?

A. Renal failure
B. Acute respiratory distress syndrome (ARDS)
C. Pneumonia
D. Cardiomyopathy

The correct answer is B: ARDS. ARDS is one of the most serious complications of pyelonephritis during pregnancy. It is a manifestation of the sepsis syndrome, occurring in 2% to 8% of patients with pyelonephritis during pregnancy. Signs and symptoms include dyspnea, tachypnea, and hypoxia. The pathophysiology of this entity is endotoxin-mediated endothelial injury and altered alveolar–capillary membrane permeability. It occurs after the initiation of antibiotic therapy, with the lysis of endotoxin-carrying bacteria. Pulmonary edema and respiratory distress can result, with some patients requiring intubation and mechanical ventilation. Patients are usually cared for in an intensive care unit setting. For milder cases, treatment is supportive and includes diuresis and supplemental oxygen. In the patient with ARDS, the chest x-ray may show pulmonary edema, pleural effusions, or diffuse parenchymal infiltrates. Renal failure (choice A) would not manifest with respiratory changes. Pneumonia (choice C) may mimic some of the findings of ARDS, but the rapid and severe course in this case suggests ARDS rather than pneumonia. Cardiomyopathy (Choice D) may present with pulmonary edema, but the chest x-ray findings would include an enlarged cardiac silhouette.

 NEED TO KNOW

Maternal and Fetal Complications of Pyelonephritis in Pregnancy

Pyelonephritis in pregnancy is associated with a number of life-threatening complications for both mother and infant (Table 3.2), including ARDS, septic shock, transient renal dysfunction, and anemia. ARDS is described above and is a manifestation of the sepsis syndrome. The pathophysiology of septic shock is similar to that of ARDS, with endotoxin-mediated endothelial activation resulting in decreased vascular resistance, subsequent changes in cardiac output and hypotension. The hypotension is further aggravated if there is dehydration due to nausea, vomiting, and fever. Most patients

TABLE 3.2

MATERNAL RISKS OF PYELONEPHRITIS. OUTCOME OF 440 CASES OF MATERNAL PYELONEPHRITIS COLLECTED IN DALLAS, TX 2000–2001

Complication	Incidence (Percentage of Women with Pyelonephritis)
Renal dysfunction	2
Respiratory insufficiency	7
Positive blood culture	10
Anemia	23
Recurrent pyelonephritis	2.7
Preterm birth	5
Low birth weight	7

Adapted from Hill JB, Sheffield JS, McIntire DD, et al. Acute pyelonephritis in pregnancy. Obstet Gynecol. 2005;105:18–23.

respond to aggressive intravenous fluid resuscitation, and vasopressors are rarely needed. Activation of the coagulation cascade, although rarely seen in severe sepsis, can be life threatening. As for ARDS, treatment is supportive.

Renal insufficiency is another complication that is usually transient, with resolution within a few days. The number of patients with serious renal dysfunction has decreased significantly over the years (approximately 5%) with early and aggressive fluid resuscitation. If renal dysfunction is identified, nephrotoxic drugs should be avoided. Anemia has been reported to occur in 25% of patients with pyelonephritis and is thought to be due to endotoxin-mediated, lipopolysaccharide-induced hemolysis. The hematocrit may be as low as 20%.

During the acute episode, the fetal condition may be affected by maternal dehydration, hypotension, hypoxemia, and fever. In addition, maternal inflammation constitutes a risk for preterm delivery and also long-term neurodevelopmental harm. Monitoring the pregnant patient with complications of pyelonephritis must often be done in an intensive care unit setting, away from the delivery room, emphasizing the importance of close coordination of the physician and nursing staffs. Tocolysis, and other interventions to benefit the fetus, must be initiated with extreme care, as beta-agonist therapy increases the likelihood of pulmonary edema and respiratory insufficiency.

The risk of an abnormal pregnancy outcome may remain elevated after treatment. A mother with a prior episode of pyelonephritis in pregnancy continues to be at high risk for preterm labor and low–birth-weight delivery and is followed more closely than a low-risk gravida.

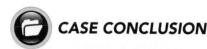 ## CASE CONCLUSION

Ms. Montoya is intubated and mechanical ventilation is continued. Aggressive diuresis is initiated, and the patient is able to be weaned off the ventilator within 24 hours. She is also monitored for preterm labor. After 48 hours, she returns to the antepartum unit and is soon discharged. Nitrofurantoin is given at a dose of 100 mg twice daily for 10 days followed by 50 mg nightly for suppression for the remainder of the pregnancy. A follow-up urine culture for test of cure is obtained in 2 weeks, followed by monthly surveillance cultures.

SUGGESTED READINGS

Cunningham FG, Lucas MJ, Hankins GD. Pulmonary injury complicating antepartum pyelonephritis. Am J Obstet Gynecol. 1987;156:797–807.

Hill JB, Sheffield JS, McIntire DD, et al. Acute pyelonephritis in pregnancy. Obstet Gynecol. 2005;105:18–23.

Millar LK, DeBuque L, Wing DA. Uterine contraction frequency during treatment of pyelonephritis in pregnancy and subsequent risk of preterm birth. J Perinat Med. 2003;31:41–6.

O'Brien BM. Pyelonephritis in pregnancy. In: Craigo S and Baker E, eds. Medical Complications in Pregnancy. New York, NY: McGraw-Hill; 2005. pp. 205–218.

Wing DA, Hendershott CM, Debuque L, et al. Outpatient treatment of acute pyelonephritis in pregnancy after 24 weeks. Obstet Gynecol. 1999;94:683–8.

Wing DA, Park AS, DeBuque L, et al. Limited utility of blood and urine cultures in the treatment of acute pyelonephritis during pregnancy. Am J Obstet Gynecol. 2000;182:1437–40.

Preeclampsia

Rizwana Fareeduddin

4

CASE PRESENTATION

You are called to the triage area of labor and delivery to evaluate Ms. Okuma, a 38-year-old G1 P0 woman who is at 34 6/7 weeks of gestation by a last menstrual period consistent with a first trimester ultrasound. She presents with a complaint of regular uterine contractions 4 minutes apart. She also relates that she has had a 2-day history of a mild headache that was relieved by acetaminophen (Tylenol). She states that this pregnancy has been uncomplicated. Review of her prenatal chart reveals that routine prenatal labs were within normal limits. As the patient is of advanced maternal age, she underwent a genetic amniocentesis at 16 weeks, resulting in a normal karyotype. However, you note that at her first prenatal visit at 7 1/7 weeks, she related a strong family history of hypertension (mother and father). Her initial blood pressure taken in the clinic was 130/85 mm Hg, but all subsequent blood pressures have been normal. She denies any significant medical, surgical, or social history. Review of the prenatal record also reveals that she has gained 5 lb in the last week.

As you complete your history and physical examination, the nurse informs you that the patient's blood pressure is 140/92 mm Hg. She has no edema and her lungs are clear. Urine analysis from a clean catch specimen shows 2+ protein. Your physical examination is completely within normal limits with a fundal height of 37 cm. On pelvic examination, the cervix is 3 cm dilated and 90% effaced, with the presenting part at −1 station. The fetal heart tracing is reactive and there are regular contractions every 4 to 5 minutes noted on the monitor.

❓ Decision 1: Diagnosis

The clinical diagnosis of preeclampsia requires elevated blood pressure (>140/90 mm Hg) and which of the following?

A. Proteinuria (>300 mg/d in a 24-hour collection or 1+ dipstick on two separate samples 6 hours apart)

B. Swelling of hands and face

C. Maternal weight gain of >2 lb in 1 week

D. All of the above

The correct answer is A: Proteinuria. Preeclampsia is defined as the new onset of hypertension after 20 weeks of pregnancy with proteinuria. Proteinuria is defined as being present if urine protein exceeds 300 mg in a 24-hour urine collection; this often correlates with a urine dipstick of 1+, and urine dipstick may be used when a 24-hour collection is not available (Table 4.1). While swelling of hands and face (Answer B) and maternal weight gain (>2 lb/wk) from fluid retention (Answer C) are common in preeclampsia, only proteinuria and hypertension are required for the diagnosis.

NEED TO KNOW

Hypertensive Disorders in Pregnancy

Preeclampsia is one of a spectrum of hypertensive disorders in pregnancy (Table 4.2). Ms. Okuma would be considered to have preeclampsia: The term gestational hypertension is reserved for new-onset hypertension in pregnancy without proteinuria. Hypertensive disorders of pregnancy complicate 6% to 8% of pregnancies and contribute significantly to maternal and neonatal morbidity and mortality. Hypertensive disorders are the second leading cause of maternal mortality in the United States, accounting for almost 15% of deaths. Hypertension is defined by the National High Blood Pressure Education Program Working Group, a consortium of academic organizations sponsored by the National Institutes of Health, as a blood pressure of 140 mm Hg systolic and/or 90 mm Hg diastolic.

The etiology of preeclampsia is not completely understood; however, some facts are available. Preeclampsia begins when the fetal trophoblast fails to fully invade and the maternal spiral arteries in the placental bed fail to fully dilate and remodel. Maternal blood flow to the placenta is reduced (Fig. 4.1). The preeclamptic

TABLE 4.1
DIAGNOSIS OF PREECLAMPSIA

- Blood pressure elevation of >140 mm Hg systolic.

OR

- Blood pressure elevation of >90 mm Hg diastolic.

- Proteinuria[a] is defined as the urinary excretion of 0.3 g (300 mg) of protein or greater in a 24-hour specimen.

- If a 24-hour urine collection is not available, then proteinuria is defined as a concentration of 30 mg/dL (at least 1+ on dipstick) in at least two random samples collected at least 6 hours apart.

[a]It is recommended that the diagnosis of proteinuria is made based on a 24-hour urine collection. Using random dipstick results or protein/creatinine ratios are not as reliable as these values may not correlate well with a 24-hour specimen.

placenta elaborates antiangiogenic, vasoactive compounds including the following: fms-related tyrosine kinase 1 (sFLIT), soluble endoglin, soluble vascular endothelial growth factor, and placental growth factor. The reason for placental release of vasoactive compounds is unknown, but it may be related to local hypoxia. The ultimate outcome is diffuse disruption of maternal vascular endothelium, with hypertension, proteinuria, and other systemic manifestations.

 CASE CONTINUES

You admit Ms. Okuma for preterm labor and preeclampsia and order the nurse to administer intravenous (IV) lactated Ringer's solution at 125 cc/hr. A 24-hour urine collection is started. You then perform a bedside ultrasound, which

reveals a vertex presentation, normal amniotic fluid index (AFI) of 12.3 cm, a biophysical profile of 8 of 8, a fundal grade II placenta without evidence of placental separation, and an estimated fetal weight of 1,965 g. Admission laboratory values are as follows: hemoglobin 13 g/dL, hematocrit 41%, white blood cell count 12,500/mm³, platelet count 98,000 × 10⁹/L, serum creatinine 0.8 mg/dL, uric acid 6.8 mg/dL, serum aspartate aminotransferase (ALT) 14 U/L, and glucose 113 mg/dL. As you discuss management options and risks to both mother and fetus from preeclampsia and prematurity with Ms. Okuma, the nurse retakes her vital signs. The blood pressure is now 165/96 mm Hg, pulse 98 bpm, respiratory rate 20 per minute, and temperature 98.3°F. Ms. Okuma also now complains of a mild persistent frontal headache. You repeat her physical examination and find that her lungs are clear and she has no abdominal pain, but has 4+ deep tendon reflexes and 2 beats of clonus at the ankles.

 Decision 2: Management

Management of the patient at this time should include

A. Aggressive tocolysis while treating with steroids for fetal lung maturation
B. Bedrest and expectant management till 37 weeks of gestation
C. Augmentation of labor with IV oxytocin
D. Cesarean section for severe and worsening preeclampsia

The correct answer is C: Augmentation of labor with IV oxytocin. This patient has severe preeclampsia based on the presence of a frontal headache, blood pressure of >160/110 mm Hg, and thrombocytopenia (<100,000 × 10⁹/L) (Table 4.3). At this time, administration of magnesium sulfate is indicated to prevent maternal seizures and oxytocin augmentation to increase uterine contractions.

TABLE 4.2
HYPERTENSIVE DISORDERS OF PREGNANCY[a]

Chronic Hypertension	Preeclampsia–Eclampsia	Preeclampsia Superimposed on Chronic Hypertension	Gestational Hypertension
Hypertension, which existed prior to pregnancy. Hypertension diagnosed prior to 20 weeks of gestation.	Pregnancy-specific syndrome involving hypertension diagnosed after the 20th week of gestation accompanied by proteinuria. Eclampsia is the occurrence of seizures in a woman with preeclampsia.	New-onset proteinuria in a patient with chronic hypertension. Sudden increase in proteinuria. Sudden increase in blood pressure in a previously well-controlled hypertensive patient.	New-onset hypertension after the 20th week of gestation WITHOUT proteinuria.

[a]As defined by the Working Group Report on High Blood Pressure in Pregnancy, National Institutes of Health, July 2000.

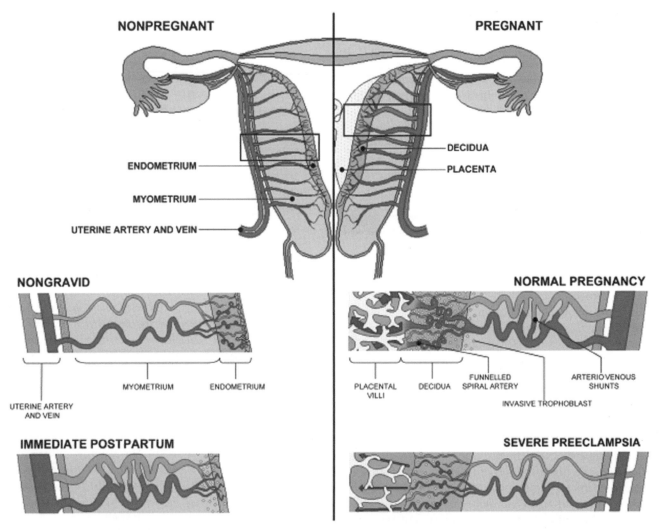

Figure 4.1 Changes in uterine vasculature in pregnancy and preeclampsia. In the nongravid state, spiral arteries have muscular walls. In pregnancy, trophoblast invades the upper third of the myometrium, remodeling the spiral arteries and abolishing the smooth muscle in their walls. The arteries become greatly dilated and develop a funneled appearance. Below the level of trophoblast invasion the arteries also become dilated, and develop arteriovenous shunts, which persist into the postpartum state. These changes are less marked in the preeclamptic placenta. (Reproduced with permission from Burton GJ, Woods AW, Jauniaux E, Kingdom JC. Rheological and physiological consequences of conversion of the maternal spiral arteries for uteroplacental blood flow during human pregnancy. Placenta. 2009;30(6):473–82.)

TABLE 4.3
CRITERIA FOR THE DIAGNOSIS OF SEVERE PREECLAMPSIA

- Blood pressure of 160 mm Hg systolic or higher or 110 mm Hg diastolic or higher on two occasions at least 6 hours apart while patient has been resting
- Epigastric or right upper quadrant pain
- Cerebral symptoms (headache)
- Impaired liver function
- Thrombocytopenia

- Proteinuria of 5 g or greater in a 24-hour urine collection or 3+or greater on two urine samples collected at least 4 hours apart
- Oliguria of <500 mL in 24 hours
- Visual symptoms (blurry vision, seeing "spots")
- Pulmonary edema
- Fetal growth restriction

Tocolysis (Answer A) in the presence of severe preeclampsia is contraindicated under this case scenario because of the risk of continuing the pregnancy. Furthermore, there is limited benefit of antenatal steroids after 34 weeks of gestation. Bedrest and expectant management (Answer B) would be the recommended therapy for mild preeclampsia. At this time, there is no indication for cesarean section (Answer D).

NEED TO KNOW

Systemic Effects of Preeclampsia

Preeclampsia is a condition of endothelial dysfunction that involves alterations in multiple maternal systems. For this reason, management of preeclampsia involves the possibility of complications anywhere in the body.

In the maternal hematologic and circulatory systems, preeclampsia is associated with increased systemic vascular resistance and decreased intravascular volume. Hemoconcentration may be a consequence, with an elevated red blood cell count, but the red blood cell volume may also be decreased due to hemolysis. Thrombocytopenia may occur in severe preeclampsia; the mechanism of this is uncertain, but it may be due to platelet activation and a low-grade intravascular coagulopathy. In conjunction with the activation of platelets, and the formation of microthrombi, there is consumption of fibrinogen and the production of fibrin degradation products. In the most severe cases, a frank coagulopathy may occur. The elevated systemic vascular resistance of preeclampsia may lead to left ventricular failure and pulmonary edema. In rare cases, there may be evidence of myocardial ischemia.

In the kidney, preeclampsia is associated with endothelial damage, with resulting decreased glomerular filtration. Glomerular function is disrupted, which contributes to the proteinuria seen in preeclampsia. The serum creatinine may increase, but if this occurs it is usually mild. The serum uric acid level may also increase, although the mechanism for this is unclear. In severe preeclampsia, oliguria may occur, as may frank renal failure, likely due to acute tubular necrosis.

The liver may be affected with evidence of periportal or subcapsular hemorrhage, centrilobular necrosis, and microvesicular fat deposition. In severe preeclampsia, liver damage may be manifested with elevations of aspartate aminotransferase (AST) and alanine aminotransferase (ALT), and rarely rupture of a subcapsular hematoma or frank liver rupture may occur.

TABLE 4.4

LABORATORY TESTS TO AID IN THE DIAGNOSIS AND MANAGEMENT OF PREECLAMPSIA

- Complete blood cell count
- Liver function tests

- Coagulation studies
- 24-hour urine collection for total protein and creatinine clearance

- Lactate dehydrogenase
- Uric acid

- Serum creatinine
- Peripheral blood smear

Placental perfusion may be impaired in preeclampsia. In severe preeclampsia, the fetus may become growth restricted, and less commonly, placental abruption may occur.

Headache and visual changes (flashes of light, scotomata, or loss of vision) are symptoms of central nervous system involvement of preeclampsia. These may be due to bleeding or vasoconstriction, either in the brain or retina, retinal detachment, or cerebral edema. Seizures may occur in about 1 in 400 and change the diagnosis to eclampsia. Rarely, cerebral edema may lead to cortical blindness and even herniation. A feared consequence of severe hypertension in preeclampsia is massive cerebral hemorrhage.

The usual laboratory evaluation for preeclampsia includes evaluation for the spectrum of possible maternal complications (Table 4.4). There is no consensus regarding the laboratory evaluation of the patient with preeclampsia, but most practitioners will evaluate for coagulopathy and liver and renal dysfunction, as alterations in these systems may change patient management.

 CASE CONTINUES

Ms. Okuma is treated with magnesium sulfate, and pitocin augmentation is begun. Her blood pressures have ranged between 145/88 and 158/105 mm Hg since magnesium sulfate was initiated. A Foley catheter was placed to monitor urine output and a repeat urine examination by dipstick reveals 3+ protein. Over the next 4 hours, the oxytocin infusion is increased to 20 mU/min. Her cervix is now found to be 5 cm dilated and 100% effaced with the vertex at zero station and in the left occiput transverse (LOT) position. Twenty minutes later, she complains of shortness of breath and right upper quadrant abdominal pain. The nurse reports that her urine output over the last hour is only 30 cc despite the IV infusion of lactated Ringer's solution at 125 cc/hr. Repeat blood pressure readings are 200/154, 195/110, and 192/102 mm Hg. Repeat labs have been obtained, and reported as hematocrit 45%, platelet count 65,000 × 10^9/L, AST 454 U/L, serum creatinine 1.4 mg/dL, magnesium 7.2 mg/dL, and uric acid 9.5 mg/ dL. Ms. Okuma's physical examination reveals rales in both lower lung fields, 3+ right upper quadrant tenderness, and absent reflexes. The fetal monitor strip reveals a fetal heart rate of 150 bpm with minimal variability and no decelerations. Uterine contractions are occurring every 3 minutes.

 Decision 3: Management

Appropriate management includes which of the following:

A. Emergency cesarean section
B. Rapid crystalloid infusion to increase intravascular volume
C. 5 mg hydralazine IV for acute reduction of blood pressure
D. Increase the MgSO$_4$ infusion rate

The correct answer is C: 5 mg hydralazine IV for acute reduction of blood pressure. Reduction of blood pressure is mandated to reduce the risk of intracerebral hemorrhage and stroke. In addition, the onset of pulmonary edema, elevated blood pressure, and oliguria suggests that afterload reduction is needed to decrease peripheral vascular resistance. Medications recommended for emergent blood pressure reduction in severe preeclampsia are noted in Table 4.5. Additional measures to consider would be a diuretic (usually furosemide) to increase urine output and mobilize fluid from the lungs and oxygen and maternal positioning, in order to improve the appearance of the fetal heart rate pattern. Emergency cesarean section (Answer A) is not indicated at this time in the face of an apparently unstable mother and a category 2 fetal heart rate tracing. Crystalloid infusion (Answer B) may be required due to intravascular volume depletion, especially if the mother requires surgery, however, in the face of rales and increased blood pressure, fluid given now may precipitate frank pulmonary edema. Magnesium sulfate is excreted by the kidneys; in the face of oliguria and diminished deep tendon reflexes magnesium overload is a real concern. In this case, increasing the magnesium infusion (Answer D) would be contraindicated.

 CASE CONTINUES

You administer hydralazine and Ms. Okuma's blood pressure stabilizes at 150/100 mm Hg. With 10 mg of furosemide, her urine output increases to 60 cc/hr. After 3 hours she is completely dilated, and after a 30-minute second stage she delivers a 2,020 g female infant with Apgar score of six and seven at 1 and 5 minutes. The baby is taken to the special care nursery, where she subsequently does well. Ms. Okuma's blood pressure remains high after delivery, and you initiate labetalol 200 mg BID for blood pressure control, with the plan to recheck her need for medication in 4 weeks. On the third postpartum day, Ms. Okuma is ready for discharge. She asks you what will happen if she gets pregnant again.

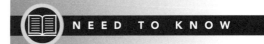
NEED TO KNOW

Recurrence of Preeclampsia

There are several known risk factors for preeclampsia including nulliparity, advanced maternal age, race, multifetal gestation, molar pregnancy, chronic hypertension, renal disease, diabetes, obesity, thrombophilias, underlying autoimmune disease (such as lupus or severe rheumatoid arthritis), conception via assisted reproductive technology, and previous pregnancy complicated by preeclampsia or family history of preeclampsia–eclampsia. It is important to note, however, that most patients have no risk factors. The patient in this scenario has two factors including advanced maternal age and nulliparity.

TABLE 4.5
MEDICATIONS FOR THE TREATMENT OF ACUTE SEVERE HYPERTENSION

Medication	Dosage	Frequency
Hydralazine	5 mg IV OR 10 mg IM	May repeat at 20-minute intervals depending upon response. If no improvement after a total dose of 20 mg IV or 30 mg IM, consider another agent.
Labetalol	20 mg slow IV push, then 40 mg IV 10 minutes later followed by 80 mg IV every 10 minutes for two additional doses.	Maximum of 220 mg. Caution in patients with asthma.

In women with or without risk factors, the reported rate of recurrent preeclampsia ranges from 11.5% to 65%. The rate of recurrence is dependent on gestational age at the onset of preeclampsia. The two highest rates, 25% and 65% occurred in those women who developed preeclampsia before 34 weeks of gestation and in those who developed the disease in the second trimester, respectively. There are some studies to suggest that recurrent preeclampsia is more likely to be severe and more likely to develop preterm as compared with women who develop preeclampsia as nulliparas. In this patient who developed preeclampsia preterm at a gestational age of 34 6/7 weeks, her risk of recurrence is about 20%.

Women with a history of a previous pregnancy complicated by preeclampsia are clearly at increased risk for preeclampsia in subsequent pregnancies. Currently there are no good interventions or preventive measures available to prevent the recurrence of preeclampsia. It is important that preexisting maternal medical conditions are optimized and well controlled. Weight loss in patients with obesity may also be beneficial.

After maternal health is optimized, the next most important key is early and frequent prenatal visits. It is important to establish gestational age as well as a baseline for blood pressure. Doppler studies of the uterine arteries in the first and second trimesters have been proposed as a screening test for preeclampsia, as abnormal velocimetry or the presence of notching may indicate a higher risk of preeclampsia. Although not standard treatment, low-dose aspirin has been used with some success and its use should be individualized. Supplementation with calcium, vitamin E, and vitamin C has been shown to be ineffective and is therefore not recommended.

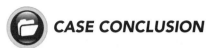 **CASE CONCLUSION**

You discuss the risk of recurrence with Ms. Okuma, and also address the potential that she has previously undiagnosed chronic hypertension, given her high blood pressure early in pregnancy and her continued hypertension postpartum. She understands the information, and at this point indicates that she does not plan any future pregnancies. You agree to see her in your office at 6 weeks postpartum for insertion of an intrauterine device (IUD) and further assessment of her blood pressure.

SUGGESTED READINGS

ACOG Committee on Obstetric Practice. ACOG Practice Bulletin No. 33. Diagnosis and management of preeclampsia and eclampsia. Int J Gynaecol Obstet. 2002;77(1):67–75.

Barton J, Sibai B. Prediction and prevention of recurrent preeclampsia. Obstet Gynecol. 2008;112:359–72.

Burton GJ, Woods AW, Jauniaux E, Kingdom JC. Rheological and physiological consequences of conversion of the maternal spiral arteries for uteroplacental blood flow during human pregnancy. Placenta. 2009;30(6):473–82. Epub 2009 Apr 17.

Cunningham FG, Leveno, KL, Bloom, SL, Hauth, JC, Rouse, DJ, Spong CY. Williams Obstetrics, 23rd ed. Pregnancy Hypertension. McGraw-Hill: New York, NY; 2010; Chapter 34, pp. 706–756.

Levine R, Lam C, Qian C, et al. Soluble endoglin and other circulating antiangiogenic factors in preeclampsia. N Engl J Med. 2006;355: 992–1005.

Roberts J, Funai E. Chapter 35 – Pregnancy related hypertension. In Creasy R, Resnik R, Iams J, editors. Maternal Fetal Medicine Principles and Practice. Philadelphia: Saunders; 2009; pp. 651–688.

Sibai B. Diagnosis and management of gestational hypertension and preeclampsia. Obstet Gynecol. 2003;102:181–92.

Spinnato J, Freire S, Pinto E Silva JL, et al. Antioxidant therapy to prevent preeclampsia – a randomized control trial. Obstet Gynecol. 2007;100:1311–8.

The National High Blood Pressure Education Program Working Group on High Blood Pressure in Pregnancy. Working Group Report on High Blood Pressure in Pregnancy, National Institutes of Health, July 2000.

Wang A, Rana S, Karumanchi SA. Preeclampsia: the role of angiogenic factors in its pathogenesis. Physiology (Bethesda). 2009;24:147–58. Review.

Chronic Hypertension and Pregnancy

5

Lisa Vasquez   Marquis Jessie

CASE PRESENTATION

You are working in the OB prenatal clinic and your first patient is Ms. Johnson, a 34-year-old G2 P1001 with a history of a previous normal spontaneous vaginal delivery 10 years ago. By last menstrual period, the patient's pregnancy is approximately 15 weeks. This is Ms. Johnson's first prenatal visit; she states that she knew she was pregnant but did not present earlier for care because she had lost her health insurance and wasn't sure where she could go. You assure her that you can help and congratulate her on initiating care. On review of the patient's history, she reports a 5-year history of hypertension and denies any other medical problems. She reports taking lisinopril (an acetylcholinesterase [ACE] inhibitor) for her hypertension since her initial diagnosis. She also says that she has been taking prenatal vitamins since taking an at-home pregnancy test.

On physical examination she is an obese (BMI of 35) woman who appears to be in no distress. Her blood pressure (BP) is 140/80 mm Hg, her pulse is 85 bpm, and she is afebrile. Her cardiac examination reveals a grade III/VI systolic murmur heard best in the left sternal border. Her lungs are clear. She has mild pedal edema. Her uterus is 15 weeks in size, and fetal heart tones are auscultated with a Doppler at 155 bpm.

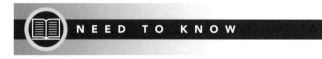

Definition of Chronic Hypertension

There are four major hypertensive conditions, which may exist in pregnancy:

- Preexisting hypertension or chronic hypertension
- Preeclampsia–eclampsia
- Preeclampsia superimposed upon preexisting hypertension
- Gestational hypertension

"Hypertension" is defined as BP of >140/90 mm Hg taken on two occasions more than 24 hours apart. Chronic hypertension (CHTN) is hypertension that is not related to the pregnancy. It is defined as hypertension present prior to the pregnancy or that is first diagnosed before the 20th week of gestation. It is also described as hypertension diagnosed during pregnancy that persists for >12 weeks after delivery. "Essential" hypertension is chronic hypertension without a known cause.

During pregnancy, hypertension can be categorized as either mild or severe. Mild hypertension is characterized by a systolic BP of <160 mm Hg and a diastolic BP of <110 mm Hg. Severe hypertension is defined by a systolic BP of >160 mm Hg or a diastolic BP of >110 mm Hg. This categorization is important for prognosis and treatment: There are no proven benefits to mother or fetus of the treatment of uncomplicated mild chronic hypertension other than a reduction in the risk of severe hypertension. This is in contrast to severe hypertension in which treatment has been shown to prevent maternal morbidity such as stroke, heart failure, and renal failure.

Decision 1: Evaluation

What work-up should be done on this patient?

- **A.** Cardiac echo on mother and fetus
- **B.** Fundoscopic examination
- **C.** 24-hour urine collection for protein
- **D.** Urine for metanephrines

The correct answer is C: 24-hour urine collection for protein. Superimposed preeclampsia on chronic hypertension occurs at earlier gestational ages and increased rates compared with preeclampsia in nonhypertensive patients. Although mild–moderate chronic hypertension may be relatively benign, preeclampsia is a leading cause of maternal mortality. Often, the preexisting hypertension makes the diagnosis unclear, and an increase in urine protein excretion may be a valuable indicator of developing preeclampsia. Establishing a baseline for urine protein as early as possible is thus an important part of the care of the hypertensive pregnant patient.

Maternal cardiac echo (Answer A) and fundoscopic examination (Answer B) may be performed in the patient with severe or long-standing CHTN to rule out end-organ damage. These investigations are seldom indicated in a hypertensive woman of childbearing age unless comorbidities such as diabetes with vascular damage are present.

It is also important to identify a possible cause of the hypertension if a previous workup has not been performed. Urine for metanephrines (Answer D) might be a part of that workup for a patient with severe or labile BP.

Maternal hypertension, in the absence of other diagnoses, is not a risk factor for fetal cardiac disease and fetal echocardiogram (Answer A) would not be indicated in this case.

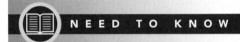

NEED TO KNOW

Etiology of Chronic Hypertension

The majority of CHTN (90% in most studies) is "essential" hypertension, with no clear etiology. Essential hypertension is associated with a number of risks, some of which, such as obesity, are subject to treatment. A small proportion of hypertension, however, is secondary to identifiable conditions that are, in many cases, treatable. Known risks and diagnoses should be considered in the hypertensive patient (not necessarily in pregnancy) to detect potentially treatable conditions.

The pathogenesis of essential hypertension is poorly understood. Some theorists consider that this condition is due to increased sympathetic neural activity, with enhanced beta-adrenergic responsiveness while others believe it to be due to increased angiotensin II activity and mineralocorticoid excess. In reality, essential hypertension is likely due to a myriad of causes including environmental and genetic factors. There are many risk factors for essential hypertension including age, race, family history, diet, obesity, and hyperlipidemia.

Nontreatable Risks for Essential Hypertension

Age and race as a risk factor for hypertension. In Caucasian women, the risk of hypertension increases from 0.6% in patients aged 18 to 29 years to 4.6% in patients aged 30 to 39 years. Although the risk at each age is greater in African-Americans, similar trends are seen with the risk increasing from 2% to 22% in the same age groups.

Family history as a risk factor for hypertension. Hypertension in mother, father, or both parents is independently associated with the development of hypertension over the course of adult life. The relative risk of developing hypertension is 1.5 with maternal hypertension only, 1.8 with paternal hypertension only, and 2.4 with hypertension in both parents, compared with patients whose parents never developed hypertension. When both parents develop hypertension before the age of 55 years, there is a 6.2-fold higher risk for the development of hypertension throughout adult life.

Treatable Risks for Essential Hypertension

Diet as a risk factor for hypertension. Hypertension is associated with sodium intake. It is likely that increased salt intake is a necessary but not sufficient cause for hypertension. Recent work has provided evidence that the current dietary intake of salt in Western societies is an important factor in the genesis of essential hypertension and may even be associated with blood pressure-independent target organ damage including renal damage.

Weight as a risk factor for hypertension. Obesity is associated with an increased incidence of hypertension, and weight gain appears to be a major determinant of the BP rise that is commonly seen with aging. As the population of pregnant women both ages and becomes increasingly obese, problems with obesity-associated hypertension will become more common in obstetrics.

Hyperlipidemia as a risk factor for hypertension. Dyslipidemia may also be associated with the development of hypertension and is independent of obesity. Drawing a baseline lipid panel should be considered in patients with long-standing hypertension especially those with metabolic syndrome (obesity, hypertension, insulin resistance, and dyslipidemia). Unfortunately, lipids are predictably increased in pregnancy, and this evaluation is better delayed until after delivery.

Secondary hypertension defines high BP that may be attributed to an identifiable cause. Some of these causes and the workup to identify them are listed in Table 5.1. It should be emphasized that not all of these investigations are appropriate in pregnancy, either due to risk to the fetus or to changes of maternal physiology with pregnancy; workup in pregnancy will be geared to excluding conditions, such as pheochromocytoma, that pose a significant short-term risk to mother or fetus.

TABLE 5.1

CAUSES OF AND EVALUATION FOR SECONDARY HYPERTENSION

The following diagnoses may be causes of secondary hypertension. Diagnostic studies available in pregnancy are as indicated.

NOTE: Secondary hypertension is more likely when:

- Hypertension is severe or difficult to treat
- The patient is less than 25 years of age
- The history or physical examination suggest an underlying cause

Coarctation of the Aorta
- Two-dimensional echocardiography
- Magnetic resonance imaging (MRI)

Cushing Syndrome
- 24-hour urinary free cortisol (elevated)

Primary Aldosteronism
- Plasma aldosterone to renin ratio (increased)

Pheochromocytoma
- Plasma catecholamines or metanephrines (increased)
- Urine catecholamines or metanephrines (increased)
- Adrenal MRI (adrenal tumor; T2-weighted MRI has characteristic appearance)

Renal Vascular Disease
- Renal duplex sonography
- Magnetic resonance angiography (renal vessel narrowing)

Renal Parenchymal Disease
- 24-hour urine protein and creatinine levels
- Renal ultrasonography (small kidney size, unusual architecture)
- Glomerular filtration rate (low)

Hyperparathyroidism
- Calcium and phosphorus levels (increased and decreased, respectively)
- Serum parathyroid hormone level (increased)

Thyroid Disease
- Thyrotropin level (suppressed in hyperthyroidism)

Adapted from Katakam R, Brukamp K, Townsend RR. What is the proper workup of a patient with hypertension? Cleve Clin J Med. 2008;75(9): 663–72.

 CASE CONTINUES

At Ms. Johnson's first prenatal visit, you discontinue her current antihypertensive medication. You explain to her that ACE inhibitors are contraindicated during pregnancy because they have been associated with neonatal hypotension, fetal growth retardation, oligohydramnios, neonatal anuria, renal failure, and neonatal death. You replace this medication with methyldopa because, as you explain to her, continued BP control during pregnancy is very important. You assure her that methyldopa has been extensively used in pregnancy and appears to be safe for both her and the fetus. In addition, you request the routine prenatal labs (complete blood cell count, blood type, HepBsAg, rubella, gonorrhea/chlamydia, and HIV status) as well as a chemistry panel and 24-hour urine collection.

 Decision 2: Risk assessment

What risks are significant for this pregnancy?

- A. Superimposed preeclampsia
- B. Placental abruption
- C. Preterm birth
- D. Intrauterine growth restriction

The answer is ABCD: All choices are correct. This patient is at increased risk for adverse outcome during this pregnancy due to her CHTN. The absolute ranges of these risks differ depending on whether the patient has mild versus severe hypertension. For mild preexisting hypertension, the rate of superimposed preeclampsia is 10% to 25%, placental abruption is 0.7% to 1.5%, preterm birth <37 weeks is 12% to 34%, and fetal growth restriction is 8% to 16%. These risks increase in women with severe preexisting hypertension in the first trimester with the risk of superimposed preeclampsia equaling 50%, placental abruption equaling 5% to 10%, preterm birth equaling 62% to 70%, and growth restriction equaling 31% to 40%.

 N E E D   T O   K N O W

Treatment of Hypertension in Pregnancy

The goal of medical treatment of hypertension during pregnancy is to lower the maternal morbidity (cerebrovascular and cardiovascular complication) and fetal morbidity (growth restriction and oligohydramnios). Treatment of uncomplicated mild essential hypertension is not recommended, as there are no proven benefits to mother or fetus, other than reduction in risk of severe hypertension. For patients who fit this profile but are already on antihypertensive therapy, tapering and even discontinuation of the agent can be considered if the patient's BPs are <120/80 mm Hg. Medications can be restarted if the patient's pressures increase to systolic pressure of >150 mm Hg or diastolic pressure of >95 mm Hg. Other reasons to restart antihypertensive therapy also include signs or symptoms of end-organ damage.

Treatment of severe hypertension in pregnancy is less controversial as there is proven benefit for both mother and infant. Treatment regimens include methyldopa (initial dosage of 250 mg taken at night and then 250 mg twice daily increasing to a maximum of 1 g twice daily). If the maximum dose is not tolerated or does not control BP, another agent may be added. Labetalol can be started as a primary or secondary agent (initial dose 100 mg taken twice daily to a maximum of 2.4 g daily in divided doses). Nifedipine may be used as a secondary agent (initial dose 10–30 mg three times daily or as 30–60 mg once daily in sustained-release form). The obstetrician should be aware that neither methyldopa nor beta-blockers are considered to be first-line drugs for the treatment of CHTN in the non-pregnant patient. Methyldopa is a relatively weak anti-hypertensive, and beta-blockers may not reduce the risk of stroke in treated patients. These drugs are used in pregnancy because of their history of safety for mother and fetus.

Target BP goals in women undergoing medical treatment should be systolic BP of 140 to 150 mm Hg and diastolic BP of 90 to 100 mm Hg if end-organ damage is not present. These thresholds are decreased to <140/90 mm Hg in women with end-organ damage.

Patients who are on ACE inhibitors or angiotensin II receptor blockers (ARBs) upon presentation to pre-natal care should have these medications discontinued and appropriately substituted. ACE inhibitors have been associated with renal dysgenesis and neonatal renal dysfunction. Similar complications have been reported with ARBs. Diuretics are used with caution during pregnancy because of the theoretical risk of maternal volume depletion due to these agents. A patient entering pregnancy on a diuretic may be continued in some cases, but diuretics are not initiated for BP control in the pregnant woman. In older studies, thiazide diuretics were associated with thrombocy-topenia in the newborn, and they, especially, should be used with caution.

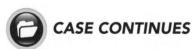

CASE CONTINUES

Ms. Johnson continues prenatal visits with you. Her fundal height growth is appropriate and her BP control remains adequate on her methyldopa. Her 24-hour urine protein excretion is 147 mg/24 hours, and her second trimester serum screen predicts a low risk for fetal

Down syndrome and trisomy 18. A fetal anatomy survey performed at 20 weeks is normal. At her 22-week visit, you notice that her BP has dropped significantly. Currently it is 110/72 mm Hg.

Decision 3: Follow up

What is the significance of a second-trimester drop in BP?

A. Worrisome—Fetal oxygenation may suffer
B. Worrisome—Mother's heart may be in failure
C. Reassuring—Hypertension may be resolving
D. Reassuring—Mother's vessels are more compliant

The correct answer is D: This is reassuring as it means that the mother's blood vessels demonstrate appropriate compliance. During the first half of normal pregnancy, a decline of both systolic and diastolic BP values occurs (Fig. 5.1). This parallels the simultaneous decrease in peripheral vascular resistance. If a woman does not demonstrate this physiologic decrease in BP, it is often a sign that she is likely to develop elevated BP later in the pregnancy. In a patient with preexisting hypertension, a failure of the BP to decline in the second trimester is also a poor prognostic sign.

Overcontrol of maternal BP is, however, associated with an increased risk of fetal growth restriction. Depending on the medication and dose, a BP of 110/72 mm Hg might prompt a reduction in antihypertensive dose.

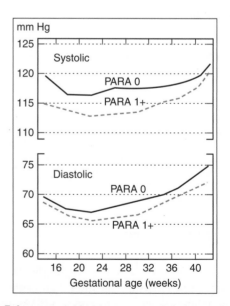

Figure 5.1 Normal blood pressure changes in pregnancy. There is a predictable decline in blood pressure in the second trimester of pregnancy with a nadir at about 22 weeks. The blood pressure then rises to term, although it should not exceed non-pregnant levels. (From: Christianson RE. Studies on blood pressure during pregnancy. I. Influence of parity and age. Am J Obstet Gynecol. 1976 Jun 15;125(4):509–13, used with permission.)

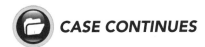

CASE CONTINUES

At the 22-week visit, Ms. Johnson is taking 250 mg of methyldopa twice daily. Given that this is a minimal dose, you elect not to change her medication at this time. At 26 weeks fundal growth is appropriate and the fetus is active. Ms. Johnson reports that her employer is requesting an estimate of the frequency of her prenatal visits, so that they can plan her duties.

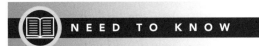

Fetal Evaluation

Infants born to mothers with a pregnancy complicated by chronic hypertension are at increased risk of sequelae of placental damage. These would include oligohydramnios, growth restriction, placental abruption, preeclampsia, and premature delivery. Follow-up for these conditions will include more frequent visits for prenatal care.

Fetal growth evaluation begins by the establishment of firm dating, preferably by first trimester ultrasound, and fetal anatomic survey between 18 and 24 weeks. Follow-up scans can be used to determine adequate incremental growth or to confirm suspicion for growth restriction as well as oligohydramnios. As growth restriction is more likely in the third trimester, ultrasound may be appropriate between 28 and 32 weeks and then at four to six intervals until delivery.

Fetal well-being is established by serial testing, although there is very limited evidence for the efficacy of the approaches used. In general, the mother can be instructed to perform self-evaluation with fetal kick counts daily beginning at 28 weeks. Fetal surveillance by modified biophysical profile (nonstress test [NST] and amniotic fluid index [AFI]) may be performed weekly after 34 weeks in a patient with mild–moderate chronic hypertension, although fetal growth restriction, worsening hypertension, or other factors may alter this schedule.

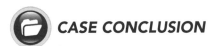

CASE CONCLUSION

Ms. Johnson continues her care and initiates weekly NST and AFI at 34 weeks of gestation. At her 39-week visit, her BP is elevated (155/96 mm Hg) and she has 2+ proteinuria. She also complains of a new headache that is not relieved with acetaminophen (Tylenol). You send her to labor and delivery for further evaluation. Her BPs continue to remain elevated while in triage. A diagnosis is made of new-onset superimposed preeclampsia, and the decision is made to induce her labor. As she is having uterine contractions every 5 to 8 minutes, the decision is made to proceed with oxytocin induction, and she is given intravenous magnesium sulfate for seizure prophylaxis. After 14 hours of induction (6 hours of active labor), Ms. Johnson delivers a 3,150-g male infant with Apgar scores of 8 and 9 at one and five minutes. Her elevated blood pressure resolves in the first 24 hours postpartum on her usual dose of methyldopa. She and the infant are discharged on the second day after delivery.

SUGGESTED READINGS

Abalos E, Duley L, Steyn DW, Henderson-Smart DJ. Antihypertensive drug therapy for mild to moderate hypertension during pregnancy. Cochrane Database Syst Rev. 2007;(1):CD002252.

ACOG Practice Bulletin. Antepartum fetal surveillance. Number 9, October 1999. Int J Gynaecol Obstet. 2000;68(2):175–85.

Katakam R, Brukamp K, Townsend RR. What is the proper workup of a patient with hypertension? Cleve Clin J Med. 2008;75(9):663–72.

Magee LA, Ornstein MP, von Dadelszen P. Fortnightly review: management of hypertension in pregnancy. BMJ. 1999;318(7194):1332–6.

Redman CW. Controlled trials of antihypertensive drugs in pregnancy. Am J Kidney Dis. 1991;17(2):149–53.

Remuzzi G, Ruggenenti P. Prevention and treatment of pregnancy-associated hypertension: what have we learned in the last 10 years? Am J Kidney Dis. 1991;18(3):285–305.

Sibai BM, Mabie WC, Shamsa F, Villar MA, Anderson GD. A comparison of no medication versus methyldopa or labetalol in chronic hypertension during pregnancy. Am J Obstet Gynecol. 1990;162(4):960–6.

Sibai BM. Chronic hypertension in pregnancy. Obstet Gynecol. 2002;100(2):369–77.

Wang NY, Young JH, Meoni LA, Ford DE, Erlinger TP, Klag MJ. Blood pressure change and risk of hypertension associated with parental hypertension: the Johns Hopkins Precursors Study. Arch Intern Med. 2008;168(6):643–8.

HELLP Syndrome

Richard Burwick

6

CASE PRESENTATION

Ms. Franklin, a 22-year-old G1 P0 at 28 2/7 weeks of gestation, is sent to labor and delivery triage by your partner for a blood pressure of 156/92 mm Hg. A spot clean catch urine in the office revealed 2+ proteinuria. She had been compliant with her prenatal care and all prior blood pressures were <140/90 mm Hg, including a blood pressure of 112/70 mm Hg at her first prenatal visit at 11 weeks of gestation. Her pregnancy dating is by last menses confirmed by a first trimester ultrasound. She denies headaches, visual disturbances, or epigastric pain.

During the triage evaluation, Ms. Franklin has blood pressures of 150/94, 148/88, and 154/92 mm Hg, 15 minutes apart, despite bedrest. Evaluation of a urine sample obtained by catheter confirms 2+ proteinuria. Laboratory work-up reveals a hemoglobin of 8.5 g/dL, hematocrit of 26.3%, platelet count of 87,000 × 10^9/L, aspartate aminotransferase (AST) of 74 U/L, alanine aminotransferase (ALT) of 56 U/L, lactate dehydrogenase (LDH) of 740 IU/L, and creatinine level of 0.9 mg/dL. A bedside ultrasound finds symmetric fetal growth, with an estimated fetal weight of 1,305 g, an amniotic fluid index of 10.4 cm, a fundal grade II placenta, and a vertex presentation. Maternal examination reveals clear lung fields, 2+ pitting edema to the knee bilaterally, and 2+ deep tendon reflexes. The fetal heart rate averages 140 bpm and is overall reassuring.

Decision 1: Diagnosis

What is the most likely diagnosis?

A. Chronic hypertension and gestational thrombocytopenia
B. Mild preeclampsia
C. Severe preeclampsia and HELLP syndrome
D. Thrombotic thrombocytopenic purpura (TTP)

The correct answer is C: Severe preeclampsia and HELLP syndrome (the syndrome of <u>H</u>emolysis, <u>E</u>levated <u>L</u>iver enzymes and <u>L</u>ow <u>P</u>latelets). The patient has a new onset of elevated blood pressures and proteinuria after 20 weeks of gestation. Her blood pressures and urine protein are in the range of mild preeclampsia (Answer B), but her laboratory abnormalities, including transaminitis and thrombocytopenia (platelet count <100,000 × 10^9/L), confirm the diagnosis of severe preeclampsia. The combination of thrombocytopenia, transaminitis, and hemolysis (diagnosed by the elevated LDH) confirms HELLP syndrome. Answer A is unlikely because this patient had a normal baseline blood pressure and the vignette gave no history of chronic hypertension. Gestational thrombocytopenia is the most common form of thrombocytopenia in pregnancy, but usually occurs in the absence of blood pressure elevations or other laboratory abnormalities. TTP (Answer D) may be confused with HELLP syndrome, and it has high maternal morbidity and mortality. Given the risk associated with TTP, this diagnosis should be considered. However, it is much less common than HELLP, and it is usually not associated with blood pressure elevations. The classic pentad of TTP includes neurologic abnormalities, fever, and kidney failure, in addition to thrombocytopenia and hemolysis, although most patients do not demonstrate all features. Other serious conditions that may be confused with severe preeclampsia or HELLP syndrome, and that should be explored in patients not responding to typical management, include systemic lupus erythematosus, hemolytic uremic syndrome, acute fatty liver of pregnancy, and idiopathic or immune-mediated thrombocytopenia.

NEED TO KNOW

Definition of HELLP Syndrome

The HELLP syndrome occurs in about 0.5% to 0.9% of all pregnancies and in 10% to 20% of cases of severe preeclampsia. It is characterized by microangiopathic hemolytic anemia in association with liver dysfunction and thrombocytopenia. HELLP syndrome has been defined (Tennessee classification) as all of the following: AST or ALT of ≥70 U/L, platelet count of ≤100,000 × 10^9/L, and LDH of ≥600 IU/L. If one of these criteria is

TABLE 6.1

MATERNAL COMPLICATIONS IN SEVERE PREECLAMPSIA, PARTIAL HELLP, AND COMPLETE HELLP SYNDROME

Maternal Complication	Complete HELLP (%)	Partial HELLP (%)	Severe Preeclampsia (%)
Blood transfusion	25[a]	4	3
DIC	15[a]	0	0
Renal failure	3	0	0
Eclampsia	9	7	9
Placental abruption	9	4	5
Pulmonary edema	8	4	3
Liver hematoma	1.5	0	0
Death	1.5	0	0

[a]$p < 0.001$.
DIC, disseminated intravascular coagulation. Adapted from Audibert F, Friedman SA, Frangieh AY, Sibai BM. Clinical utility of strict diagnostic criteria for the HELLP (hemolysis, elevated liver enzymes, and low platelets) syndrome. Am J Obstet Gynecol. 1996;175(2):460–4.

not met, the condition is partial HELLP syndrome. Clinical outcomes with partial HELLP syndrome are comparable to severe preeclampsia and are more favorable than those seen with the complete HELLP syndrome (Table 6.1).

In the alternative Mississippi classification, HELLP syndrome is classified by the degree of thrombocytopenia: class I ($<50,000 \times 10^9$/L), class II ($50–100,000 \times 10^9$/L), or class III ($100–150,000 \times 10^9$/L), in the setting of AST or ALT of $\geq$70 U/L and LDH of $\geq$600 IU/L. For class III HELLP syndrome, the criterion for AST or ALT is lowered to $\geq$40 U/L. Utilizing this classification system, a relationship between HELLP class and maternal morbidity has been reported. The clinical symptom most predictive of HELLP class severity is right upper quadrant or epigastric pain, seen in 50% of patients with class I HELLP syndrome.

While HELLP syndrome is a triad of hemolysis, elevated liver enzymes, and low platelets, usually in a patient with preeclampsia, it can occur in the absence of hypertension and proteinuria. In the absence of frank preeclampsia, other clinical signs such as excessive weight gain, pulmonary edema, oliguria, fetal growth restriction, or oligohydramnios may help establish the diagnosis. This presentation is unusual; for patients without preeclampsia, and with a clinical picture atypical for HELLP syndrome, it would seem prudent to reevaluate the diagnosis.

For management purposes, HELLP is considered as a variant of preeclampsia and treatment is generally the same as in severe preeclampsia with special attention to the triad mentioned above. When remote from term and when the patient is relatively stable, expectant management for 48 hours may be attempted to allow for steroid administration while the patient is being treated with

magnesium sulfate to provide seizure prophylaxis. Contraindications to expectant management include maternal hemodynamic instability (i.e., shock), nonreassuring fetal heart monitoring, severe hypertension unresponsive to antihypertensive medication, eclampsia, pulmonary edema, renal failure, disseminated intravascular coagulation, and abruption placenta.

 CASE CONTINUES

Following admission to labor and delivery for severe preeclampsia and HELLP syndrome, Ms. Franklin is treated with IV magnesium sulfate to prevent maternal seizures and with betamethasone to induce fetal lung maturity. The plan is to deliver the fetus after 48 hours by labor induction. A Foley catheter is placed in the bladder and a 24-hour urine collection is started with strict input and outputs recorded. Ms. Franklin's fetal heart rate pattern is devoid of abnormal characteristics and she is not experiencing uterine contractions.

You are called 12 hours later by the nurse for a critical platelet value of $24,000 \times 10^9$/L. Upon evaluation, you also find that Ms. Franklin now has a frontal headache and the urine output has decreased to approximately 30 cc/hr. The fetal heart rate pattern remains reassuring. There are no uterine contractions, although her cervix is 3 cm dilated, 50% effaced, and the vertex is at −2 station.

 Decision 2: Management

What is the best management for this patient's low platelets at delivery?

A. Platelet transfusion at the time of cesarean delivery (if indicated)
B. Corticosteroids now
C. Plasmapheresis prior to cesarean delivery
D. Intravenous immunoglobulin (IVIG) now

The correct answer is A: Platelet transfusion at the time of cesarean delivery (if indicated). The patient's condition appears to be deteriorating, suggesting that delivery is now appropriate. Excessive bleeding during surgery is uncommon unless the platelet count is $<50,000 \times 10^9$/L. Thus, to ensure hemostasis at cesarean delivery platelet transfusion should be given if a Cesarean is performed. Platelet transfusion would only be recommended at vaginal delivery if there were bleeding complications. With HELLP syndrome the best method is to transfuse the platelets in the operating room at the time of surgery, as the survival of transfused platelets is diminished. Anesthesia choices are also limited by the thrombocytopenia, some anesthesiologists require platelet counts of 75,000 to $100,000 \times 10^9$/L for an epidural to be offered, and some may not feel comfortable with regional anesthesia in this patient under any circumstances. Although there is little data regarding the risk of regional anesthesia in the patient with HELLP, the standard of care is to avoid neuraxial anesthesia in the patient with a significant coagulopathy. If Cesarean delivery is planned, a general anesthetic may be required. Corticosteroids (Answer B) have been utilized by some authors for HELLP syndrome and may increase platelet counts by decreased splenic sequestration and destruction. However, the response is relatively slow, making corticosteroids more useful in the nonacute setting, such as in women undergoing expectant management remote from term or in the postpartum period. Of note, plasma exchange is another alternative that has been utilized in severe or atypical HELLP syndrome, which has failed to abate within 72 hours following delivery. Plasmapheresis (Answer C) is the preferred therapeutic choice in TTP, while IVIG (Answer D) may be used in the treatment of other conditions such as immune thrombocytopenic purpera, but neither is routinely used for the thrombocytopenia associated with HELLP syndrome.

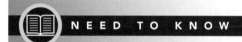

Mode of Delivery in HELLP Syndrome

In HELLP syndrome the optimal route of delivery has not been studied in clinical trials. However, it is clear that vaginal delivery is preferable to cesarean delivery if maternal and fetal health is not compromised. A review of women with severe preeclampsia found that immediate cesarean section showed no clear benefit in maternal or fetal morbidity when compared with labor induction, regardless of initial cervical examination. In addition, the group with immediate cesarean section had higher rates of newborn respiratory distress syndrome.

There is general agreement that cesarean section is indicated for the usual obstetric indications such as breech presentation, placenta previa, nonreassuring fetal heart tracing, or arrest of labor. If vaginal delivery is not anticipated shortly, other indications for cesarean section may include uncontrolled severe hypertension, eclampsia, pulmonary edema, placental abruption, oliguria unresponsive to treatment, persistent severe headache, visual disturbances or epigastric pain, worsening thrombocytopenia, or deterioration of renal function.

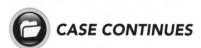

CASE CONTINUES

After coordination with nursing staff, anesthesia, and pediatrics, oxytocin is begun to induce labor. Platelets and red blood cells are ordered to be crossmatched. One

hour later, Ms. Franklin begins experiencing significantly increased right upper quadrant pain. Vital signs reveal a blood pressure of 140/85 mm Hg, pulse of 125 bpm, respiratory rate of 24/min, temperature of 97.8°F. Results of the labs drawn at initiation of induction reveal a hemoglobin level of 5.6 g/dL, hematocrit of 23.6%, platelets count of 18,500 × 10⁹/L, creatinine level of 1.1 mg/dL, AST of 656 U/L. The urine output during the last hour was 10 cc.

Decision 3: Management

All of the following treatments are indicated at this time except?

- **A.** Transfusion of packed red blood cells
- **B.** Infusion of crystalloid
- **C.** Continued oxytocin induction of labor
- **D.** Emergency cesarean section under general anesthesia

The correct answer is C: Continued oxytocin induction of labor. The clinical presentation strongly suggests that in addition to HELLP syndrome the patient has ruptured her liver capsule. Cesarean section and exploratory laparotomy under general anesthesia (Answer D) are indicated because of the altered vital signs that suggest acute bleeding. In addition to prompt cesarean delivery, resuscitation with crystalloid (Answer B) and red blood cells (Answer A) is indicated with the diagnosis of early hemorrhagic shock. Continued attempts to achieve vaginal delivery (Answer C) are unwarranted at this point because of the likelihood of liver rupture and maternal distress.

Complications of HELLP Syndrome

The most common maternal complications seen with HELLP syndrome are transfusion of blood products (packed red blood cells, platelets, or fresh frozen plasma), disseminated intravascular coagulopathy, placental abruption, and acute renal failure. The most common fetal or neonatal complications include intrauterine growth restriction, prematurity, fetal or neonatal demise, and neonatal thrombocytopenia. A compilation of published complication rates in HELLP syndrome is seen in Table 6.2.

CASE CONCLUSION

An emergency cesarean section and exploratory laparotomy are performed under general anesthesia, with delivery

TABLE 6.2

COMPLICATIONS REPORTED IN THE HELLP SYNDROME

Maternal Complications	Incidence (%)
Eclampsia	4–9
Placental abruption	9–20
DIC	15
Acute renal failure	3–7
Severe ascites	4–11
Cerebral edema	1–8
Pulmonary edema	3–10
Subcapsular liver hematoma	Between 0.9% and <2%
Liver rupture	about 1.8%
Retinal detachment	1
Cerebral infarction	Few case reports
Cerebral hemorrhage	1.5
Maternal death	1

Fetal/Neonatal Complications

Perinatal death	7.4–20
IUGR	38–61
Preterm delivery	70 (15% <28 gestational weeks)
Neonatal thrombocytopenia[e]	15–50
RDS	5.7–40

Note: some studies have found much higher rates of complications is selected populations.
Data from Sibai BM. Diagnosis, controversies, and management of the syndrome of hemolysis, elevated liver enzymes, and low platelet count. Obstet Gynecol. 2004 May;103(5 Pt 1):981–91.
Haram K, Svendsen E, Abildgaard U. The HELLP syndrome: clinical issues and management. A Review. BMC Pregnancy Childbirth. 2009 Feb 26;9:8.
DIC, disseminated intravascular coagulation; IUGR, intrauterine growth restriction; RDS, respiratory distress syndrome.

of a 1,295-g male infant, with Apgar scores of 6 and 7 at 1 and 5 minutes. Following the delivery of the fetus, a 3 × 3 cm rent in the right lobe of the liver is identified. A general surgeon provides intraoperative consultation and surgical repair of the liver rupture is successful. Following transfusion of platelets and red blood cells, the patient stabilizes and is discharged from the hospital after 1 week.

SUGGESTED READINGS

ACOG practice bulletin: Thrombocytopenia in pregnancy. Number 6, September 1999. Clinical management guidelines for obstetrician-gynecologists. American College of Obstetricians and Gynecologists. Int J Gynaecol Obstet. 1999;67(2):117–28.

Audibert FA, Sibai BM, et al. Clinical utility of strict diagnostic criteria for the HELLP syndrome. Am J Obstet Gynecol. 1996;175: 460–4.

Chames MC, Haddad B, Barton JR, et al. Subsequent pregnancy outcome in women with a history of HELLP syndrome at <28 weeks of gestation. Am J Obstet Gynecol. 2003;188:1504–8.

Coppage KH, Polzin WJ. Severe preeclampsia and delivery outcomes: is immediate cesarean delivery beneficial? Am J Obstet Gynecol. 2002;186:921–3.

Ertan AK, Wagner S, Hedrik HJ, Tanriverdi HA, Schmidt W. Clinical and biophysical aspects of HELLP syndrome. J Perinat Med. 2002; 30:483–9.

Haddad B, Sibai BM. Expectant management of severe preeclampsia: proper candidates and pregnancy outcome. Clinical Obstet Gynecol. 2005;48(2):430–40.

Haram K, Svendsen E, Abildgaard U. The HELLP syndrome: clinical issues and management. A review. BMC Pregnancy Childbirth. 2009;9:8.

Martin JN Jr, Blake PG, Perry KG Jr, et al. The natural history of HELLP syndrome: patterns of disease progression and regression. Am J Obstet Gynecol. 1990;76:737–41.

Martin JN Jr, Rinehart BK, May WL, Magann EF, Terrone DA, Blake PG. The spectrum of severe preeclampsia: comparative analysis by HELLP syndrome classification. Am J Obstet Gynecol. 1999;180: 1373–84.

Martin JN Jr, Rose CH, Briery CM. Understanding and managing HELLP syndrome: The integral role of aggressive glucocorticoids for mother and child. Am J Obstet Gynecol. 2006;195:914–34.

Sibai BM. The HELLP syndrome (hemolysis, elevated liver enzymes and low platelets): much ado about nothing? Am J Obstet Gynecol. 1990;162:311–6.

van Pampas MG, Wolf H, Mayruhu G, et al. Long-term follow-up in patients with a history of (H)ELLP syndrome. Hypertens Pregnancy. 2001;20:15–23.

Gestational Diabetes

Jeotsna Grover

CASE PRESENTATION

Ms. Creech, a 32-year-old Pima Indian female G4 P3003 is seen in the prenatal clinic for her first visit at 12 weeks of pregnancy. Ms. Creech's obstetrical history is significant for three uncomplicated vaginal deliveries with birth weights of 3,563, 3,850, and 4,200 g. Her medical history is negative for significant medical problems and is specifically negative for diabetes or hypertension. Her surgical history is noncontributory. The family history is significant for presence of diabetes mellitus in her grandfather and hyperthyroidism in her mother. No other family members are reported to have diabetes or other medical problems. On further interrogation, she acknowledges that she herself is a smoker, using half a pack of cigarettes per day. She denies use of illicit drugs but reports occasional alcohol use. Her own weight at birth was about 9½ lbs.

On physical examination, her blood pressure is 120/65 mm Hg, her pulse is 85 bpm, and her respiratory rate is 12/min. She weighs 205 lb and is 5′2″ tall. Her body mass index (BMI) is 37.5. The remainder of her physical examination is within normal limits.

Decision 1: Diagnosis

Which of the following are predictors of diabetes in this patient?

A. BMI
B. Ethnic background
C. Prior delivery of 4,200-g fetus
D. Maternal age

The correct answers are A and B: BMI and B: ethnic background. Her overweight is a significant risk factor: about 90% of type 2 diabetes has been attributed to obesity, and women with obesity have a 2.5-fold higher risk of gestational diabetes. Her ethnic background is also a risk factor for diabetes, as the Pima Indians have one of the highest risks of diabetes in the world with as many as 50% of adult Pima being diabetic. The Fifth International Workshop

Conference on Gestational Diabetes regarded severe obesity, a strong family history, and a prior history of gestational diabetes mellitus (GDM) as the highest risk factors for GDM in the current pregnancy (Table 7.1).

In contrast, the history of a prior 4,200-g fetus (Answer C) is of little predictive value if the patient screened negative for diabetes in that pregnancy. A maternal age above 25 years (Answer D) puts the patient in an average risk category, but does not indicate an elevated risk for GDM.

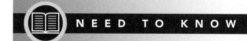

NEED TO KNOW

The definition of gestational diabetes (GDM) is glucose intolerance of varying degrees of severity with onset or first recognition during pregnancy. GDM affects about 7% of pregnancies in the United States per year (i.e., affecting 200,000 cases per year). The Northern California Kaiser Permanente study reported the prevalence rate of GDM at 6.9% in 2000, although the rate differs markedly by ethnicity (Fig. 7.1).

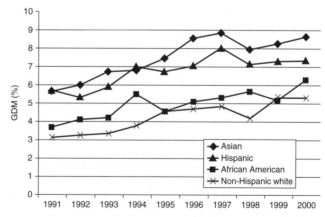

Figure 7.1 Prevalence of GDM by ethnicity. Northern California Kaiser Permanent. (Data from Ferrara A, Kahn HS, Quesenberry CP, Riley C, Hedderson MM. An increase in the incidence of gestational diabetes mellitus: Northern California, 1991–2000. Obstet Gynecol. 2004 Mar;103(3):526–33.)

TABLE 7.1

SCREENING STRATEGY FOR DETECTING GESTATIONAL DIABETES MELLITUS (GDM)

GDM risk assessment: Should be ascertained at the first prenatal visit
- Low risk: Blood glucose testing is not routinely required if *all* of the following characteristics are present:
  - Member of an ethnic group with a low prevalence of GDM
  - No known diabetes in first-degree relatives
  - Age <25 yr
  - Weight normal before pregnancy
  - Weight normal at birth
  - No history of abnormal glucose metabolism
  - No history of poor obstetric outcome
- Average risk: For patients not meeting criteria for either low or high risk, perform blood glucose testing at 24–28 wk (see Table 7.2)
- High-risk: Perform blood glucose testing as soon as feasible, if one or more of these are present:
  - Severe obesity
  - Strong family history of type 2 diabetes
  - Previous history of: DGM, impaired glucose metabolism, or glucosuria. If GDM is not diagnosed, blood glucose testing should be repeated at 24–28 wk or at any time a patient has symptoms or signs that are suggestive of hyperglycemia.

 CASE CONTINUES

Although not required by standard care, the patient undergoes a screening test for diabetes at her first visit, a 50-g, 1-hour glucose tolerance test (GTT). This result is reported to be 126 mg/dL. Since this is a normal result, the patient is given the usual instructions on healthy eating and dietary requirements in pregnancy. She is advised to get the test repeated at 24 to 28 weeks. The next screening test at 25 weeks yields a result of 176 mg/dL. She then undergoes the diagnostic test, a 100-g, 3-hour GTT after a preparation period of high-carbohydrate diet and an overnight fast. The results are as follows:

Fasting	110 mg/dL
1-hour	176 mg/dL
2-hour	166 mg/dL
3-hour	160 mg/dL

The patient has three abnormal values and is diagnosed with gestational diabetes.

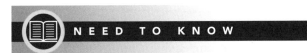

Diagnosis of GDM

The following are the screening and diagnostic methods and their normal values employed to screen and diagnose diabetes in pregnancy (Table 7.2).

Although random glucose (>200 mg/dL) and fasting (>126 mg/dL) plasma glucose values have been utilized, they are not established diagnostic tests for gestational diabetes.

TABLE 7.2

TESTS FOR DIAGNOSIS OF GESTATIONAL DIABETES

A. Two-step test: 50 g oral glucose, 1-hour screen followed by GTT if screen abnormal
B. One-step test: 75 g oral glucose, 2-hour GTT (recommended by the World Health Organization [WHO])

50 g Oral Glucose Screen

	Carpenter & Coustan	Fourth/Fifth International Workshop for GDM
Value	130 mg/dL	140 mg/dL
Blood	Plasma	Plasma
Sensitivity	>90%	80%

100 g, 3-hour GTT:

Timing	Carpenter & Coustan mg/dL	Glucose mmol/L
Fasting	95	5.3
1-hour	180	10.0
2-hour	155	8.6
3-hour	140	7.8

Test positive if two abnormal values or fasting hyperglycemia
75 g, 2-hour GTT: Recommended by WHO

Timing	75 g Glucose mg/dL	75 g Glucose mmol/L
Fasting	95	5.3
1-hour	180	10.0
2-hour	155	8.6

Test positive if two abnormal values or fasting hyperglycemia
GDM, gestational diabetes mellitus; GTT, glucose tolerance test.

 CASE CONTINUES

Now that the diagnosis is made, Ms. Creech is classified (Table 7.3) as a class A (gestational) diabetic. At the present time she is class A1 (diet controlled) and will initially be placed on a diabetic diet and exercise program for the first 2 weeks. She is advised to monitor her capillary blood glucose at home, including fasting and 2-hour postprandial values after breakfast, lunch, and dinner using the glucometer she is prescribed. She is advised to bring her blood glucose log back for review in 2 weeks. At that time based on her blood sugar results, her regimen will be adjusted to achieve

TABLE 7.3
CLASSIFICATION OF DIABETES COMPLICATING PREGNANCY

Class	Age of Onset (year)	Duration (year)	Vascular Disease
A$_1$	Any	Gestational controlled by diet	
A$_2$	Any	Gestational requiring medication	
B	>20	<10	None
C	10–19	10–19	None
D	Before 10	>20	Benign retinopathy
F	Any	Any	Nephropathy
R	Any	Any	Proliferative retinopathy
H	Any	Any	Heart

target blood glucose. Regardless of the treatment, target plasma or blood glucose goals are typically lower than that of the nonpregnant diabetic (Table 7.4).

You discuss with the patient the importance of glucose control during pregnancy, including effects of hyperglycemia on the growing fetus, newborn, and the mother.

TABLE 7.4
TARGETS FOR GLUCOSE CONTROL IN GESTATIONAL DIABETES

State	Glucose Level
Fasting	60–90 mg/dL
1-hour postprandial	130–140 mg/dL
2-hour postprandial	<120 mg/dL
Nocturnal	60–120 mg/dL

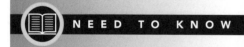

Risks of GDM

Gestational diabetes carries a risk for maternal and fetal adverse events. The fetus of a mother with GDM is at risk for macrosomia (see Chapter xx) and hyperbilirubinemia, as well as shoulder dystocia and birth injuries. Infants of normal birth weight have a relative increase in body fat compared to the infants of non diabetic mothers. If the mother actually has undiagnosed pregestational diabetes, the fetus may also be at risk for congenital abnormalities. GDM also involves maternal risks including an increased rate of preeclampsia, and an increased incidence of cesarean delivery.

 CASE CONTINUES

The patient returns in 2 weeks at approximately 28 weeks of gestation. She had followed her 2,200-calorie American Diabetes Association (ADA) diet and has been walking for 30 minutes a day. She brings her blood glucose and dietary log. More than 25% of her fasting and postprandial blood glucose values are elevated. Given these findings, she is placed on glyburide, 2.5 mg twice daily. At 34 weeks, she is begins antenatal testing using a modified biophysical profile, twice a week.

At 36 weeks, an ultrasound shows the fetus to have accelerated growth, with the abdominal circumference in the 95th percentile and an estimated fetal weight of 4,200 g.

Decision 2: Management

What is the best course of action given an estimated fetal weight of 4,200 g at 36 weeks?

   A. Immediate cesarean section
   B. Immediate induction of labor
   C. Cesarean section at term
   D. Vaginal delivery at term

The correct answers are C or D: Cesarean section at term or vaginal delivery at term. There is no indication for preterm delivery either by cesarean section or vaginal delivery. Delivery at this time would incur a risk of late preterm birth for the newborn. Furthermore, studies indicate no benefit of induction of labor to reduce the cesarean section rate resulting from impending macrosomia. Because of the risk of shoulder dystocia, GDMs with estimated fetal weights of >4,500 g may be offered an option of an elective cesarean section at term or at the time of spontaneous labor. Although the fetal weight is currently <4,500 g, you could counsel the patient that she ultimately may be offered a cesarean section, as the fetus will gain approximately

TABLE 7.5

RISK OF SHOULDER DYSTOCIA BY BIRTH WEIGHT IN DIABETIC AND NONDIABETIC PREGNANCIES

Weight	Nondiabetic (%)	Diabetic (%)
3,750–4,000	0.2	0.5
4,000–4,250	2.6	3
4,250–4,500	5	6.9
4,500–4,750	7.5	21.8
4,750–5,000	12.9	35.7
>5,000	8.9	38.5

250 g/wk during the remaining pregnancy. Despite the fact that she had an uncomplicated normal delivery of a 4,200-g baby in her last pregnancy, she was also not diabetic at the time. The body habitus of an infant of a diabetic mother is often marked by increased adiposity. Thus, compared with the prior infant, the current fetus may have an increased risk of shoulder dystocia (Table 7.5).

 CASE CONTINUES

The patient returns at 37½ weeks of gestation with ruptured membranes. Based upon the prior ultrasound, you estimate the fetal weight at 4,500 g. After discussion with the patient, she opts for an elective cesarean section with bilateral tubal ligation. Her admission blood glucose level is 105 mg/dL. She is started on Ringer's lactate solution, and blood glucose is monitored every 2 hours until surgery. She undergoes a primary cesarean delivery of a male infant, weighing 4,656 g with Apgar scores of 8 and 9 at one and five minutes.

 Decision 3: Management

How is the patient managed postpartum?

- **A.** Continue diabetic diet and GTT at 6 to 12 weeks
- **B.** Continue glyburide, diabetic diet, and blood sugar checks
- **C.** Advise regular diet and GTT at 6 months

The best management is A: Continue diabetic diet, GTT at 6 to 12 weeks. Postoperatively, it is best to continue the ADA diet. If the patient is breastfeeding she can

remain on the same diet, if not she will require a calorie prescription based on her ideal body weight. Fasting and postprandial blood glucose checks may be performed in the hospital to exclude the patient with severe preexisting diabetes who requires ongoing medical therapy. Insulin or oral hypoglycemic agents are typically withheld, as glucose tolerance returns to prepregnancy levels. A postpartum GTT should be performed as following pregnancy 5% to 10% women with GDM are found to have diabetes. Furthermore, gestational diabetics have a 40% to 60% chance of developing diabetes within 5 to 10 years. Due to this risk, it has been recommended that a patient with a history of GDM be tested for diabetes on a regular basis as a part of their routine health care.

 CASE CONCLUSION

You discharge Ms. Creech with her baby with an appointment to return to your office in 6 weeks for a checkup and an oral GTT.

SUGGESTED READINGS

American College of Obstetricians and Gynecologists Committee on Practice Bulletins–Obstetrics. ACOG Practice Bulletin. Clinical management guidelines for obstetrician-gynecologists. Number 30, September 2001. Gestational diabetes. Obstet Gynecol. 2001; 98(3):525–38.

Carpenter MW, Coustan DR. Criteria for screening tests for gestational diabetes mellitus. Am J Obstet Gynecol. 1982;144: 768–73.

Committee on Obstetric Practice. ACOG Committee Opinion No. 435: postpartum screening for abnormal glucose tolerance in women who had gestational diabetes mellitus. Obstet Gynecol. 2009;113(6):1419–21.

Ferrara A, Kahn HS, Quesenberry CP, Riley C, Hedderson MM. An increase in the incidence of gestational diabetes mellitus: Northern California, 1991–2000. Obstet Gynecol. 2004;103:526–33.

HAPO Study Cooperation Research Group. Hyperglycemia and adverse pregnancy outcomes. N Engl J Med. 2008;358:1991–2002.

Lucas MJ, Leveno KJ, Williams ML, Raskin P, Whalley PJ. Early pregnancy glycosylated hemoglobin, severity of diabetes and fetal malformations. Am J Obstet Gynecol. 1989;161:426–31.

O'Sullivan JB, Mahan CM. Criteria for the oral glucose test in pregnancy. Diabetes. 1964;13:278–85.

Rowan JA, Hague WM, et al. Metformin versus insulin for the treatment of gestational diabetes. N Engl J Med. 2008;358:2003–15.

Diabetes in Pregnancy

Dotun Ogunyemi

 CASE PRESENTATION

Ms Francis presents to your office for prenatal care because of a positive home pregnancy test. She is 37 years old, G6 P4014, and her last menstrual period was 8 weeks ago. Her first, second, and third pregnancies occurred 12, 10, and 8 years ago; all had uneventful prenatal courses with spontaneous vaginal deliveries and neonatal birth weights of 3,800, 4,000, and 4,200 g, respectively. In her fourth pregnancy, which occurred 5 years ago, she was diagnosed with gestational diabetes. She was treated with a diabetic diet and had a term vaginal delivery with neonatal weight of 4,400 g. After that pregnancy, she subsequently developed type 2 diabetes and has been treated with glyburide 10 mg twice daily for the last 4 years. Her body mass index is 40, and her general examination is within normal limits. Transvaginal ultrasound reveals a viable pregnancy compatible with dates. A glcosylated hemoglobin obtained is 7.5 mg/dL. Her fasting blood glucose is 119 mg/dL, and her 2-hour postprandial blood glucose is 185 mg/dL.

 Decision 1: Initial management

What should be done to manage this patient's blood glucose?

A. Initiate a weight loss diet
B. Increase glyburide dosage
C. Add metformin
D. Start insulin

The correct answer is D: insulin. Insulin is the accepted therapy for glucose control in pregnant women who have diabetes predating the pregnancy. Answers B and C are less correct since both hypoglycemic agents are not yet the standard of care for treatment of pregestational diabetics in pregnancy. They are most commonly used for women with gestational diabetes who fail to control their blood glucose with diet and exercise. Answer A is not correct. Although weight control is desirable, current obstetrical practice does not support weight loss in pregnancy.

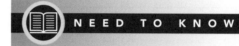 **NEED TO KNOW**

Natural History of Diabetes in Pregnancy

Pregestational diabetes is present in about 1% of pregnancies. The natural history of pregestational diabetes in pregnancy is related to the duration of diabetes, presence of microvascular disease, and glycemic control. The Priscilla White classification categorizes diabetes in pregnancy on the basis of duration and complications of diabetes and has been shown to correlate with pregnancy outcomes (see Table 8.1).

Some diabetic complications may worsen in pregnancy. Proliferative retinopathy is related to the duration of the disease and is present in the majority of those with diabetes for longer than 20 years. Women with diabetes predating pregnancy my benefit from a ophthalmological fundoscopic examination since pregnancy may worsen proliferative retinopathy. Pregnancy clearly increases the risk of mortality in diabetic women with heart disease, thus pregnancy may be contraindicated in these individuals. Diabetic ketoacidosis occurs in about 1% of diabetic pregnancies. Diabetic ketoacidosis is associated with poor compliance, as well as pregnancy-specific risk factors such as hyperemesis gravidarum, tocolysis with β-sympathomimetic drugs, infections, and use of corticosteroids for fetal lung maturation. It is associated with poor pregnancy outcome (Fig. 8.1). Hypoglycemia is also more common in pregnancy because of the tighter glycemic control attempted during pregnancy as compared to nonpregnant conditions. Diabetic nephropathy does not seem to be worsened during pregnancy.

Diabetes also increases obstetrical complications. Pyelonephritis and vaginal candidal infections occur more commonly. Diabetic neuropathy may present as gastroparesis. This is associated with nausea, vomiting and malabsorption which can result in difficult glucose control and nutritional deficiencies in pregnancy. The risk of preeclampsia is increased and is greater with

TABLE 8.1

CLASSIFICATION OF DIABETES COMPLICATING PREGNANCY

Class	Age of Onset (year)	Duration (year)	Vascular Disease
A_1	Any	Gestational controlled by diet	
A_2	Any	Gestational requiring medication	
B	>20	<10	None
C	10–19	10–19	None
D	Before 10	>20	Benign retinopathy
F	Any	Any	Nephropathy
R	Any	Any	Proliferative retinopathy
H	Any	Any	Heart

longer duration of diabetes, presence of preexisting hypertension, renal disease, or other microvascular diseases. The risk of placental abruption is also increased in those who develop preeclampsia, especially if renal disease is present with elevated serum creatinine levels. Polyhydramnios is more common and is usually a sign of suboptimal glycemic control, likely a consequence of fetal glycosuria. Infants of pregestational diabetics may be large (as may occur with gestational diabetes) and thus expose the mother to increased risk of genital trauma with vaginal delivery, and to an increased risk of cesarean delivery.

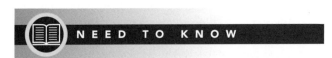

NEED TO KNOW

Calculation of Insulin Dose

Insulin is the only current therapy used in the management of pregestational diabetes in pregnancy. Both short-acting and intermediate-acting insulin are used. Rapid-acting insulin analogs such as lispro or aspart may produce better postprandial control with less hypoglycemia compared with the use of premeal regular

insulin. Injections should be in the abdomen or hips for consistency of absorption (Table 8.2).

The insulin dose is calculated on the basis of maternal weight as follows: 0.7 units/kg in the first trimester, 0.8 units/kg in the second trimester, and 0.9 units/kg in the third trimester. Compared with prepregnancy, insulin requirement may decrease in the first trimester by 10% to 25%. Overall during pregnancy, insulin requirement may increase by 10% to 20% in type 1 diabetes and by 30% to 90% in type 2 diabetes. Two thirds of the calculated insulin dosage is usually given prior to breakfast using intermediate-acting and short-acting insulin in a ratio of 2:1. One third of the calculated insulin dosage is given prior to dinner using an intermediate-acting and short-acting insulin in a ratio of 1:1. To reduce fasting hyperglycemia, the evening intermediate-acting insulin may be given at bedtime. If persistent elevated glucose levels are present after lunch, short-acting insulin maybe given with lunch. It is recommended that patients monitor their blood glucose at home and maintain the recommended levels (Table 8.3).

CASE CONTINUES

The patient is started on subcutaneous insulin twice daily. Her fasting blood glucose levels are 90 mg/dL, and 1 hour postprandial glucose levels are below 120 mg/dL. Pregnancy progresses to 18 weeks. She is followed every 2 weeks by her obstetrician. At 18 weeks of gestation,

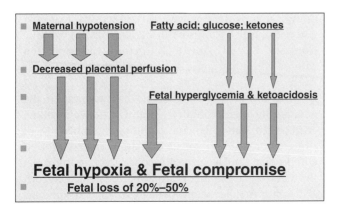

Figure 8.1 Diabetes ketoacidosis fetal consequence.

TABLE 8.2

INSULIN TYPE

Insulin Type	Onset	Peak Action	Duration
Humalog lispro	10 minutes	1 hour	2 hours
Regular insulin	20 minutes	2 hours	4 hours
NPH Insulin	1–2 hours	4 hours	8 hours

TABLE 8.3

PATIENT-MONITORED CAPILLARY BLOOD GLUCOSE GOALS IN DIABETIC PREGNANCIES

Specimen	Blood Glucose (mg/dL)
Fasting	60–95
Premeal	60–105
Postprandial 1 hour	100–120
Postprandial 2 hours	130–140
0200–0600 hours	60–120

she is referred to the perinatologist for consultation. A level II ultrasound is performed. She is also seen by the genetic counselor.

Decision 2: Management

What laboratory values will the genetic counselor need?

A. Mean corpuscular volume (MCV)
B. Blood type
C. HgbA$_{1c}$
D. Platelet count

The correct answer is C: HgbA1c. Elevations in the maternal HgbA1c are associated with an increased risk of fetal anomalies (see below). Although the genetic counselor may request the MCV (answer A) and the blood type (answer B) neither these nor the platelet count (answer D) are used to assess the risk of congenital anomalies in diabetic pregnancies.

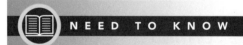

Effect of Diabetes on Fetus and Neonate

Maternal hyperglycemia is associated with fetal and neonatal complications; conversely optimum maternal glycemic status is associated with good pregnancy outcome. Glucose is transported across the placenta by facilitated diffusion with resultant fetal hyperglycemia (in cases of maternal hyperglycemia), which stimulates fetal pancreatic β-cell insulin production. Fetal hyperglycemia in early pregnancy is associated with first trimester abortions, embryonic delays, and during embryogenesis with birth defects. Caudal regression syndrome is pathognomonic of diabetic fetopathy, but congenital cardiac lesions, central nervous defects, and urinary tract anomalies are more common. There is a

TABLE 8.4

BIRTH DEFECT RISK BASED ON HBA$_{1c}$

HbA$_{1c}$ <7%	Low risk
HbA$_{1c}$ 7.2%–9.1%	14% Risk
HbA$_{1c}$ 9.2%–11.1%	23% Risk
HbA$_{1c}$ >11.2%	25% Risk

direct correlation between birth defects in diabetic pregnancies and increasing glycosylated hemoglobin levels (HbA$_{1c}$) in the first trimester (Table 8.4).

Preterm delivery is increased in pregestational diabetic pregnancies; one cause is polyhydramnios causing uterine overdistension. Preeclampsia, renal disease, and abruption also increase the risk of both spontaneous and induced preterm delivery in the diabetic pregnancy. Thus the neonate is also at greater risk for the sequelae of preterm birth, including respiratory distress syndrome and intraventricular hemorrhage. Stillbirth is also increased in diabetic pregnancies. Mechanisms of fetal death may include fetal acidosis from ketones, maternal hypotension from osmotic diuresis causing decreased uteroplacental perfusion, hypoxia from increased fetal metabolism of the excessive glucose load, microvascular disease affecting uterine vessels, or edema of the chorionic villi limiting placental transfer.

Fetal hyperglycemia and hyperinsulinism may cause excessive fetal growth, and fetal macrosomia is present in 20% to 50% of diabetic pregnancies. Infants of diabetic mothers may have increased adiposity, muscle mass, and organomegaly. The head is not affected; thus there is a disproportionate increase in shoulders and trunk resulting in asymmetric macrosomia. This may increase the risk of a traumatic vaginal delivery including shoulder dystocia and neonatal injury such as Erbs' palsy. Although controversial, macrosomic fetuses may be at increased risk of respiratory distress syndrome because insulin inhibits type II pneumocytes in fetal lung decreasing the production of surfactant. After delivery, islet cell hypertrophy with hyperinsulinism is present in these neonates and with the clamping of the umbilical cord there is loss of the excessive maternal glucose supply with resultant neonatal hypoglycemia. Conversely, fetal growth restriction can occur in women with longstanding diabetes with microvascular disease.

Other metabolic derangements that may occur in the neonate include hypocalcemia and hypomagnesemia. Polycythemia and neonatal jaundice occur because of chronic intrauterine hypoxia that stimulates erythropoietin production. Hypertrophic congestive cardiomyopathy that may be a cause of cardiac failure in the newborn also occurs in macrosomic neonates of diabetic mothers with poor glucose control in pregnancy. A major public

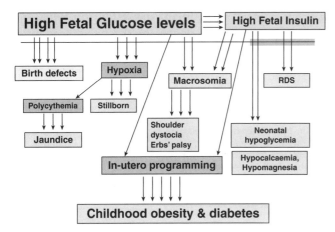

Figure 8.2 Pathogenesis of fetal and neonatal consequences from maternal diabetes.

 Decision 3: Follow up

How is the patient managed postpartum?

- **A.** Advise two third of the present insulin dose, current diabetic diet, blood glucose checks
- **B.** Advise glyburide, regular diet, blood glucose checks
- **C.** Advise continue present insulin, regular diet, glucose tolerance test at 6 weeks
- **D.** Advise glyburide, current diabetic diet, glucose tolerance test at 6 weeks

The correct answer is A: reduce the insulin dose and continue the diabetic diet and blood glucose checks. Answers B, C, and D are incorrect because patient should continue a diabetic diet, the insulin dosage should be reduced, as the patient is expected to become less insulin resistant after delivery, and postpartum glucose tolerance testing is not indicated since the patient is a known diabetic.

health concern is the increased risk of obesity and diabetes in the infants of diabetic mothers because of in utero programming (Fig. 8.2).

Fetal surveillance is indicated in pregestational diabetic pregnancies because of the risk of birth defects, macrosomia, stillbirth, and fetal hypoxia. All pregestational diabetic pregnancies should have a second trimester level II ultrasound performed to exclude major birth defects. A fetal echocardiography should be considered since cardiac defects are among the most common. The fetal abdominal circumference measured in the second or third trimester can predict excessive fetal growth and has been used to modify insulin therapy. An ultrasound or clinical estimated fetal weight at delivery, which exceeds 4,500 g would require counseling as to the risk/benefit of an elective cesarean delivery. Twice weekly fetal biophysical profiles are usually initiated between 32 and 34 weeks of gestation. This may be initiated at an earlier gestational age if there is evidence of fetal or obstetrical complications such as fetal growth restriction or preeclampsia.

 CASE CONTINUES

Ms Francis is followed in prenatal clinic. Her level II ultrasound is normal. Her insulin dosage requires adjustment to maintain good glycemic control. Biweekly fetal testing using modified biophysical profiles is initiated at 34 weeks of gestation. At 39 weeks of gestation, the patient presents in spontaneous labor. An estimated fetal weight done at the bedside is approximately 4,000 g, and labor is allowed to continue. Ms Francis has normal vaginal delivery of a male infant with a birth weight of 4,200 g and Apgar scores of 9 and 9 and one and five minutes.

📖 **N E E D   T O   K N O W**

Intra and Postpartum Management

In general, delivery is recommended in pregestational diabetic pregnancies by 38 to 39 weeks, because of the increased risk of stillbirth at term in these pregnancies. Counseling regarding cesarean delivery is recommended if estimated fetal weight is >4,500 g because of the risk of shoulder dystocia. Lung maturity amniocentesis should be considered before 38 weeks of gestational age if delivery is elective and there is no concern of fetal compromise. Delivery maybe indicated at an earlier gestational age if there is evidence of maternal or fetal compromise.

During labor, maternal euglycemia should be established and maintained. Continuous infusion of regular insulin is utilized and plasma glucose levels are measured frequently. The insulin dosage is adjusted to maintain a plasma glucose level of 80 to 120 mg/dL. Maternal euglycemia in labor reduces the risk of neonatal hypoglycemia.

Many insulin-dependent patients may not require insulin for the first 48 to 72 hours postdelivery, as the insulin requirements may drop from 50% to 30%. Plasma glucose levels should be obtained serially and regular insulin should be given if the glucose is elevated. Patients can be restarted on two thirds of the prepregnancy insulin dosage, with adjustments as indicated. Contraception and breastfeeding should be discussed and encouraged. Breastfeeding has been linked to decreased incidence of diabetes in offspring of diabetic mothers. If the patient is breastfeeding she may continue on the same diet; if not she should have her calories calculated based on her ideal body weight.

 ## CASE CONCLUSION

Ms Francis' insulin is decreased by one third. She establishes breastfeeding and contraception counseling is performed. The patient elects to receive medroxyprogesterone acetate (Depo-Provera) deep intramuscular injection. Her blood glucose is controlled. On postpartum day 3, both the mother and infant are discharged home. You arrange follow-up for the mother within your office in 1 week to check her glucose control. In addition, she is given a follow-up appointment with an endocrinologist for continued management of her diabetes.

SUGGESTED READINGS

Castro LC, Ogynyemi D: Common medical and surgical conditions complicating pregnancy in Hacker NF, Moore JG, Gambone JC, editors. Essentials of Obstetrics and Gynecology. 5th ed. Philadelphia, PA: Elsevier Saunders; 2009; Chapter 16, pp. 191–218.

Cunningham FG, Leveno KJ, Bloom SL, Hauth JC, Rouse D and Spong C. Williams Obstetrics, 23rd ed. New York, NY: McGraw-Hill; 2005. Chapter 52, pp. 1104–1125.

Fraser R and Farrell T: Diabetes in James DK, Steer PJ, Weiner CP, Gonik B, editors. High Risk Pregnancy: Management Options, 4th ed. Philadelphia, PA: Elsevier Saunders; 2010. Chapter 45; pp. 795–812.

Moore TR, Catalano P: Diabetes in pregnancy in Creasy RK, Resnik R, editors. Maternal-Fetal Medicine: Principles and Practice. 6th ed. Philadelphia, PA: Saunders; 2009. Chapter 46; pp. 953–93.

RBC Alloimmunization

Steven A. Laifer

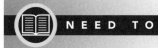

CASE PRESENTATION

Ms. Greene, a 24-year-old G2 P0010 presents at 12 weeks of gestation for prenatal care. Her medical history is unremarkable; she has no chronic illnesses, has never had surgery, has no allergies, takes no medications, and has never received a blood transfusion. She is a graduate student in psychology and does not smoke or use recreational drugs, although prior to pregnancy she used alcohol socially. She is married; her husband is 25 years old and healthy. She had a miscarriage of an unplanned pregnancy as a teenager but never sought medical care for that event. She has had no abnormal Papanicolaou test and reports no history of sexually transmitted infections. The patient reports mild nausea but no vomiting; she has had no vaginal bleeding.

The physical examination shows a blood pressure of 110/70 mm Hg and a maternal weight of 130 lb (body mass index [BMI] 24). The uterine size is consistent with 12 weeks. The remainder of the examination is unremarkable. Ms. Greene has an ultrasound to confirm gestational age and for early aneuploidy screening. The nuchal translucency measurement is 1.7 mm and aneuploidy screening is negative (adjusted risk of trisomy 21 <1:10,000, adjusted risk of trisomy 18 <1:10,000).

Routine prenatal tests and labs are also obtained; they are remarkable for a maternal blood type of A−, and an antibody screen positive for anti-D at a titer of 1:16.

The patient returns with her husband at 14 weeks for counseling regarding red blood cell (RBC) alloimmunization.

NEED TO KNOW

Red Blood Cell Alloimmunization

RBC alloimmunization refers to exposure and sensitization of the immune system to foreign RBC antigens stimulating the production of antibodies. Exposure to foreign RBCs can occur with transfusion, pregnancy (both during pregnancy and at the time of delivery), and less commonly with organ transplantation and sharing of needles. In this case the patient, who is Rh (D)-negative, was probably exposed at the time of her prior spontaneous miscarriage to Rh-positive RBCs and as a result developed antibodies to the Rh (D) antigen. This is probably an avoidable event, as most cases of Rh (D) alloimmunization can be prevented with the proper use of Rh immune globulin.

RBC alloimmunization poses no risk to a woman if she is not pregnant. During pregnancy, however, anti-RBC IgG antibodies can cross the placenta and, if present in sufficient concentration, hemolyze antigen-positive fetal RBCs. Many fetuses can tolerate a minor amount of hemolysis and compensate by producing additional RBCs. However, if the antibody concentration is high, the amount of hemolysis may exceed the ability of the fetus to compensate and the fetus may become anemic. If the anemia becomes severe, the fetus recruits nonmarrow sites to produce RBCs (extramedullary hematopoiesis), and the combination of anemia and extramedullary hematopoiesis can lead to hypoproteinemia, hypoxemia, hydrops, and fetal death (Fig. 9.1).

In general, the hemolytic anemia and other fetal consequences of RBC alloimmunization tend to be less severe in first-affected pregnancies. With the anamnestic response seen with repeat exposure to the foreign antigen, subsequent pregnancies may be complicated by higher maternal antibody titers and more severe hemolysis and anemia.

In addition to Rh(D), fetal anemia and hydrops can result from maternal antibodies to other antigens (Table 9.1). In general, severe fetal anemia is not associated with anti-ABO or anti-Lewis antibodies; these antibodies are usually of the IgM type and do not easily cross the placenta.

? Decision 1: Evaluation

What additional evaluation should be done immediately?

- **A.** Ultrasound for fetal hydrops
- **B.** Paternal blood typing
- **C.** Amniocentesis for fetal blood type
- **D.** Maternal antibody titer

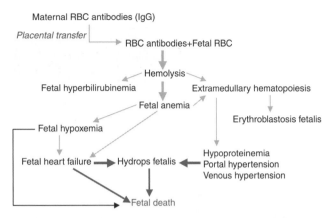

Figure 9.1 Pathophysiology of red blood cell (RBC) alloimmunization.

The correct answer is B: Paternal blood typing. The goals of managing a pregnancy complicated by RBC alloimmunization are the following:

1. to determine if the fetus is at risk for anemia
2. to closely monitor the at-risk fetus for severity of anemia
3. to provide treatment to the severely anemic fetus and prevent hydrops and fetal death.

Only a fetus that is antigen positive will be at risk for hemolytic anemia caused by antibodies directed against that antigen. Determining the fetal blood type (i.e., is the fetus antigen positive), therefore, is the key to determining whether the fetus is at risk for anemia. If paternity is known, evaluating the paternal blood type and zygosity is the first step in determining if the fetus is antigen positive.

TABLE 9.1

ATYPICAL ANTIBODIES ASSOCIATED WITH FETAL HYDROPS

Blood Group System	Antigens Related to Hemolytic Disease
Kell	K
	K
	Ko
	Kp^a
	Kp^b
	Js^a
	Js^b
Rh (non-D)	E
	C
	C
Duffy	Fy^a
	Fy^b
	By^3

Note: Alloimmunization is possible with many other blood group antigens; these have not been demonstrated to cause hydrops.
Adapted from ACOG Practice Bulletin No. 75. Obstet Gynecol. 2006; 108(2):457–64.

If the father is antigen negative (Rh negative in this case), the fetus will be Rh negative and not at risk for anemia. If the father is antigen positive (Rh positive) and heterozygous for the gene coding for the antigen, there is a 50% chance that the fetus will be antigen positive and at risk for anemia. If the father is antigen positive and homozygous for the gene coding for the antigen, the fetus is definitely antigen positive and therefore at risk for hemolytic anemia from RBC antibodies directed against the antigen. In the case of Rh sensitization, blood banks are able to predict zygosity in the father by using a combination of antisera to all of the antigens coded on the Rh locus (D, C/c, E/e) and race-based gene frequency tables, or it may be possible to directly examine the paternal genes of interest using DNA techniques.

In cases where the father is heterozygous or if the father is not available for testing or paternity is uncertain, fetal DNA testing, using either amniocytes (Answer C) or chorionic villi, can be performed. Polymerized chain reaction amplification of fetal DNA from the Rh gene on chromosome one can reliably identify the fetus who is antigen positive or antigen negative. In order to limit the small inaccuracies that may occur as a result of inaccurate paternity or gene rearrangements and from Rh pseudogenes, most labs request a maternal and paternal blood sample (if available) for comparison with the fetal DNA specimen. Using techniques similar to those being studied for prenatal diagnosis of aneuploidy, fetal blood type and antigen status can also be determined experimentally using free fetal DNA found in the maternal circulation. Once refined, this technique may obviate the need for chorionic villus sampling or amniocentesis with their associated risks.

Although ultrasound may be useful in the diagnosis of fetal hydrops (Answer A), hydrops is unlikely to be present at 14 weeks in a first sensitized pregnancy. Maternal antibody titer (Answer D) is useful in predicting the likelihood of fetal harm from alloimmunization with an at-risk fetus, but antibody titers are not useful in determining fetal antigen status.

 CASE CONTINUES

Ms. Greene's husband agrees to have zygosity testing; the results indicate that he is heterozygous for the D antigen. The fetus therefore has a 50% chance of being D antigen positive and potentially at risk for fetal anemia. Ms. Greene consents to an amniocentesis for fetal Rh typing. At 16 weeks, an amniocentesis is performed with special attention to avoid penetrating the placenta (which can lead to a fetal-to-maternal bleed and potentially worsen the alloimmunization). The patient's antibody titer, which was initially 1:16 is now 1:64. The results indicate that the fetus is Rh (D)-positive and therefore at risk for hemolytic anemia.

Based on DNA testing that revealed the fetus to be Rh positive and the antibody titer of 1:64, the patient and her husband are counseled that their fetus is at risk for severe anemia and that more intensive monitoring is required.

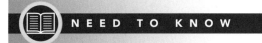

NEED TO KNOW

Monitoring of the Pregnancy at Risk for Fetal Anemia

If the fetus is identified as being antigen positive and at risk for hemolytic anemia due to maternal Rh alloimmunization, the first stage of monitoring may be the maternal antibody titer. The antibody concentration (antibody titer) is directly related to the severity of the hemolytic anemia. In anti-D alloimmunization, the critical antibody titer (the antibody concentration at which the fetus is at risk for severe anemia and hydrops) is laboratory dependent, and is between 1:8 and 1:16 in most centers. As long as the antibody titer remains stable and subcritical, severe fetal disease is unlikely. In a patient with a subcritical antibody titer, maternal antibody titers may be monitored approximately every 4 weeks. A one-fold increase in titer (e.g., 1:4 to 1:8) may reflect laboratory variation, but a two-fold or greater increase in titer is most consistent with increased antibody concentration. The increased titer most likely indicates maternal exposure to antigen-positive RBCs and increased maternal antibody production, and it may require increased fetal surveillance. Once a critical titer is reached, more complex fetal monitoring is required to evaluate the fetus for severity of anemia. In a mother with a prior history of an affected fetus, or in non–anti-D alloimmunization, antibody titers are not sufficiently predictive, and primary fetal surveillance is undertaken by means of ultrasound (see below).

The most accurate and direct method for evaluating the severity of anemia is to measure the hemoglobin and hematocrit. In a fetus, however, this requires the skill and expertise associated with the procedure of percutaneous umbilical blood sampling (PUBS), which carries a procedure-associated mortality of approximately 1% to 2%. Therefore, less invasive but indirect methods are used to evaluate the severity of fetal anemia, and fetal blood sampling is reserved for confirmation of severe anemia and treatment.

Spectral analysis of amniotic fluid bilirubin (obtained by amniocentesis) was the mainstay of evaluation of severity of anemia for many years. Bilirubin is a breakdown product of RBCs; higher amounts of bilirubin in amniotic fluid indirectly indicate a greater degree of RBC hemolysis and a more severe degree of fetal anemia. Bilirubin absorbs light at a wavelength of 450 nm; the difference in the optical density reading at 450 nm (ΔOD450) between the patient and normal values (dependent upon gestational age) reflects the amount of bilirubin in the amniotic fluid. A high ΔOD450, therefore, suggests a more severe fetal anemia. Spectral analysis generally requires serial amniocenteses to identify a trend; the ΔOD450 values are graphed and displayed against gestational age. Two graphs have been used to evaluate ΔOD450: the Liley curve (Fig. 9.2) evaluated

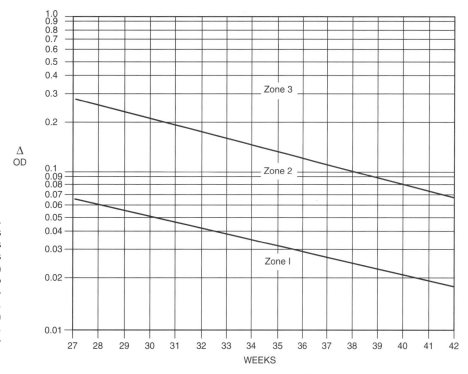

Figure 9.2 Liley curve for ΔOD450. The increase in absorbance at 450 nm is plotted against gestational age. Patients in zone 1 have no evidence of hemolysis and are considered normal. Patients in the lower part of zone 2 are also likely to be normal, but require enhanced surveillance, including repeat amniocentesis. Patients in the upper part of zone 2 or in zone 3 are likely to have RBC hemolysis, and require further evaluation and possibly treatment.

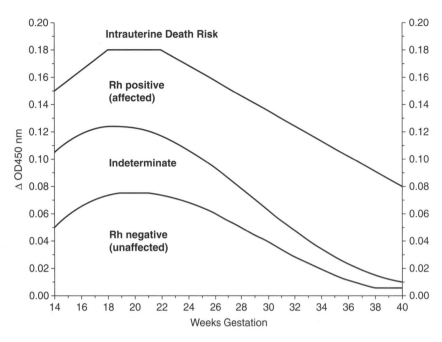

Figure 9.3 Queenan curve for ΔOD450. Queenan's curve is useful in the management of pregnancies earlier than 27 weeks, but the categories of risk are similar, with Liley's zone 2 explicitly divided into two zones (Indeterminate and Rh positive [affected]). Published in Queenan JT, Tomai TP, Ural SH, King JC. Deviation in amniotic fluid optical density at a wavelength of 450 nm in Rh-immunized pregnancies from 14 to 40 weeks of gestation: a proposal for clinical management. Am J Obstet Gynecol 1993;168:1370–6.

pregnancies from 27 weeks until term and is divided into three zones. Fetuses with values in high zone 2 or zone 3 were at risk for severe anemia, hydrops, and death. Because of improved neonatal survival at earlier gestational ages and the many advances in ultrasound technology that allowed for more accurate fetal imaging and earlier diagnostic and therapeutic interventions, Queenan introduced a modified curve that included ΔOD450 values for earlier gestational ages and consisted of four zones (Fig. 9.3). Values in the high affected or intrauterine death risk zones indicate a fetus at high risk for severe anemia, hydrops, or death.

Although spectral analysis of amniotic fluid is still available for the management of RBC alloimmunization and has proved to be a valuable technique that provides reasonably accurate diagnosis and treatment of severely anemic fetuses (as well as identification of the unaffected or minimally affected fetus), it has several disadvantages. Interpretation of the analysis can be impacted by other pigments or contaminants in the amniotic fluid. In addition, serial procedures are required that are each associated with risks of preterm labor, amniorrhexis, and infection, and worsening of the immune process if the needle traverses the placenta.

In current practice, the mainstay for evaluating severity of anemia in the RBC alloimmunized patient is the noninvasive Doppler evaluation of the fetal cerebral circulation. In a landmark publication, Mari et al. demonstrated that the peak velocity in the middle cerebral artery (MCA), a vessel that is able to be visualized and interrogated with contemporary ultrasound equipment (Fig. 9.4) correlated accurately with fetal anemia. These investigators demonstrated that all fetuses with moderate or severe anemia had peak velocities in the MCA of >1.5 multiples of the median (MOM, sensitivity of 100%, false-positive rate of 12%). In a follow-up study that directly compared Doppler evaluation of MCA with amniocentesis and spectral analysis of amniotic fluid, investigators found that Doppler evaluation of the MCA was more accurate than spectral analysis of amniotic fluid for identifying severely anemic fetuses.

In most centers, therefore, the noninvasive technique of Doppler evaluation of the MCA has replaced spectral analysis of amniotic fluid as the preferred method for evaluating severity of anemia in antigen-positive fetuses. If the patient is followed with subcritical antibody titers, Doppler evaluation of MCA is undertaken when a critical

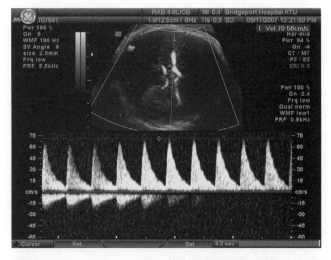

Figure 9.4 Doppler interrogation of MCA and measurement of peak systolic velocity.

Rh Alloimmunization: Management

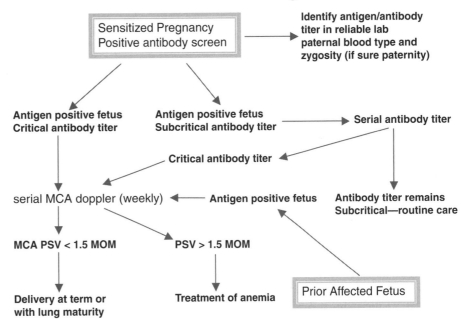

Figure 9.5 Algorithm for management of Rh alloimmunization. Note that, with a prior affected fetus, maternal antibody titers are not used. In addition, maternal antibody titers are not useful with sensitization to other antigens such as Kell. Antigen-negative fetus reverts to normal Ob care. MCA, middle cerebral artery; PSV, peak systolic velocity; MOM, multiples of the median.

antibody titer is reached. In a patient in whom antibody titers are not useful, Doppler evaluation of MCA is performed on a weekly basis beginning at approximately 20 weeks of gestation. As long as the MCA peak velocity remains below 1.5 MOM, adjusted for gestational age, the fetus is not severely anemic. These patients can be safely followed and delivered at term or with evidence of fetal lung maturity. If the peak velocity exceeds 1.5 MOM, the fetus may be severely anemic and at risk for hydrops or fetal death and treatment is indicated. An algorithm that describes the general management scheme of patients with RBC alloimmunization is described in Figure 9.5.

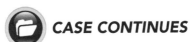 **CASE CONTINUES**

A comprehensive ultrasound for the evaluation of fetal anatomy is performed at 18 weeks. Fetal growth is appropriate, the anatomic survey is normal, the placenta is anterior-fundal, and the placental cord insertion is visualized. Beginning at 20 weeks, Ms. Greene comes in weekly for Doppler evaluation of the MCA. Serial evaluation reveals MCA peak velocities <1.5 MOM (Fig. 9.6). At 31 weeks of gestation, the MCA nears 1.5 MOM. At $31^{3/7}$ weeks of gestation, the MCA peak velocity is 1.5 MOM, and at 32 weeks the MCA peak velocity

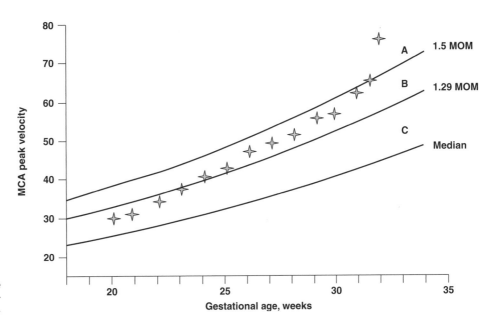

Figure 9.6 Graph of middle cerebral artery (MCA) peak velocities. MOM, multiples of the median.

exceeds 1.5 MOM. Severe fetal anemia is now suspected. The estimated fetal weight is 1,850 g and the amniotic fluid index is 19. Biophysical profile (BPP) score is 8/8, and there is no evidence of fetal hydrops on the ultrasound.

Decision 2: Management

Which of the following is the most appropriate response to elevated MCA velocity?

A. Immediate delivery
B. Fetal intraperitoneal transfusion
C. Nothing (await hydrops)
D. PUBS for fetal hematocrit and intravascular transfusion if anemic

The correct answer is D (PUBS for fetal hematocrit and intravascular transfusion if anemic). The immediate threat to the fetus is severe anemia and its consequences (Fig. 9.1), and the most effective immediate treatment is blood transfusion. This can be accomplished by delivery of the fetus and transfusion of the neonate in the intensive care unit or by transfusing the fetus in utero. Intrauterine transfusions are performed when, as in this patient, the additional risks and complications of prematurity are considered greater than the risks of intrauterine transfusion. At this gestational age, and without evidence of fetal lung maturity, the best option is intrauterine therapy, and not to proceed to immediate delivery (Answer A). Fetal hydrops represents the end stage of fetal anemia and implies a considerably increased risk of fetal loss. Awaiting hydrops before treatment (Answer C) would never be a recommended course of action. Fetal intraperitoneal transfusion (Answer B) could be a correct answer, but this management plan would require fetal treatment based on the suspicion of anemia alone, without confirmation.

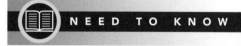

Intrauterine Transfusion

In current practice, intrauterine transfusions are most commonly performed by the intravascular route through the umbilical cord. Under direct ultrasound guidance, a needle is inserted percutaneously into the umbilical vein at the insertion site of the cord into the placenta. A sample of blood is obtained for a complete blood cell count, and a short-acting paralytic agent may be infused to prevent fetal movement from dislodging the needle. If severe anemia is confirmed on rapid eval-uation, tightly packed, O negative, cytomegalovirus negative, leukoreduced, and irradiated RBCs crossmatched to the mother are transfused to the fetus. The blood is prepared in this fashion to minimize risks to the fetus of infection, volume overload, and graft-versus-host disease. The volume of blood to be transfused is dependent on the starting hematocrit, desired posttransfusion hematocrit, and the gestational age and estimated fetal blood volume.

Depending upon the gestational age at the initial intrauterine transfusion, additional transfusions may be required to maintain an adequate fetal hematocrit and to suppress fetal erythropoiesis. One common practice is to transfuse every 14 days until fetal erythropoiesis is suppressed, as determined by obtaining a fetal blood sample and failing to demonstrate fetal hemoglobin. The schedule for further transfusions may vary and depends on the volume that was transfused, the final hematocrit that was achieved, and the expected daily 1% decline in the hematocrit after a transfusion. In addition, some centers perform combined intravascular/intraperitoneal transfusions, in order to increase the mass of RBCs transfused and reduce the needed frequency of transfusions. Because of technical factors that may impact the success of fetal therapy (maternal habitus, placental location) cases need to be individualized.

The complication rate associated with each intrauterine transfusion is approximately 3%. Complications include amniorrhexis, infection, fetal bradycardia, cord hematomas, cord bleeding, and fetal death. The gestational age at which delivery and neonatal therapy becomes more advantageous and beneficial than fetal therapy is debated. Some argue that delivery with evidence of lung maturity is appropriate while others advocate transfusion until 35 weeks with delivery at 37 to 38 weeks. Fetal outcome after intrauterine transfusion is favorable, with >90% survival in nonhydropic fetuses.

 CASE CONTINUES

Your counsel Ms. Greene and her husband that therapy for suspected fetal anemia is necessary. The options include fetal therapy with intravascular transfusion or delivery with neonatal (exchange) transfusion. In view of the early gestational age and likelihood of additional prematurity complications, fetal therapy is recommended and accepted by the patient.

Because of the risk of complications requiring delivery, the transfusion is performed in the hospital in the delivery room. Under ultrasound guidance, a needle is advanced into the umbilical vein as it exits the placenta. Fetal hematocrit is found to be 25%, consistent with marked anemia. Fetal transfusion is performed.

After transfusion, Ms. Greene is followed with twice-weekly modified BPPs and MCA Doppler. Fetal testing is reassuring and the MCA peak velocities remain below 1.5 MOM. An amniocentesis for evaluation of fetal lung maturity is performed at 34 2/7 weeks to determine if an additional fetal transfusion is appropriate. The amniocentesis reveals that the fetal lungs are mature. The patient does not want a trial of labor and a primary cesarean delivery is performed at 34 3/7 weeks. A 2,250-g female infant is delivered without complications. The cord hematocrit is 30% and the initial total bilirubin is 15 mg/dL. The neonate is on room air and requires no ventilatory support. Because of an increasing bilirubin, a single volume exchange transfusion is performed and for several days supplemental phototherapy is used. The baby has mild temperature instability but no other complications. The mother's recovery is uneventful, and the baby is discharged to home on day of life 15.

On visiting your office for her postpartum checkup, Ms. Greene asks if there is any way for her to avoid another sensitized pregnancy.

Decision 3: Counseling

What options does the mother have in her next pregnancy?

A. Adopt
B. Artificial insemination with Rh-negative donor
C. Intravenous immunoglobulin (IVIG)
D. Steroids

The correct answers are A and B. Either adoption (Answer A) or artificial insemination with an Rh-negative donor (Answer B) would avoid another sensitized pregnancy.

Whether either of these is an option for an individual patient is a personal decision. IVIG (Answer C) has been used in limited cases to ameliorate fetal sensitization, but the reports concern treatment of mothers with previous severe alloimmunization, including fetal death. Steroids (Answer D) have not been shown to prevent fetal harm with an alloimmunized mother.

 ## CASE CONCLUSION

After considering her options, Ms. Greene elects to attempt another pregnancy with her husband. As he is a heterozygote, she has a 50% chance of having an Rh-negative fetus, without any sensitization risk.

SUGGESTED READINGS

ACOG Practice Bulletin No. 75. Management of alloimmunization during pregnancy. Obstet Gynecol. 2006;108(2):457–64.
Bowman JM. Hemolytic disease. In: Creasy RK, Resnick R, editors. Maternal Fetal Medicine: Principles and Practice. 2nd ed. Philadelphia, PA: W.B. Saunders Company; 1989, pp. 613–55.
Mari G, Deter RL, Carpenter RL, et al. Noninvasive diagnosis by Doppler ultrasonography of fetal anemia due to maternal red cell alloimmunization. Collaborative Group for Doppler Assessment of the Blood Velocity of Anemic Fetuses. N Engl J Med. 2000; 342(1):9–14.
Moise KJ. Hemolytic disease of the fetus and newborn. In: Creasy RK, Resnick R, Iams JD, editors. Maternal Fetal Medicine: Principles and Practice. 6th ed. Philadelphia, PA: Saunders Elsevier; 2009, pp. 477–99.
Moise KJ. Management of rhesus alloimmunization in pregnancy. Obstet Gynecol. 2008;112:164–76.
Oepkes D, Seaward PG, Vandenbussche FP, et al. Doppler ultrasonography versus amniocentesis to predict fetal anemia. N Engl J Med. 2006;355(2):156–64.

Pelvic Mass in Pregnancy

10

Samuel S. Im

 CASE PRESENTATION

You are asked to consult on Ms. Francis, a 24-year-old G2 P0 who is at 9 weeks of gestation by her last menstrual period. One week ago, at her initial prenatal care visit, the midwife felt that her uterine size was not appropriate for gestational age. An ultrasound was ordered to confirm the gestational age, and it showed an apparently normal 9-week intrauterine pregnancy and a 12-cm complex right ovarian mass. She is extremely concerned about her pregnancy and the mass.

Ms. Francis denies any pain or vaginal bleeding. She has begun to have some morning nausea but has only vomited twice. This is her second pregnancy after one prior first trimester loss. Ms. Francis denies any significant past medical history. She reports that her mother has a history of diabetes and hypertension and that her husband's aunt died of ovarian cancer, but she denies any family history of birth defects or recurrent pregnancy losses.

On physical examination, Ms. Francis' blood pressure is 120/70 mm Hg, and her pulse is 85 bpm. Her weight is 165 lbs. She is afebrile. Her abdominal examination is nontender, with a palpable fullness in the lower midabdomen. On pelvic examination, there is a palpable, nontender 12- to 15-cm soft mass in the midline and behind the uterine fundus, which is 9 weeks' size. Ms. Francis asks you whether you think that she has a cancer.

 NEED TO KNOW

Common Ovarian Neoplasms in Young Women

Ovarian masses and cysts may be reported as an incidental finding at first trimester ultrasound in as many as 8% of patients. The majority of these are small, functional cysts, and 70% to 90% will resolve by the second trimester without treatment. Masses that persist into the second trimester may still be physiologic cysts, such as a persistent corpus leutea, or they may be benign

neoplasms. The incidence of malignancy in an adnexal mass found in the second trimester is about 2% (Table 10.1). When a malignancy is found, the cell type is consistent with ovarian malignancies found in nonpregnant women of similar age. Compared with postmenopausal patients, the incidence of tumors of low malignant potential is higher, as is the rate of germ cell tumors (Table 10.2).

? **Decision 1:** Workup

What is your next step?

A. Immediate surgery to prevent torsion
B. Draw tumor markers: human chorionic gonadotropin (hCG), CA-125, CEA, alpha-fetoprotein (AFP), lactate dehydrogenase (LDH)
C. Follow-up ultrasound
D. Schedule surgery at 15 to 20 weeks of gestational age

The correct answer is C: Follow-up ultrasound. Most adnexal cysts and masses found in early pregnancy will resolve spontaneously. Scheduling a repeat ultrasound evaluation is prudent both to ascertain whether the cyst has persisted into the second trimester and to evaluate the risk of malignancy. Although the possibility of ovarian torsion is a concern with an adnexal mass in pregnancy, the likelihood of torsion is probably about 3%, which would not justify the risks of surgery in an asymptomatic patient (Answer A). It is prudent to inform the patient to seek care immediately if she develops acute lower abdominal pain or a sudden increase in nausea or vomiting.

In pregnancy, many of the common tumor markers are elevated and do not serve to differentiate a malignancy (Answer B). In particular, CA 125 levels are elevated during the first and third trimesters of pregnancy. Other tumor markers such as AFP and hCG are elevated throughout pregnancy. Only LDH remains constant during pregnancy. If the adnexal mass is >5 cm in size and persists through the early second trimester of pregnancy, then surgical resection is usually recommended (Answer D). The surgery is often scheduled between 16 and 18 weeks of gestation. At this

TABLE 10.1

PATHOLOGIC DIAGNOSIS OF ADNEXAL MASSES PERSISTING TO THE SECOND TRIMESTER OF PREGNANCY

	Pathology	Percentage of Masses
Benign	Persistent corpus luteum	17%
	Benign cystic teratoma	37%
	Cystadenoma	24%
	Luteoma of pregnancy	Rare
	Endometrioma	5%
	Paraovarian cyst	5%
	Leiomyoma	5%
	Other	4.8%
Malignant		2.2%

time fetal organogenesis has been completed and most physiologic cysts have resolved, but the uterus is relatively small and resistant to contractions, and the fetus is previable.

 CASE CONTINUES

Ms. Francis has normal first and second trimester screening for aneuploidy, including a normal maternal serum AFP and hCG. A repeat ultrasound at 16 weeks reveals a normally grown fetus and the fetal anatomy survey is unremarkable. The ultrasound also shows a persistent right adnexal cystic mass. It is complex, 10 cm in size with two thin septations. No excrescences or papillations are noted and the Doppler pulsatility index is 1.2.

TABLE 10.2

HISTOLOGY OF OVARIAN MALIGNANCIES OCCURRING IN CALIFORNIA WOMEN 1991 TO 1999

Histology	Number
Low malignant potential	117 (57%)
Serous	83
Mucinous	34
Malignant	89 (43$)
Serous	14
Mucinous	10
Endometrioid	5
Clear cell	3
Other epithelial	14
Pseudomyxoma peritonei	8
Germ cell	34
Granulosa cell	1
Total	**206**

She has had no complaints since her last visit. The patient asks if she should have an operation.

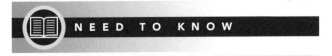 **NEED TO KNOW**

Predictors of Malignancy

The great majority of adnexal masses found during pregnancy will be benign; however, the concern for malignancy is the factor driving surgical intervention in the asymptomatic patient. Assessment of an adnexal mass for possible malignancy is difficult, and it is especially challenging during pregnancy because tumor markers are unreliable. Ultrasound characterization of an ovarian mass can help predict malignancy (Table 10.3). The presence of solid nodules, thick internal septations, or papillary projections inside the cyst (Fig. 10.1) heightens the concern for malignancy. In addition, color Doppler evidence of flow within the septations increases the risk. In the nonpregnant patient, a Doppler pulsatility index of >1 in uterine, ovarian, or intratumor vessels has a negative predictive value of 0.93 for ovarian malignancy; however, this cutoff has not been validated in pregnancy. In cases in which the ultrasound is not sufficiently reassuring, a magnetic resonance imaging (MRI) may provide additional diagnostic information.

In addition to the ovarian findings, free fluid or ascites in the abdomen and pelvis, or evidence of metastatic disease on an imaging study also increases the concern for malignancy.

 CASE CONTINUES

You discuss the ultrasound findings with Ms. Francis. You let her know that her risk for malignancy is low, but that the persistence of the cyst, the ovarian size, and presence of multiple septations are of some concern. You offer her MRI scan to further elucidate the findings but concede

TABLE 10.3

ULTRASOUND CHARACTERIZATION OF PELVIC MASSES

Favor benign cyst	Simple cyst Thin internal septation Doppler pulsatility index >1
Favor malignant cyst	Multiple thick septations Solid internal nodules Papillary projections Internal blood flow on color Doppler

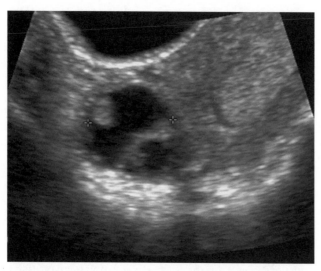

Figure 10.1 Papillary projection and a thick septum in an ovarian cyst (a borderline tumor). (From Chiang G, Levine D. Imaging of adnexal masses in pregnancy. J Ultrasound Med. 2004;23(6):805–19.)

Figure 10.2 Blood flow within the ovarian septum detected by Doppler sonography. Pulsatiity index is 0.72. Both findings are suspicious for malignancy; this cyst was a cystadenocarcinoma. From Pascual MA, Tresserra F, Grases PJ, Labastida R, Dexeus S. Borderline cystic tumors of the ovary: gray-scale and color Doppler sonographic findings. J Clin Ultrasound. 2002 Feb;30(2):76–82. Used with permission.

that no imaging procedure will completely eliminate the chance that she has an ovarian cancer. She is very fearful about cancer and would like to have surgery as soon as possible. You discuss surgical options with her, including laparotomy, laparoscopy, ovarian cystectomy, oophorectomy, and the risk that she will have a miscarriage or hysterectomy as a consequence of the procedure. After much discussion, you agree to perform a laparoscopy at 18 weeks of gestation, with the plan to remove the cyst laparoscopically if possible. She agrees to undergo oophorectomy, if examination of the pelvis indicates a high suspicion for ovarian cancer, but she does not agree to undergo hysterectomy (and therefore abortion) unless her life is in danger. She understands that the size or position of the mass may make a laparotomy necessary.

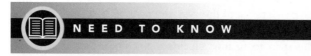

NEED TO KNOW

Risks of Surgery in Pregnancy

Surgery during pregnancy involves risks to both mother and fetus. The mother assumes the usual surgical risks of pain, bleeding, infection, and damage to other organs. If regional anesthesia is performed, there are additional risks of spinal headache, central nervous system infection, and excessive block, causing respiratory arrest. With general anesthesia the risk is greater, including the risk of bronchospasm with failure to intubate/failure to ventilate, the risk of aspiration pneumonitis, and the risk of a reaction to one of the

drugs used. Aspiration pneumonitis may be a particular concern in the pregnant woman, as relaxation of the esophageal sphincter and the slower gut transit time may increase the risk of reflux of stomach contents. Although all of these risks have been reported in pregnant women, the likelihood of maternal mortality with adnexal surgery in pregnancy is very low: the maternal mortality related to anesthesia for cesarean delivery (the most common surgical procedure on pregnant women) is estimated to be 1.3 to 2.8 per million live births, and there is no reason to think that anesthesia-related deaths with elective maternal abdominal surgery would be higher. There are limited numbers of reports of the consequences of adnexal surgery in pregnancy and maternal deaths have not been reported. The risk of maternal death after all nonobstetric abdominal procedures has been reported to be 6 per 100,000 procedures.

For the fetus, maternal abdominal surgery has been associated with an increased risk of miscarriage, premature delivery, and low birth weight. These risks appear to be most prominent in patients with acute events such as appendicitis or ovarian torsion. The rate of miscarriage or fetal death after a nonemergent procedure appears to be 1% to 2%, whereas the rate of prematurity is reported to be 8% to 9%. These risks may be higher in patients undergoing surgery after 23 weeks of gestation. In terms of anesthetic risk, regional anesthesia may induce hypotension, which may be associated with reduced placental perfusion and fetal hypoxemia. Although no commonly used anesthetic agents are proven teratogens, lack of teratogenic potential is difficult to prove.

In terms of the surgical technique, there has been persistent concern regarding possible fetal harm associated with laparoscopy. Specific concerns have been that the pneumoperitoneum may alter uterine blood flow and that the uterus will be injured during the insertion of trochars. Case series have not demonstrated any difference in fetal outcome between laparoscopy and laparotomy, and maternal outcome, in terms of pain and hospital stay is clearly improved with laparoscopy. At this point, laparoscopy can be considered for adnexal surgery on the pregnant patient if the lesion is felt not to be malignant and if the uterus is not so large as to obstruct visualization.

 Decision 2: Management

What is the most appropriate management of the pregnancy during surgery?

- **A.** Tocolysis with magnesium sulfate
- **B.** Continuous fetal and uterine monitoring during the procedure
- **C.** Pregnancy termination at the time of surgery
- **D.** Indomethacin tocolysis after the procedure

The correct answer is D: Indomethacin tocolysis after the procedure. Although the benefit of tocolysis is uncertain in this situation, many practitioners will utilize a brief (24–48 hours) course of indomethacin after surgery in the second trimester. It would be equally correct to use no tocolytic. Tocolysis with magnesium sulfate during the procedure (Answer A) may be problematic; magnesium sulfate is known to potentiate neuromuscular blockade in patients undergoing general anesthesia, and it is used to reduce blood pressure in some surgical settings. Given these risks, magnesium intraoperatively is not recommended. Continuous fetal monitoring (Answer B) is not appropriate in an 18-week fetus, given the fetal size and nonviable status. Pregnancy termination (Answer C) would be inappropriate, as the patient has stated her desire to continue the pregnancy.

 CASE CONTINUES

Ms. Francis undergoes an attempted laparoscopic resection of her ovarian mass. The procedure is converted to a laparotomy because of an inability to mobilize the mass secondary to adhesions. At surgery, the abdomen appears to be free of peritoneal implants, and the surface of the mass is smooth. An ovarian cystectomy is performed; frozen section performed at the time of surgery is read as mucinous cystadenoma, and this is confirmed by the final

pathology. Fetal heart tones are recorded before and after the procedure.

On the third postoperative day, Ms. Francis is discharged home with Ob follow-up. She has normal fundal height growth and feels well. At 24 weeks she has a 1-hour glucose screen of 110 mg/dL; an ultrasound reveals a normally grown fetus and confirms absence of the adnexal cyst. However, at 26 weeks of gestation, she presents to your office with an acute onset of abdominal pain.

 Decision 3: Diagnosis

What is the most likely diagnosis of abdominal pain 8 weeks postsurgery?

- **A.** Sudden wound dehiscence due to pressure from the uterus
- **B.** Bleeding from pedicles
- **C.** Thrombosed ovarian vein
- **D.** Preterm labor

The correct answer is D: Preterm labor. Although the surgical incision site may not be 100% healed by 8 weeks postsurgery, wound strength increases with time from the surgery and would be predicted to be about 50% of normal at 8 weeks. Under normal conditions, the slow growth of the gravid uterus should not result in sudden wound dehiscence (Answer A). Similarly, bleeding from surgical pedicles (Answer B) would most often occur immediately after surgery. Thrombosis of an ovarian vein (Answer C) following the removal of an ovarian mass is a possibility. However, this is a rare event and frequently, these patients are asymptomatic.

During the late second trimester, especially after 24 weeks of gestation, preterm labor should always be considered in a patient with abdominal pain. In addition, when the patient presents with acute abdominal pain, other potential causes for her pain, including appendicitis, cholecystitis, and various gastrointestinal conditions may be considered.

 CASE CONCLUSION

Ms. Francis is found to have preterm contractions without any evidence of cervical change. She is also noted to have a urinary tract infection. After treatment of the infection and observation for cervical change she is discharged home with close follow-up. The remainder of the pregnancy is uneventful; at 39 weeks of gestation she delivers vaginally a 3,200-g female with Apgar score of 9 and 9 at 1 and 5 minutes. Mother and baby are discharged on the second postpartum day.

SUGGESTED READINGS

American College of Obstetricians and Gynecologists. ACOG Practice Bulletin. Management of adnexal masses. Obstet Gynecol. 2007; 110(1):201–14.

Bisharah M, Tulandi T. Laparoscopic surgery in pregnancy. Clin Obstet Gynecol. 2003;46(1):92–7.

Chiang G, Levine D. Imaging of adnexal masses in pregnancy. J Ultrasound Med. 2004;23(6):805–19.

Cohen-Kerem R, Railton C, Oren D, Lishner M, Koren G. Pregnancy outcome following non-obstetric surgical intervention. Am J Surg. 2005;190(3):467–73.

Giuntoli RL II, Vang RS, Bristow RE. Evaluation and management of adnexal masses during pregnancy. Clin Obstet Gynecol. 2006;49(3): 492–505.

Leiserowitz GS. Managing ovarian masses during pregnancy. Obstet Gynecol Surv. 2006;61(7):463–70.

Schmeler KM, Mayo-Smith WW, Peipert JF, Weitzen S, Manuel MD, Gordinier ME. Adnexal masses in pregnancy: surgery compared with observation. Obstet Gynecol. 2005;105(5 Pt 1):1098–103.

Van De Velde M, De Buck F. Anesthesia for non-obstetric surgery in the pregnant patient. Minerva Anestesiol. 2007;73(4):235–40.

Venous Thromboembolism

Steven A. Laifer

 ## CASE PRESENTATION

You are called to the emergency department to consult on Ms. Miner, a 27-year-old G1 P0 who has presented to the emergency department at 24 weeks of gestation with complaints of sudden onset of shortness of breath.

Her past medical history is significant for obesity (her body mass index is 38); she has been overweight since she was a teenager. She had a laparoscopic cholecystectomy at the age of 25 years. She has no allergies, takes no medications, and has never received a blood transfusion. She is a nursing assistant, and she does not smoke, drink, or use recreational drugs. She is single; her partner is 35 years old and is also obese. Her mother died of breast cancer at the age of 50 years, and her father is hypertensive and has had an angioplasty for coronary artery disease. She has one sister who recently suffered a stillbirth during her pregnancy. She has had no abnormal Papanicolaou tests and reports no history of sexually transmitted infections.

Ms. Miner's pregnancy has been uncomplicated thus far. Her prenatal labs were unremarkable. Serum aneuploidy screening was negative; an MSAFP (maternal serum alpha fetoprotein) was in the normal range. An ultrasound at 20 weeks revealed consistent fetal measurements and normal fetal anatomy.

Ms. Miner states that fetal activity is normal. She has no abdominal pain or cramping and no vaginal bleeding. She was feeling well until the morning of presentation when she noticed some occasional discomfort with a deep breath. Over the next few hours, she has developed increasing shortness of breath. She has no cough. She has no gastrointestinal or urinary symptoms.

Her temperature is 37.6°C, pulse is 120 bpm, respiratory rate is 24/min, blood pressure is 140/80 mm Hg, and oxygen saturation is 96%. Her physical examination reveals an obese Caucasian woman in mild distress. Her lungs are clear to auscultation and percussion; her cardiac examination reveals a rapid S_1 and S_2 with no murmurs or gallops appreciated. On abdominal examination, her fundal height is 26 cm; the uterus is nontender. No abdominal masses are appreciated. There is 1+ pitting edema bilaterally at the ankles, with no calf or thigh tenderness, the calf and thigh diameters are equal on the right and left, and there is no skin erythema or hyperemia. The pelvic examination is deferred.

 ### Decision 1: Diagnosis

What is your first diagnostic test in this patient?

A. Pulmonary function testing
B. Chest x-ray
C. Ultrasound of the lower extremity
D. Plasma fibrinogen

The best answer is C: Ultrasound of the lower extremity. This patient's presentation raises concern for a venous thromboembolism (VTE), specifically a pulmonary embolism (PE). The symptoms of deep venous thrombosis (DVT) include pain, swelling, and discoloration of the involved extremity. Signs and symptoms of PE include dyspnea, pleuritic chest pain, cough, hemoptysis, tachycardia, tachypnea, and rales. Some of the more common of these signs and symptoms (lower extremity edema, dyspnea, tachycardia) can also be seen during the course of normal pregnancy. It is essential, therefore, to maintain a high index of suspicion and low threshold for initiating a diagnostic evaluation, as PE is a life-threatening condition. Compression ultrasound of the lower extremity has approximately a 95% sensitivity and specificity for the diagnosis of symptomatic thrombosis of the proximal lower extremity. It is also without risk to the patient, making it an excellent initial test in the workup of the patient with suspected VTE. Although a normal study virtually excludes the diagnosis, some centers may repeat a negative study within a week if the patient's symptoms persist. In addition, a negative test does not exclude a clot in another location, such as a more proximal pelvic vein. If the study is equivocal, or the clinical suspicion for a DVT remains high, an alternative study such as magnetic resonance angiography or contrast venography can be obtained (Fig. 11.1). Pulmonary function testing (Answer A) and chest x-ray (Answer B) are not helpful in making this diagnosis, although the chest x-ray may be of benefit in excluding other pulmonary pathology. Although plasma fibrinogen (Answer D) may be decreased in the presence of extensive

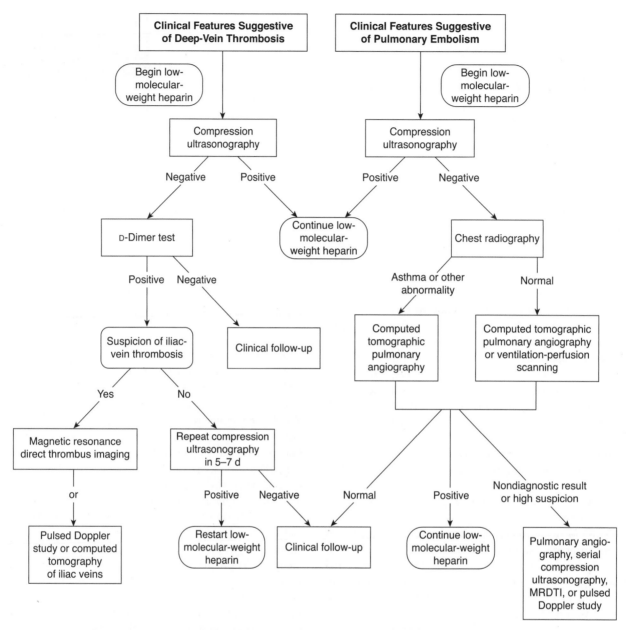

Figure 11.1 Algorithm for diagnosing deep venous thrombosis (DVT). (Reproduced with permission from Marik PE, Plante LA. Venous thromboembolic disease and pregnancy. N Engl J Med. 2008;359: 2025–33.)

clot formation, the normal amount of fibrinogen is so variable between patients as to make the test meaningless for this diagnosis.

In addition to compression ultrasound, D-dimer is a useful diagnostic test in the initial evaluation of patients with suspected VTE in nonpregnant patients. Its use in pregnancy, however, is controversial as concentrations of D-dimer increase during normal pregnancy. While some authorities incorporate the measurement of D-dimer into their diagnostic algorithms, it is more useful when negative, and many centers are not using D-dimer measurements in the diagnosis of pregnant patients with suspected VTE.

Diagnostic testing for PE involves radiologic imaging of the lung. Although ventilation perfusion (VQ) scanning provides accurate diagnosis of PE, especially for younger patients who are not likely to have pulmonary comorbidities, it has largely been replaced by computed tomography pulmonary angiography (CTPA) as the method of choice for diagnosing PE. CTPA is often more readily available, can identify atypical pneumonias or other findings that may confound the findings in VQ scanning, and newer CTPA scanners are able to identify emboli in smaller peripheral and subsegmental vessels. An additional advantage in pregnancy is that CTPA exposes the fetus to lower doses of ionizing radiation than does the VQ scan. Although the radiation exposure to the fetus from either VQ or CTPA is small, because of the concern about any radiation exposure, some centers initially use compression ultrasound to evaluate the extremities, and presumptively treat for PE when a patient with pulmonary symptoms has a clot in the extremity. Compression ultrasonography may be a reasonable diagnostic test in some cases, especially while waiting for CTPA as well as an additional evaluation for patients in whom the results of CTPA are nondiagnostic or equivocal. However, this approach does not provide any information on location or size of the PE.

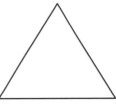

Hypercoaguability
Increased clotting factors
Decreased anticoagulants
Decreased fibrinolysis

Venous Stasis
Uterine compression
Immobilization

Vascular injury
Vaginal delivery
Cesarean delivery
Preeclampsia

Figure 11.2 Virchow's triad in pregnancy.

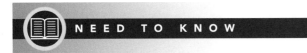

NEED TO KNOW

Thromboembolic Disease in Pregnancy

Venous thromboembolic disease is a leading cause of maternal mortality world wide. It is the number one cause of maternal deaths in the United Kingdom and, though statistics vary from state to state, it is the second leading cause of maternal death in the United States after hemorrhage. Although unusual sites of venous thrombosis have been reported in pregnant patients, most events in pregnancy are pulmonary emboli and thromboses that involve the veins of the pelvis and lower extremity (iliac, femoral, and calf veins). DVT and PE are considered to be components of the same pathologic process. As many as 40% of patients with a DVT, but without pulmonary symptoms, are found to have pulmonary emboli and approximately 30% of patients with pulmonary emboli are found to have abnormalities in the veins of the lower extremities. Timely diagnosis and treatment of VTE is important to prevent the potential consequences associated with PE (mortality) and DVT (chronic venous insufficiency, postphlebitic syndrome).

In simplistic terms, the coagulation system can be viewed as a delicate balance between the procoagulant clotting factors and the endogenous anticoagulants and fibrinolytic system. A deviation in either system can lead either to bleeding or thrombosis. Pregnancy is considered a hypercoagulable condition. Normal physiologic changes that occur in the coagulation system during pregnancy include an increase in hepatically synthesized clotting factors (fibrinogen, factors II, VII, VIII, X, XII) as well as a decrease in endogenous anticoagulant and fibrinolytic activity (decreased protein S levels, increased plasminogen activator inhibitor-1), resulting in a tipping of the balance toward clotting. The net effect of the coagulation changes is promotion of clot formation, extension, and stability. These changes provide the pregnant woman with some protection against hemor-

rhage, perhaps in preparation for delivery, but also make her more susceptible to pathologic thrombosis. Studies show that pregnant women are five times more likely than age-matched nonpregnant women to experience a thrombosis.

In addition to the hypercoagulable state of pregnancy, the other elements of Virchow's triad, that is stasis and endothelial or vascular damage, are also present during pregnancy and especially after delivery. Stasis may be caused by uterine compression, which impedes venous return, and if patients are immobilized for other pregnancy complications. Vascular injury may occur during pregnancy but more commonly occurs at the time of vaginal or cesarean delivery (Fig. 11.2).

Most cases of DVT during pregnancy occur prior to delivery; approximately 75% occur in the antepartum period and approximately 50% occur before the early second trimester. Interestingly, most DVTs are left sided; this may be related to the relationship of the uterus and the iliac veins at the level of the pelvic brim. In contrast, most cases of PE occur in the postpartum period; this is likely secondary to vascular injury that occurs with delivery and especially with cesarean delivery.

Other risk factors that are associated with the increased risk of VTE associated with pregnancy include advanced maternal age, obesity, cesarean delivery, prior VTE, and thrombophilias.

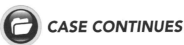

CASE CONTINUES

The emergency department physician ordered a compression sonogram of the lower extremities on Ms. Miner, which showed normal flow with no suspicion of a thrombosis. A chest radiograph (with abdominal shielding) was unremarkable. Despite the normal lower extremity ultrasound, your colleague is suspicious for a PE and you are consulted about the safety of CTPA in this patient.

After your discussion with the emergency physician and your evaluation of the patient, a CTPA is performed. Bilateral peripheral pulmonary emboli are identified. The patient is admitted to the obstetric service for treatment and begun on low–molecular-weight heparin.

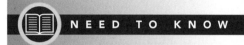 **N E E D   T O   K N O W**

Treatment of Thromboembolism

If the diagnosis of DVT or PE is confirmed, the initial treatment objective will depend on the patient's condition, the size and extent of the thrombosis, and in pregnant patients, the gestational age and presence of associated obstetric complications. In hemodynamically stable patients with no additional obstetric complications, the objective is to stabilize the clot and prevent further embolization; this is accomplished with anticoagulation therapy.

The standard model for anticoagulation therapy for VTE in the nonpregnant patient is initial therapy with heparin followed by chronic maintenance therapy with oral anticoagulants (warfarin) for approximately 6 months. The maintenance therapy is intended to prevent recurrence of thrombosis. The treatment model differs in the pregnant patient because of concerns about fetal exposure to warfarin. Warfarin crosses the placenta and may lead to the warfarin embryopathy after exposure during early pregnancy (weeks 6–9). Use of warfarin in the second and third trimesters may result in fetal bleeding and is associated with an increased risk of central nervous systems abnormalities. Therefore, the treatment model for anticoagulation therapy for VTE in pregnancy includes the use of heparin for chronic maintenance therapy. The maintenance therapy should be continued for the duration of pregnancy and for at least 6 weeks postpartum (and longer if necessary to complete 6 months). After delivery, warfarin can be used for maintenance therapy.

The use, dosage, and monitoring of heparin in thromboembolism is undergoing a change. The American College of Obstetricians and Gynecologists supports the use of both low–molecular-weight and unfractionated heparin, but some published guidelines include recommendations only for low–molecular-weight heparin. Low–molecular-weight heparin may be advantageous as there is a lower risk of heparin-associated thrombocytopenia, osteoporosis, and bleeding as compared with unfractionated heparin in nonpregnant individuals. Limited data suggest that there may be similar advantages to the use of low–molecular-weight heparin in pregnancy, but unfractionated heparin remains an acceptable alternative at the present time. Unfortunately,

TABLE 11.1

HEPARIN PROTOCOLS FOR THE TREATMENT OF ACUTE VENOUS THROMBOEMBOLISM IN PREGNANCY[a]

- Unfractionated heparin
  - Bolus of 80 U/kg
  - Initial maintenance dose 18 U/kg/hr
  - Adjust dose to maintain aPTT of 1.5–2.5 of control
- Low–molecular-weight heparin
  - *Either*
    - Enoxaparin: 1 mg/kg SQ BID
    - Tinzaparin 175 U/kg SQ QD
  - Maintain peak anti–factor-Xa levels at 0.6–1.2 U/mL

[a]Other protocols and other low–molecular-weight heparins have been used in some centers.
aPTT, activated partial thromboplastin time.

there are also limited data to guide therapy for the pregnant patient requiring full anticoagulation in pregnancy, and monitoring of the level of anticoagulation is easier with unfractionated heparin. In a pregnant patient, therefore, anticoagulation can be initiated either with adjusted-dose unfractionated heparin or with adjusted-dose low–molecular-weight heparin, utilizing a weight-based calculation (Table 11.1).

In hemodynamically unstable patients or in the setting of a very large clot, lysing or removing the clot is appropriate and this is accomplished with thrombolytic therapy or surgical thrombectomy. In patients with contraindications to anticoagulation, for example, those who require surgery or delivery, then preventing primary or secondary embolization is paramount and this may be accomplished with inferior vena cava filters.

 Decision 2: Workup

What additional diagnostic testing would be indicated?

A. Maternal estrogen levels
B. activated partial thromboplastin time (aPTT)
C. Factor V Leiden mutation
D. Maternal echocardiography

The correct answer is C: Factor V Leiden mutation. Women with a history of thromboembolism have a higher risk of an inherited or acquired thrombophilia, and testing may be justified (Table 11.2). Women with a thrombophilia and a history of VTE may require full anticoagulation with any future pregnancy, depending on their specific abnormality. Although elevated maternal estrogen levels (Answer A) will increase the risk for VTE, determining the estrogen level does not assist with diagnosis or therapy. Although aPTT (Answer B) is useful in the management of the patient

TABLE 11.2
RECOMMENDED TESTING FOR THROMBOPHILIA[a]

	Testing Unreliable in Pregnancy	Testing Unreliable with Anticoagulation
Acquired Thrombophilias		
Lupus anticoagulant		
Anticardiolipin antibodies		
Inherited Thrombophilias		
Factor V Leiden mutation		
Prothrombin G20210 A mutation		
MTHFR mutation/fasting homocysteine (only a risk with hyperhomocysteinemia)		
AT-III antigen activity levels		X
Protein C antigen activity levels	X	X
Protein S antigen activity levels	X	X

[a]In some cases, testing is difficult or impossible in pregnancy or while the patient is anticoagulated: due to this difficulty, and to the reduced chance that thromboembolism is related to AT-III or protein S or C deficiency, ACOG recommends that these only be tested for if other tests are negative.
Adapted from American College of Obstetricians and Gynecologists. ACOG practice bulletin No. 19, Thromboembolism in Pregnancy, August 2000, reaffirmed 2008.

treated with unfractionated heparin, it is not useful as a diagnostic test in this setting. Maternal echocardiography (Answer D) may be used to diagnose right heart dysfunction in the setting of a large PE, or to diagnose an intracardiac or central clot, but it is not useful in distal disease when a diagnosis has already been made.

 CASE CONTINUES

Ms. Miner undergoes testing for thrombophilias and is found to be a heterozygote for factor V Leiden. She does well on subcutaneous doses of low–molecular-weight heparin and is discharged from the hospital with the plan to continue anticoagulation for 6 months (and at least 6 weeks postpartum). As you are discussing her discharge plan with her, she expresses concern that she will have a stillbirth, like her sister. You consider how to manage the remainder of the pregnancy.

 Decision 3: Follow-up

What management (in addition to heparin) will give the best outcome in this pregnancy?

A. Aspirin 81 mg PO daily, deliver at term
B. NST three times weekly, deliver at 34 weeks with evidence of fetal lung maturity
C. Bedrest for the remainder of pregnancy, deliver at 36 weeks
D. Continued antepartum surveillance, deliver at term

The correct answer is D: Continued antepartum surveillance, deliver at term. Numerous reports have identified an association between inherited thrombophilias and a variety of poor perinatal outcomes, including severe preeclampsia, recurrent pregnancy loss, fetal growth restriction, and stillbirth. However, there is no good evidence that this association is causal. In addition, the association has not been consistently demonstrated when women without a history of prior pregnancy complications have been screened for thrombophilias. Should pregnancy complications (e.g., growth restriction, preeclampsia) occur during prenatal care, the clinician should institute appropriate treatment. Recommendations have been made that patients with inherited thrombophilias be treated with anticoagulation, either with heparin or aspirin, or both, to improve pregnancy outcome. Although early reports suggested that these treatments were helpful in patients with a history of pregnancy complications, there is no evidence of efficacy in randomized, controlled trials. Given that the use of aspirin (Answer A), early delivery (Answers B and C), and prolonged bedrest (Answer C) have not been shown to be effective, and may be harmful, there is no justification for these interventions in this patient.

 CASE CONTINUES

Ms. Miner returns home and continues to use low–molecular-weight heparin throughout pregnancy. An ultrasound performed at 29 weeks of gestation reveals normal fetal growth with no abnormalities seen. At 37 weeks of gestation, Ms. Miner is seen in your office for a prenatal visit. At this time she complains of possible passage of her mucous plug. An examination reveals that her cervix is 80% effaced and 1 cm dilated with the vertex at 0 station. She asks when she should come to the hospital for delivery.

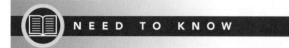

Delivery Planning in the Anticoagulated Patient

Labor and delivery in the anticoagulated patient are complicated by two issues: the blood loss expected at delivery, especially if a cesarean delivery is required, and the risk of epidural hematoma if regional anesthesia (epidural or spinal) is performed. The blood loss at delivery can often be managed with careful operative technique, but the use of regional anesthesia in an anticoagulated patient involves a risk for epidural hematoma. This is a potentially catastrophic complication, and regional anesthesia is contraindicated in most anticoagulated obstetric patients. The most common response to these issues is to perform a planned delivery, with discontinuation of anticoagulation. The published recommendations regarding the required delay from the last use of heparin until regional anesthesia can safely be used are seen in Table 11.3. In a patient with a need for continuous anticoagulation, it may be advisable to transition the patient to intravenous unfractionated heparin for delivery and/or consider the placement of an inferior vena cava filter. However, in most patients heparin can safely be discontinued for 24 hours prior to a scheduled cesarean delivery or planned pregnancy induction. The decision about when to schedule an elective induction of labor in a primigravida involves more art than science; the aim is to schedule the delivery when the induction will proceed smoothly and be successful, but prior to the time that spontaneous labor occurs. Necessary conditions would include a mature fetus and a favorable cervix, but the ability to predict successful labor induction is limited. Attempting the delivery too early would involve the risk of iatrogenic prematurity, and the risk of recurrent maternal thrombosis due to prolonged bedrest without anticoagulation. Delaying the delivery too long involves the risk of the patient going into labor while anticoagulated. There is no right answer to this issue, and the range of choices would include a scheduled primary cesarean delivery to control delivery timing.

 CASE CONCLUSION

You elect to schedule Ms. Miner for labor induction no earlier than 38.5 weeks of gestation, and plan to see her in your office then to examine her cervix and assess her readiness for induction. One day prior to this visit, she is admitted to labor and delivery with premature rupture of the

TABLE 11.3

RECOMMENDATIONS FOR NEURAXIAL (REGIONAL) ANESTHESIA IN PATIENTS TAKING HEPARIN PREPARATIONS[a]

Agent/Dose	Hours After Last Heparin Dose Before Needle Insertion	Hours (After Needle Insertion) Before Next Heparin Dose
Unfractionated heparin		
■ Prophylactic dose SQ (twice daily)	No recommendation (not contraindicated when used for acute thromboprophylaxis)	1 hour after needle insertion. Remove catheter 2–4 hours after dose and 1 hour prior to next dose
■ Treatment dose SQ (three times daily)	No recommendation	
■ Treatment dose IV	6 hours (with normal aPTT)	
LMW heparin		
■ Prophylactic dose SQ (once daily)	10–12 hours	6–8 hours postoperatively and 2 hours after catheter removal. Catheter may be left in place, but is removed 10–12 hours after dose
■ Treatment dose SQ	24 hours	Delay 24 hours postoperatively, and at least 2 hours after catheter removal. Catheter removal prior to first heparin dose

[a]The recommendations are based largely on data from nonpregnant patients. These recommendations are for patients not taking antiplatelet drugs (aspirin) and with normal platelet counts.
aPTT, activated partial thromboplastin time; LMW, low molecular weight.
Adapted from American Society of Regional Anesthesia and Pain Medicine Evidence-Based Guidelines. 3rd ed.

membranes. At this point, she is 8 hours after her last heparin injection. You discontinue heparin and await spontaneous labor; after 14 hours of ruptured membranes Ms. Miner begins to have active labor. She asks for, and receives, intravenous narcotics for pain relief, and after 5 hours of active labor she delivers a 3,600-g female infant with Apgar score of 8 and 9 at 1 and 5 minutes. Her blood loss at delivery is 700 ml, and she has a small perineal hematoma that responds to local measures. She is ambulating 2 hours after the birth, and is restarted on her low–molecular-weight heparin 8 hours after delivery, with the plan to transition to warfarin for the first 6 weeks postpartum.

SUGGESTED READINGS

American College of Obstetricians and Gynecologists. ACOG practice bulletin No. 19, Thromboembolism in Pregnancy, August 2000, reaffirmed 2008.

Bates SM, Greer IA, Pabinger I, Sofaer S, Hirsh J. Venous thromboembolism, thrombophilia, antithrombotic therapy, and pregnancy. Chest. 2008;133;844S–86S. DOI 10.1378/chest.08–0761.

Duhl AJ, Paidas MJ, Ural SH, et al. Antithrombotic therapy and pregnancy: consensus report and recommendations for prevention and treatment of venous thromboembolism and adverse pregnancy outcome. Am J Obstet Gynecol. 2007;197:457.e1–457.e21.

Horlocker TT, Wedel DJ, Rowlingson JC, Enneking FK, Kopp SL, Benzon HT, et al. Regional Anesthesia in the Patient Receiving Antithrombotic or Thrombolytic Therapy: American Society of Regional Anesthesia and Pain Medicine Evidence-Based Guidelines (Third Edition). Reg Anesth Pain Med. 2010;35(1):64–101.

Lockwood CJ. Thromboembolic disease in pregnancy. In: Creasy RK, Resnick R, Iams JD, editors. Maternal Fetal Medicine: Principles and Practice. 6th ed. Philadelphia, PA: Saunders Elsevier; 2009. pp. 855–65.

Marik PE, Plante LA. Venous thromboembolic disease and pregnancy. N Engl J Med. 2008;359:2025–33.

Pabinger I. Thrombophilia and its impact on pregnancy. Thromb Res. 2009;123(Suppl 3):S16–21. Review.

Said JM, Higgins JR, Moses EK, et al. Inherited thrombophilia polymorphisms and pregnancy outcomes in nulliparous women. Obstet Gynecol. 2010;115(1):5–13.

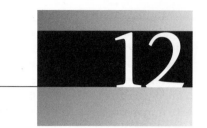

Trauma in Pregnancy

Martin L. Gimovsky   Elena Bronshtein

 CASE PRESENTATION

Your patient, Ms. Jones, an 18-year-old primigravida, is on her way to her prenatal appointment. While walking toward the medical office entrance, she is struck from behind by an out-of-control SUV. When the EMTs arrive, they find a young woman, about 5 months pregnant, lying on the sidewalk. She is not conscious. Her initial vital signs include a pulse of 120 bpm and regular, blood pressure of 150/60 mm Hg supine, respiratory rate of 24/min, and temperature of 99.9°F. A neck brace is fitted and a 16-gauge IV is started. During transport to the emergency department (ED), she regains consciousness and complains of a headache. You are paged to see and evaluate her on admission.

Ms. Jones is lying supine and is complaining of a severe occipital headache. Her vital signs are pulse of 80 bpm and regular, blood pressure of 166/68 mm Hg, respiratory rate of 28/min, temperature of 100.4°F. She is alert, oriented, and responsive. She reports that her last menstrual period was 27 weeks ago. Her past medical history is significant for sickle cell anemia with multiple transfusions. Her past surgical history and gynecology history are negative. She denies medications, drug allergies, or relevant family history. She is a 1 pack per day smoker and denies alcohol or substance abuse.

 Decision 1: Workup

Assuming that the patient remains hemodynamically stable, what is the next best step?

- **A.** Lab tests: Rh and antibody screen
- **B.** Pregnancy test
- **C.** Cervical examination
- **D.** Ultrasound

The correct answer is D: Ultrasound. Since the patient herself is stable, attention can be directed to her fetus. The patient has been subjected to significant trauma and once hemodynamic stability has been ascertained, evaluation

must be made of gestational age and fetal status. Given the witnessed loss of consciousness and the complaint of a severe headache, a computed tomography scan of the patient's head would also be part of her initial appraisal. The patient's blood type and antibody screen are of secondary importance, although an assessment of the patient's hemoglobin and hematocrit would certainly be advisable. A pregnancy test is not indicated based upon your physical examination findings. Cervical examination should await the ultrasound findings.

 N E E D   T O   K N O W

Evaluation of a Potentially Viable Gestation After Maternal Trauma

Concerns for the fetus after maternal trauma include fetal trauma, premature labor and placental abruption. The occurrence of a placental abruption post–minor trauma resulting in fetal death is uncommon (~1%); however, the likelihood of abruption is increased in the presence of severe and/or direct abdominal trauma. Most cases of abruption occur within 24 hours of traumatic injury; however, abruption posttrauma has been reported up to 72 hours after the event. Abruption signs and symptoms may include, but are not limited to

1. Persistent uterine tenderness
2. New-onset vaginal bleeding
3. Nonreassuring fetal heart rate tracing
4. Spontaneous premature rupture of membranes
5. Development of coagulopathy

All women >24 weeks of gestation subjected to abdominal trauma should have an ultrasound as soon as possible after admission. The scan should visualize (if possible) and document the following:

1. Number and viability of fetus(es)
2. Fetal biometry to determine gestational age

3. Placental location
4. Amniotic fluid volume
5. Biophysical profile

Following the scan, a careful speculum examination may be undertaken. The presence of blood may suggest an abruption, although the absence of vaginal bleeding does not exclude it, as concealed abruption may occur. Pooling of amniotic fluid or prolapse of the umbilical cord or of a fetal extremity are less likely findings, but they indicate rupture of the membranes, and likely preterm labor and imminent delivery.

Continuous fetal and uterine monitoring with external fetal heart rate monitor and tocodynamometer should be performed to assess for preterm contractions and/or abruption for a minimum of 4 hours. The presence of vaginal bleeding, signs of coagulopathy, frequent uterine contractions, or uterine irritability should signal increased concern for premature labor and/or underlying placental abruption and necessitates a lengthier course of fetal monitoring surveillance, as does evidence of fetal compromise.

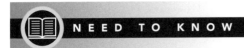

NEED TO KNOW

Maternal and Fetal Trauma

Trauma is a significant cause of injury in women of childbearing age and the leading cause of maternal death. Significant accidental injury has been estimated to occur in up to 10% of all pregnancies, and 3 to 4 pregnant women per 1,000 sustained injuries sufficiently severe to require hospitalization. Motor vehicle accidents are responsible for approximately two thirds of all maternal trauma cases although violent assault, suicide, physical abuse, and sexual assault are also major contributors to traumatic injury during pregnancy. In assault victims, the pregnant abdomen is a common target site for injury.

Major trauma in pregnancy may result in serious or fatal maternal injury associated with hemorrhage and shock, fractures, cerebral contusion or intracerebral hemorrhage, or visceral injury. In a motor vehicle accident or other blunt trauma, the direction of impact can determine the pattern of injuries. A frontal collision involves an abrupt stop, causing the patient to collide with the windshield, air bag, dashboard, and/or steering wheel. A blunt force trauma may ensue, and in rare circumstances, a puncture wound

may also be seen. In the worst-case scenario, an unrestrained patient may be ejected from the moving vehicle. Common front-end collision injuries include lower extremity fracture or dislocation as well as head, cervical spine, or torso blunt trauma. During a side-impact collision, the patient may be accelerated (and rapidly decelerated) side-to-side and either thrown across the vehicle or even expelled from the vehicle. Common injuries with side-to-side collision may include pelvic fracture, pulmonary contusion, solid organ injury, and diaphragmatic rupture. Rear-end collisions may also result in whiplash with concomitant head and spinal cord injuries. Immobilization at the scene of the accident is important in lessening the extent of injury.

In pregnancy, blunt injury may also result in uterine rupture or the dehiscence of a scar from prior surgery. Uterine rupture occurs in 0.6% of cases and is almost always secondary to major abdominal trauma; severe injury and fetal death may result. Indirectly, blunt trauma may result in an acute deceleration phenomenon with rapid changes in the size and shape of organs, leading to shearing of blood vessels. This is thought to be the mechanism for the placental abruptions observed after trauma.

During late pregnancy, the uterus fills the abdomen and displaces the abdominal viscera up and laterally. This may protect a pregnant woman from the effects of abdominal trauma, as the uterus absorbs the force. In addition to the anatomic changes of pregnancy, physiologic changes may modulate the response to trauma. The 35% to 45% increase in blood volume protects a pregnant woman from shock due to hypovolemia. Because of placental abruption, disseminated intravascular coagulation (DIC) may be more frequently associated with severe trauma in pregnancy. Diagnosis of DIC may pose a problem, since fibrinogen levels during pregnancy are normally twice that of the nonpregnant state. A fibrinogen level that is normal for a nonpregnant woman may be indicative of the onset of DIC during gestation. In addition, the presence of a low titer of fibrin split products (FSPs) is common during pregnancy and thus is not necessarily indicative of embolism or DIC.

Management

The initial management of trauma in pregnancy is similar to that in the nonpregnant state. On arrival at the ED, the patient should be immediately assessed for airway, breathing, and circulation. Further workup depends on the initial findings (Fig. 12.1). The teratogenicity of certain medications and imaging techniques is considered in Chapter 24: Teratogens.

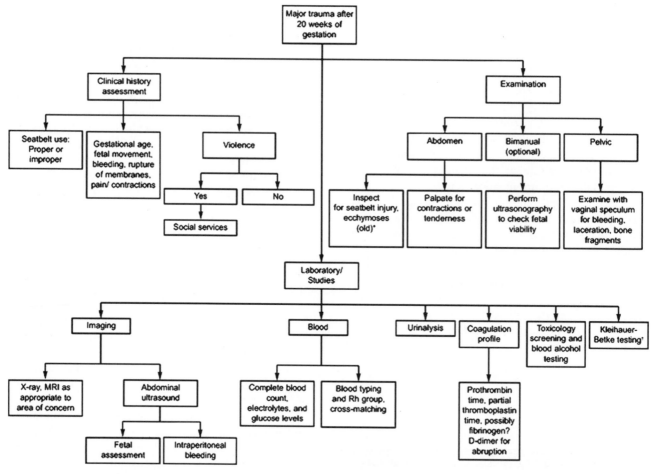

Figure 12.1   Acute management of the pregnant trauma patient. Maternal status is assessed first and acute resuscitation begun if needed. When the mother is stable, the fetal condition is addressed. (Adapted from Grossman NB blunt trauma in pregnancy. American Family Physician. 2004 70(7) 1303-10. Accessed online 12/13/10.)

Fetal and Neonatal Consequences

The risk of fetal death subsequent to trauma correlates with the following circumstances:

1. Direct fetal or placental injury
2. Maternal shock
3. Maternal pelvic fracture
4. Maternal head injury
5. Maternal hypoxemia
6. Maternal death
7. Maternal age, history of smoking, and history of alcohol use
8. Absence of maternal seat belt use

The effect of trauma on the fetus depends on the gestational age of the fetus, the type and severity of the trauma to the mother, and the extent of disruption to the normal uterine and fetal physiology. Maternal trauma in the first trimester does not usually cause fetal trauma because the maternal pelvis protects the uterus. First trimester fetal harm is most likely in cases complicated by profound maternal hypotension or serious maternal pelvic injuries. In later gestation, the uterus becomes an abdominal organ, and direct and secondary fetal harm becomes more frequent.

It is estimated that 1,300 to 3,900 fetal deaths each year result from maternal trauma. Overall, the most common causes of fetal demise are maternal death, maternal shock, and placental abruption. Less frequent causes are uterine rupture or laceration or direct fetal injury. The fetal death rate approaches 80% in the case of maternal shock. During hypovolemic shock, the maternal autonomic nervous system shunts blood from the uterus, extremities, and other nonessential organs to maintain core perfusion. The resulting decrease in perfusion and oxygenation may result in intrauterine fetal demise (IUFD), premature labor, and/or placental abruption.

Fetal death may be seen with complete or partial placental abruption. It is important to note that placental abruption is the most common cause of fetal death in motor vehicle accidents, occurring in 30% to 50% of major traumatic injuries. The key signs to be noted post-trauma are increased uterine contractions and/or irritability and abnormalities of fetal heart rate patterns. These are usually the earliest sign of this condition, and abruption rarely occurs in their absence.

Direct fetal injury may be seen in about one out of five motor vehicle accidents with pregnant occupants. Head trauma is the most common direct fetal injury. A traumatic head injury can occur when the fetal head has become engaged in the maternal pelvis. With the rapid deceleration of a motor vehicle accident, the fetal body moves forward, while the head is fixed in place, leading to a basal skull fracture. Fetal head injury may also result from a *contrecoup* effect if the fetus is free floating.

Fetomaternal hemorrhage is rare; it is typically detected after abdominal trauma when an anterior placenta and/or a tender uterus are present. Complications associated with fetomaternal hemorrhage include anemia, fetal death, and Rh isoimmunization.

Work in animal models demonstrates a profound reduction in both maternal and fetal injury with the proper use of seat belts. The American College of Obstetricians and Gynecologists recommends the use of three-point restraint seat belts during travel by automobile. Proper use of seat belts in pregnancy is described in Table 12.1.

CASE CONTINUES

Ultrasound reveals a live male fetus in a breech presentation. Fetal biometry is consistent with the gestational age of 27 weeks 2 days. The estimated fetal weight is 1,057 g, which is 50th percentile for gestational age. The amniotic fluid volume is normal, with an amniotic fluid index of 10 cm. The placenta is anterior and appears unremarkable. The initial laboratory results are all within normal limits. The patient is noted to have some contractions on the monitor. The trauma team finishes their workup and decides that Ms. Jones has no evidence of serious maternal trauma requiring surgery or intensive care. They clear her for admission to labor and delivery.

On labor and delivery, the nurse notes blood in the Foley catheter and a repeat set of coagulation parameters are obtained. Fibrinogen is 150 mg/dL, platelet count is 100,000/mm³, activated partial thromboplastin time is mildly prolonged at 42 seconds, and the prothrombin

TABLE 12.1

PREVENTION OF MATERNAL AND FETAL INJURIES DUE TO MOTOR VEHICLE ACCIDENTS

1. Always fasten and keep seat belt fastened
2. Sit at least 10 inches from the steering wheel
3. Position lap belt below prominence of the pregnant abdomen
4. Place shoulder harness to the side of the uterus, between the breasts and over the midline of the clavicle
5. Tilt the steering wheel toward the chest, away from the abdomen
6. Do not disable the air bags

time is normal. FSPs are positive at a 1:8 dilution. The urinalysis demonstrates gross blood.

 Decision 2: Diagnosis

What obstetrical complications might be the cause of this patient's coagulopathy?

   A. Fetal demise
   B. Placental abruption
   C. Preeclampsia
   D. Amniotic fluid embolism

The correct answer is B: Placental abruption. Placental abruption with significant bleeding results in a consumptive coagulopathy on an acute basis. Fetal demise as a cause of coagulation defects generally requires a longer time course (i.e., weeks, not days or hours). The patient does have a headache and systolic hypertension on a single measurement, but the timing of events makes preeclampsia less likely as a diagnosis. An amniotic fluid embolus (AFE) could conceivably occur with traumatic injury and a coagulopathy ensue, but cardiovascular collapse usually precedes a coagulopathy associated with AFE, and in its absence, AFE is unlikely.

 CASE CONTINUES

You are paged stat to the labor room. Ms. Jones has suffered a cardiac arrest. Upon arriving, you see a fetal heart rate of 60 bpm on the monitor. Ms. Jones has an oxygen mask on and the nurse is palpating for a carotid pulse. She reports that no pulse is present. A code is called and the team assembles outside of the patient's room. You note the presence of a large pool of dark blood on the bed, the source of which appears to be vaginal.

Decision 3: Management

What is the best obstetric management?

A. Airway, breathing, and chest compressions (ABC). Resuscitate the mother, her needs take precedence
B. Resuscitate the fetus with position change, intravenous fluids, and a tocolytic if indicated
C. Cesarean delivery only if the mother is judge nonresuscitable
D. Maternal resuscitation and cesarean delivery on an emergent basis

The correct answer is D: Maternal resuscitation and cesarean delivery. In the scenario above, a woman at 27 weeks of gestation has suffered a witnessed cardiac arrest in the hospital setting. In the second half of pregnancy, the size of the gravid uterus will interfere with resuscitation efforts by blocking cardiac return and greatly diminishing cardiac output. Intubation, oxygenation, and cardiac compressions will have limited efficacy. Thus, rapid delivery of the infant can facilitate the effort to save the life of both. A limited trial of resuscitation (3–4 minutes) is warranted while setting up to perform a perimortem cesarean delivery (Table 12.2). While the mother's needs are of primary concern, cardiopulmonary resuscitation without delivery is suboptimal due to the presence of the gravid uterus during the second half of gestation. The ultimate success of maternal resuscitation efforts cannot be judged until after the fetus has been delivered, which will enhance maternal circulation. In the present case, the presence of both an abruption and resultant coagulopathy further complicate the situation. Clearly, correction of the clotting deficiency would be preferable prior to surgical intervention were time available. In this case, both will need to be performed concurrently. In terms of answer B, interventions designed to alleviate the fetal bradycardia will not be effective when maternal cardiac arrest has occurred.

When maternal cardiac arrest has been witnessed, the best results are obtained with delivery within 4 to 5 minutes. If maternal resuscitation with oxygenation, chest compressions, and intravenous hydration is ongoing, fetal survival may ensue with longer intervals. When the gestational age is <24 to 25 weeks, a more aggressive trial of resuscitation may be undertaken before emptying the uterus. Prior to 24 weeks, the presumptive maternal benefits to be derived from delivering the fetus may be minimal, with a corresponding decrease in neonatal survival due to extreme prematurity. When the duration of arrest is uncertain, as with injury out-of-hospital or unwitnessed arrest, best practice remains uncertain and care must be individualized.

 NEED TO KNOW

Cardiopulmonary Resuscitation (CPR) in Pregnancy

Survival of the mother and infant when a pregnant woman suffers cardiac/respiratory arrest requires an experienced team familiar with advanced cardiac life

TABLE 12.2

TECHNIQUE FOR PERIMORTEM CESAREAN SECTION

1. Decision by most experienced physician available
2. Stat page for anesthesia, pediatrics, or technician
3. Midline abdominal incision
4. Vertical uterine incision
5. Deliver and handoff with long cord segment
6. Cord blood, cord gases
7. Uterotonics, broad spectrum antibiotics
8. If mother is pronounced dead, bulk closure of abdominal wall
9. If resuscitation is to continue, uterine closure prior to bulk closure of the abdominal wall
10. Thoughtful and complete documentation
11. Discussion with family

TABLE 12.3

AMERICAN HEART ASSOCIATION RECOMMENDATIONS FOR CPR IN PREGNANCY

CPR is to be performed as per usual protocols with the following modifications
- Insure venous return from the lower body
  - Patient on angled surface
         Or
  - Wedge under righ hip
         Or
  - Manually displace the uterus

ACLS to be performed as per usual protocols with the following modifications
- Insure oxygenation/protect the airway
  - Use 100% O_2
  - Be aware of the increased risk of failed intubation
  - Be aware of more rapid development of hypoxemia in pregnancy
- Prepare for perimortem Cesarean delivery

Adapted from the American Heart Association, 2005 American Heart Association Guidelines for Cardiopulmonary Resuscitation and Emergency Cardiovascular Care: Cardiac Arrest Associated with Pregnancy. Circulation. 2005;112(IV):150–153.

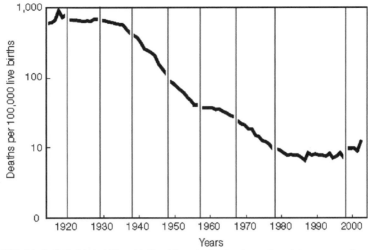

Figure 12.2 Maternal Mortality, United States, 1915–2003 (From National Center for Health Statistics. *Vital Health Stat* 2007;3(33))

support (ACLS) protocols as well as the special needs of the pregnant women. The first step is to evaluate the airway, breathing, and circulation of the mother (ABC), and to assure appropriate intervention to promote ventilation and circulation. The American Heart Association recommendations for modification of resuscitation protocols in pregnancy are summarized in Table 12.3.

CPR and ACLS protocols should be maintained as long as possible while preparations are made for perimortem cesarean section to maximize maternal and placental perfusion.

and is discharged home to her boyfriend's mother after 106 days in the hospital. His neurologic status is "guarded."

United States maternal mortality (pregnancy-related mortality) rates have decreased steadily over the past century. Although there is an increase since about 1990 (Fig. 12.2), maternal mortality rates are 10-11 per 100,000 births, meaning that a pregnant woman in the US is more likely to die of a cause not directly related to the pregnancy. This is not true world-wide: the maternal mortality rate in sub-Saharan Africa is more than 6000/100,000 making pregnancy by far the greatest risk to the life of a young woman.

 ## CASE CONCLUSION

The code team begins the ACLS protocol. You call for blood, fresh frozen plasma, cryoprecipitate, and the neonatal intensive care unit (NICU) resuscitation team. You initiate a perimortem cesarean section, and at minute 6 of the code Ms. Jones delivers a 1,060-g male infant with Apgar scores of one and three at one and five minutes. The infant is taken to the NICU.

Ms. Jones receives 6 units of packed red blood cells, and 2 units of fresh frozen plasma. The cryoprecipitate must be thawed and is delayed. Despite this she does not respond to attempts at resuscitation and is pronounced dead after a total of 95 minutes of resuscitation. You leave the operating room to inform her family.

An autopsy reveals that Ms. Jones has experienced an intracranial bleed from a basal skull fracture, exacerbated by the severe coagulopathy. Her child survives

SUGGESTED READINGS

American College of Obstetricians and Gynecologists. Automobile passenger restraints for children and pregnant women. ACOG Technical Bulletin No. 151, 1991.

American College of Obstetricians and Gynecologists. Obstetric aspects of trauma management. Educational Bulletin No. 251, September, 1998.

American Heart Association Guidelines 2005 for cardiopulmonary resuscitation and emergency cardiovascular care. ACLS 2005. Circulation. 2005;112(24 Suppl):IV1–203.

Atta E, Gardner M. Cardiopulmonary resuscitation in pregnancy. Obstet Gynecol Clin North Am. 2007;34(3):585–97.

Goldman SM, Wagner LK. Radiologic ABCs of maternal and fetal survival after trauma: when minutes count. Radiographics. 1999; 19(5):1349–57.

Mallampalli A, Powner DJ, Gardner MO. Cardiopulmonary resuscitation and somatic support of the pregnant patient. Crit Care Clin. 2004;20(4):747–61.

O'Grady JP, Fitzpatrick TK. Cesarean delivery and surgical sterilization. In: O'Grady JP, Gimovsky ML, editors. Operative Obstetrics. 2nd ed. New York, NY: Cambridge University Press; 2008, Chapter 18:509–607.

Pearlman MD, Klinich K, Schneider LW. A comprehensive program to improve safety for pregnant women and fetuses in motor vehicle crashes: a preliminary report. Am J Obstet Gynecol. 2000;182: 1554–64.

Shapiro JM. Critical care of the obstetric patient. J Intensive Care Med. 2006;21(5):278–86.

Stone IK. Trauma in the obstetric patient. Obstet Gynecol Clin North Am. 1999;26(3):459–71.

Weiss HB, Songer TJ, Fabio A. Fetal deaths related to maternal injury. JAMA. 2001;286(15):1863–8.

Sexually Transmitted Diseases in Pregnancy

Neil Silverman

CASE PRESENTATION

Ms. Shaw, a 23-year-old G1 P0 woman, presents to your office at 12 weeks of gestation for her first prenatal visit. She reports no significant past medical history, and her review of systems and physical examination are unremarkable.

The patient had her first sexual intercourse at the age of 20 years, and reports two sexual partners prior to her current partner, who is the father of the pregnancy. She had her first and only gynecologic examination 2 years ago through the student health service at her community college. Since leaving school, she has not seen a need for medical follow-up. She reports that she was told that all of her tests, including a Papanicolaou test, from that prior examination were "normal," though she does not recall all of the specific tests that were ordered.

Decision 1: Testing

What, if any, screening for sexually transmitted diseases (STDs) should be performed at this patient's initial prenatal visit?

A. HIV infection and syphilis
B. HIV infection, syphilis, and chlamydia
C. HIV infection, syphilis, chlamydia, gonorrhea, and hepatitis B
D. HIV infection, syphilis, chlamydia, and gonorrhea

The correct answer is C: HIV infection, syphilis, chlamydia, gonorrhea, and hepatitis B. All five of the infections listed are sexually transmitted and are listed by the Centers for Disease Control and Prevention (CDC) as those which are recommended prenatal screening tests, to be performed at the first obstetric visit. STDs can have serious effects on pregnant women, their partners, and their fetuses. Initiation of care for pregnancy is frequently the first point of entry into the medical care system for otherwise healthy, sexually active young women who may be at increased risk

for STDs. By definition, spontaneous pregnancy implies at least one episode of unprotected sexual intercourse. All pregnant women and their partners should be asked about STDs, counseled about the risk of perinatal infections, and given access to any indicated treatment.

NEED TO KNOW

STD Screening and Treatment (Including Management of High-Risk Groups)

HIV

Pregnant women in the United States should be offered testing for HIV infection as early in the pregnancy as possible. Testing should be conducted after the woman is notified that she will be tested for HIV as part of a routine prenatal, unless she declines the test (opt-out screening). Women who decline tsting because they have had a previous negative test should be instructed in the importance of retesting during each pregnancy. Testing pregnant women as they access medical care is important for both the health of the woman herself as well as for fetal well-being, since both medical and obstetric interventions have been shown to significantly lower the risk of perinatal (vertical) transmission of HIV.

Retesting for HIV in the third trimester (ideally before 36 weeks of gestation) is recommended for women at high risk for acquiring infection (women who use illicit drugs, who have multiple sex partners and/or are sex workers, or who have HIV-infected partners). Rapid HIV testing should be performed on women who present in labor with undocumented HIV status. If a rapid HIV test result is positive, antiretroviral prophylaxis (with consent) should be initiated during labor without waiting for the results of the confirmatory test. Management and treatment of the pregnant woman with HIV infection is covered in Chapter 15.

Syphilis

A serologic test for syphilis should be performed on a pregnant women at the first prenatal visit. The most commonly employed screening tests are the rapid plasma reagin (RPR) test and the venereal disease research laboratory (VDRL) test; when positive, screening tests need to be confirmed by a treponemal-specific test, either the fluorescent treponemal antibody absorption test (FTA-ABS) or the microhemagglutination assay for treponema pallidum (MHA-TP). In populations with a high prevalence of syphilis, or for high-risk patients, screening should also be considered at 28 to 32 weeks and at delivery, given the risks of undiagnosed congenital syphilis, as well as the long-term risks of untreated syphilis for the woman (and her partner).

Syphilis is defined by the stage of infection. *Primary syphilis* is characterized by the presence of the chancre, a painless genital ulcer. In women, the chancre may never be recognized, since the majority are intravaginal. *Secondary syphilis* occurs a few weeks to several months after the primary infection in the absence of treatment, with systemic symptoms that are related to the hematogenous and lymphatic spread of the disease. A characteristic rash on the palms and soles can be seen at this time. *Latent syphilis*, either early (<1 year) or late latent (>1 year) is when the untreated infection exists asymptomatically within the body. When a patient presents with a positive serum test for syphilis without preceding symptoms, she is presumed to be in the latent stage. In one third of patients, latent syphilis can progress to *tertiary syphilis*, with involvement of skin, bones, central nervous system, and heart.

The treatment of choice for all stages of syphilis during pregnancy is parenteral (intramuscular) benzathine penicillin G. Penicillin, unlike other treatment options for nonpregnant adults such as erythromycin, readily crosses the placenta and treats the fetus as well. Primary and secondary syphilis are treated with a single course of 2.4 million units of benzathine penicillin (1.2 million units in each buttock). Early latent syphilis may be treated the same way, but late latent syphilis (syphilis lasting for more than a year, or an inability to determine when the infection occurred) is treated with 2.4 million units once weekly for 3 consecutive weeks.

Chlamydia

Chlamydial genital infection is the most frequently reported infectious disease in the United States, and its prevalence is highest among persons younger than 25 years of age. Pelvic inflammatory disease (PID), ectopic pregnancy, and tubal infertility can result from untreated chlamydial infections in women. Annual screening of all sexually active women 25 years or younger is recommended, as is screening of older women with sexual risk factors. The benefits of *Chlamydia trachomatis* screening in women have been demonstrated in areas where screening programs have reduced both the prevalence of infection and rates of PID. Prenatal screening (and appropriate treatment) for chlamydia during pregnancy can prevent both gynecologic sequelae in the woman as well as chlamydial infection and its sequelae among neonates. Infected untreated neonates are at risk for both ophthalmitis and pneumonia. Prenatal treatment of maternal infection has been shown to be the most efficient method for preventing neonatal infection.

Pregnant women can be treated with azithromycin or erythromycin for chlamydial infection. Erythromycin is poorly tolerated because of the gastrointestinal side effects, and investigators have established the safety and efficacy of azithromycin. Azithromycin also has the advantage of being a single 1-g oral dose. Azithromycin and doxycycline are listed as recommended regimens for chalmydial infection in the most recent CDC STD Treatment Guideline, however doxycycline generally is contraindicated in pregnancy. Erythromycin is listed as an alternative regimen.

Gonorrhea

Gonorrhea is the second most commonly reported STD in the United States. Because gonococcal infections among women are frequently asymptomatic, screening continues to be an essential component of gonorrhea control. The U.S. Preventive Services Task Force recommends that clinicians screen all sexually active women, including those who are pregnant, for gonorrhea infection. Left untreated, gonorrhea results in high rates of PID and tubal scarring that can lead to infertility or ectopic pregnancy. Nucleic acid hybridization tests (NAATs) are currently available for both gonorrhea and chlamydia and have superior sensitivity and specificity to older culture- or antigen-based tests. NAATs are FDA approved for use with endocervical swabs, vaginal swabs, male urethral swabs, and female and male urine, allowing for noninvasive screening (e.g., without use of speculum examinations). However, nonculture tests cannot provide antimicrobial susceptibility results, so that in cases of persistent gonococcal infection after treatment, clinicians should perform both culture and antimicrobial susceptibility testing.

Patients infected with *Neisseria gonorrhoeae* are frequently coinfected with *C. trachomatis*; this finding has led to the recommendation that patients treated for gonococcal infection also be routinely treated with a regimen that is also effective against chlamydia. However, patients with a negative chlamydial NAAT result at the time of treatment of gonorrhea do not need to be treated for chlamydia as well.

Treatment of gonorrhea has been an evolving challenge, since the bacterium has become resistant to an increasing number of effective antibiotics, including penicillin and quinolones. Treatment of gonorrhea in nonpregnant adults with single-dose ciprofloxacin, for example, has not been recommended since 2003 to 2004. Currently, for uncomplicated infections of the cervix, urethra, and rectum, the recommended regimens are (1) ceftriaxone 125 mg intramuscularly (IM) in a single dose or (2) cefixime 400 mg orally in a single dose. For pharyngeal infections, only ceftriaxone is currently recommended. Spectinomycin, 2 g IM in a single dose, has been recommended as an alternative by the CDC in the face of documented penicillin allergy; however, it is currently unavailable in the United States and does not treat pharyngeal infection. Alternatively, if a true penicillin allergy (anaphylaxis) is documented, then antibiotic susceptibility testing for a quinolone may be requested on a culture specimen, and single-dose treatment can cautiously be administered, even during pregnancy.

Hepatitis B

In an individual chronically infected with hepatitis B, the virus is widely present in body fluid, so that hepatitis B is efficiently transmitted sexually, and is viewed as an STD. Perinatal transmission is a particularly efficient method of viral infection; 90% to 95% of infants born to chronically infected women will themselves become chronic hepatitis B carriers in the absence of effective neonatal immunoprophylaxis. Therefore, screening for hepatitis B infection is currently an established component of routine prenatal testing in the United States: all women are screened, not just those in high-risk categories. Screening consists of a blood test for the presence of the hepatitis B surface antigen (HBsAg).

Identification of chronic HBsAg carriers during pregnancy permits their newborns to receive both hepatitis B immune globulin (HBIG) and the first dose of the hepatitis B vaccine series within the first 12 hours after birth. This combination protocol has been demonstrated to be up to 95% effective in preventing vertical infection of newborns. Screening of other household members should also be performed, and hepatitis B vaccination is strongly encouraged for uninfected family members.

Treatment of pregnant women with antiviral medications against hepatitis B to lower the risk of perinatal transmission is currently not recommended.

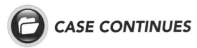

CASE CONTINUES

Ms. Shaw's initial test results are significant for a positive RPR, with a titer of 1:8. All other tests, including HIV, are negative. The patient is contacted to return to the office prior to her next scheduled visit to review these results and to have her partner come with her. The patient appears for this appointment, but her partner is "unavailable." She is informed of the positive RPR test result, and the need to treat with IM penicillin for three doses. She reports a significant penicillin allergy: she required hospitalization as a child after receiving a penicillin-like antibiotic for an ear infection. She remembers difficulty breathing "like her throat was closing up," and needed to be treated in an emergency department. Her mother was told that she was close to requiring mechanical ventilation, and that she should never take penicillin in the future. Desensitization to penicillin to treat her syphilis during pregnancy was discussed.

Decision 2: Treatment

Why is penicillin desensitization needed in this case?

A. Some syphilis is resistant to other antibiotics
B. Other effective antibiotics may not prevent fetal disease and are riskier during pregnancy
C. Other effective antibiotics may not prevent maternal recurrence
D. Desensitization is actually controversial in this setting, and treatment should wait until after delivery

The correct answer is B: Other antibiotics are expected to be effective in the mother but may not prevent fetal infection. In nonpregnant adults, while penicillin is clearly the best-established and most efficacious treatment of syphilis, other regimens are acceptable if (1) a history of severe penicillin allergy is documented (skin testing should be performed if uncertain) and (2) the patient is not HIV infected, since alternate regimens have not been validated in this population, and they are at particularly increased risk of serious sequelae of untreated or undertreated syphilis. Doxycycline (100 mg orally BID for 28 days) and tetracycline (500 mg orally QID for 28 days) are regimens that have been used for latent syphilis in such individuals.

For pregnant patients with syphilis and a penicillin allergy (and for all HIV-infected individuals), tetracycline is not an acceptable or proven alternative to penicillin. In addition, the tetracycline class of antibiotics is contraindicated for use during pregnancy because of fetal toxicities. Therefore, both for maternal and fetal indications, penicillin is the only indicated treatment of syphilis during pregnancy and should be administered after acute desensitization takes place.

Rate (per 100,000 live births)

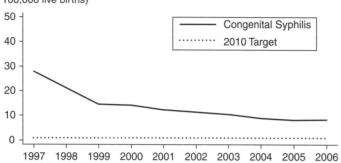

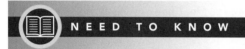

Figure 13.1 Congenital syphilis—rates for infants <1 year of age: United States, 1997 to 2006 and the Healthy People 2010 objective. Note: The Healthy People 2010 objective for congenital syphilis is 1.0 case per 100,000 live births (Courtesy of CDC at www.cdc.gov/std/stats06/slides.htm. Accessed on December 17, 2010.)

NEED TO KNOW

Congenital Syphilis and Penicillin Treatment

The incidence of congenital syphilis in 2002 was 11.2/100,000 live births, a 21% decline from 2000; since that time, the rate of congenital syphilis has plateaued (Fig. 13.1). Syphilis spirochetes can cross the placenta at any time during pregnancy. Clinical manifestations of congenital syphilis include hydrops, growth restriction, hydrocephalus, and skeletal abnormalities. Intrauterine fetal death can also occur, particularly with primary and secondary stage infections. Between 50% and 100% of untreated pregnant women with primary syphilis will transmit it to the fetus, and 50% of those infants will have clinical manifestations of congenital syphilis. Up to 50% of infants with congenital syphilis will be stillborn or deliver prematurely. Early latent syphilis transmission rates are approximately 40%, though only 20% result in a preterm delivery or perinatal mortality. Late latent and tertiary syphilis have a frequency of transmission of 10%, and there is no increase in preterm delivery or perinatal mortality. Treatment is crucial, as only 1% to 2% of infants born to adequately treated women will have congenital syphilis.

No proven alternatives to penicillin are available for treating congenital syphilis, or syphilis in pregnant women. Of the adult U.S. population, 3% to 10% have experienced an IgE-mediated allergic response to penicillin, such as urticaria, angioedema, or anaphylaxis (upper airway obstruction, bronchospasm, or hypotension). Readministration of penicillin to these patients can cause severe, immediate reactions. Because anaphylactic reactions to penicillin can be fatal, every effort should be made to avoid administering penicillin to penicillin-allergic patients, unless they undergo acute desensitization to eliminate anaphylactic sensitivity.

The results of many studies indicate that skin testing with the major and minor determinants of penicillin can reliably identify persons at high risk for penicillin

reactions. Skin testing using the major determinants will only miss 3% to 10% of allergic patients. Skin testing is not contraindicated during pregnancy.

Patients who have a positive skin test to one of the penicillin determinants can be desensitized and safely treated. This is a straightforward, safe procedure that can be performed orally or intravenously. Patients should be desensitized in a hospital setting because serious IgE-mediated allergic reactions can occur. The desensitization is usually undertaken by an allergy–immunology specialist. Desensitization can usually be completed in approximately 4 hours, after which the first dose of penicillin can be administered. For patients who require three weekly doses of penicillin for latent syphilis, a small daily oral dose of penicillin (usually 500 mg/d) is given as maintenance until all three doses have been administered, to prevent resensitization to penicillin between the weekly doses. One oral desensitization protocol used during pregnancy is shown in Table 13.1.

Treatment of syphilis during pregnancy can be complicated by the Jarisch–Herxheimer reaction. During pregnancy, this reaction has been reported to occur in 100% of treated primary infections, 60% of treated secondary infections, and in no treated latent infections. The reaction typically consists of fever, chills, myalgia, headache, and accentuation of any cutaneous lesions. It usually occurs within several hours after treatment and resolves in 24 to 36 hours. The reaction is thought to result from a cytokine cascade initiated by the immune response to the dying spirochetes' cellular components, as it is more common in the earlier the stage of infection, when there is a higher rate of spirochetemia. No proven prophylactic measures are available, although pretreatment with acetaminophen has been recommended. During pregnancy, the reaction can precipitate uterine contractions (67%) and decreased fetal movement (67%) along with the fever (73%). Some experts recommend fetal monitoring and ultrasound evaluation of the fetus (in the third trimester) if primary or secondary syphilis is being treated on an ambulatory basis.

TABLE 13.1
ORAL DESENSITIZATION PROTOCOL FOR PATIENTS WITH A POSITIVE SKIN TEST[a]

Penicillin V Suspension Dose[b]	Amount[c] (Units/mL)	mL	Units	Cumulative Dose (Units)
1	1,000	0.1	100	100
2	1,000	0.2	200	300
3	1,000	0.4	400	700
4	1,000	0.8	800	1,500
5	1,000	1.6	1,600	3,100
6	1,000	3.2	3,200	6,300
7	1,000	6.4	6,400	12,700
8	10,000	1.2	12,000	24,700
9	10,000	2.4	24,000	48,700
10	10,000	4.8	48,000	96,700
11	80,000	1.0	80,000	176,700
12	80,000	2.0	160,000	336,700
13	80,000	4.0	320,000	656,700
14	80,000	8.0	640,000	1,296,700

Note: Observation period: 30 minutes before parenteral administration of penicillin.
[a]Reprinted with permission from the *New England Journal of Medicine* (Wendel GO Jr, Stark BJ, Jamison RB, Melina RD, Suliivan TJ. Penicillin allergy and desensitization in serious infections during pregnancy. N Engl J Med. 1985;312:1229–32).
[b]Interval between doses, 15 minutes; elapsed time, 3 hours and 45 minutes; cumulative dose, 1.3 million units.
[c]The specific amount of drug was diluted in approximately 30 mL of water and then administered orally.

CASE CONTINUES

Ms. Shaw is admitted at 14 weeks of gestation for penicillin desensitization and receives appropriate treatment for presumed late latent syphilis consisting of three weekly injections of benzathine penicillin. Fetal surveillance via ultrasound is normal. At 28 weeks of gestation, a repeat RPR test is drawn to monitor response to therapy and is again positive, now at a titer of 1:32. The patient reports no symptoms or lesions.

Decision 3: Management

How should the patient be managed at this point?

A. Re-treat and notify public health authorities to contact partner

B. Do not re-treat and notify patient to come in with partner for joint treatment

C. Re-treat with a second antibiotic

D. Do not re-treat and check an FTA

The correct answer is A: Re-treat and report the infection; public health authorities will then contact the partner.

Screening test (RPR and VDRL) titers usually correlate with disease activity, and results are reported quantitatively. A fourfold change in titer, equivalent to a change of two (2) dilutions (e.g., from 1:4 to 1:16 or from 1:8 to 1:32) is considered necessary to show a clinically significant difference between two serial tests that were performed using the same methodology. RPR and VDRL tests are not interchangeable for serial surveillance. These tests will usually become nonreactive over time after appropriate treatment. However, in some patients, nontreponemal antibodies can persist at a low titer (1:1 to 1:2) for a long period of time, sometimes for the life of the patient. This response is referred to as the *serofast* reaction.

In contrast, treponemal-specific antibody tests (FTA, MHA-TP), which are used to confirm reactive RPR/VDRL tests, will, in most cases, remain reactive for the remainder of the patient's life. Therefore, serial surveillance of these tests to monitor adequacy of therapy is not indicated. The only reported loss of these antibodies has been in individuals treated during the **primary** stage of syphilis; 15% to 25% of these patients may revert to serologically nonreactive for a treponemal test after 2 to 3 years.

Since the patient received documented appropriate therapy for presumed late latent syphilis, the fourfold rise in her titer 14 weeks after treatment is indicative of reinfection rather than treatment failure. No other antibiotic regimens have been shown to be more efficacious than benzathine penicillin. Treatment failure has been reported in HIV-infected individuals, and a repeat HIV test is indicated, since the presumption here is that there has been sexual activity with a high-risk individual. If this patient were found to also be HIV infected, lumbar puncture and evaluation of cerebrospinal fluid for evidence of neurosyphilis would be indicated before re-treatment.

Assuming that the patient is HIV uninfected, she should be re-treated for primary syphilis and the appropriate public health authorities notified. Her treatment should not be delayed while awaiting her sexual partner to present for treatment, since the risk of untreated primary syphilis producing congenital syphilis in the fetus is too high. She should be counseled to avoid all sexual activity with that individual until he has been appropriately treated. The timing of maternal therapy in preventing congenital syphilis is critical: if the mother receives treatment <4 weeks before delivery, more extensive neonatal workup and treatment regimen are indicated.

 ## CASE CONCLUSION

Ms. Shaw acknowledges ongoing sexual contact with the father of the pregnancy, who has not presented to any medical facility for syphilis testing or treatment. She expresses understanding of her probable reinfection through him, and promises to see that he is treated and to avoid any sexual contact until he has been treated completely. Her repeat HIV test result is negative. The patient is readmitted for penicillin desensitization and, after completing the protocol, receives a single course of IM benzathine penicillin G, 2.4 million units. The pregnancy is monitored with serial fetal ultrasounds with no

evidence of fetal growth restriction or other fetal developmental abnormalities appreciated.

Her repeat RPR test at 36 weeks decreases to a titer of 1:8. At 38 weeks, the patient delivers a healthy baby girl weighing 3,260 g with Apgar score of 7 and 9 at one and five minutes after spontaneous labor. The infant has a normal newborn physical examination, and her RPR test result (obtained via heel stick sample) is 1:4. The newborn receives treatment with a single course of IM benzathine penicillin G at a dose of 50,000 units/kg.

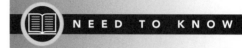

Evaluation of Infants at Risk for Congenital Syphilis

Infants born to mothers diagnosed with and/or treated for syphilis before delivery need to have a quantitative nontreponemal serologic test (RPR or VDRL) performed on infant serum, because umbilical cord blood can be contaminated with maternal blood and yield a false-positive result. Ordering a treponemal-specific test is not necessary, and no IgM testing is recommended. These infants are also examined thoroughly for evidence of congenital syphilis (nonimmune hydrops, jaundice, hepatosplenomegaly, rhinitis, skin rash, and/or

TABLE 13.2

CDC RECOMMENDATIONS FOR TREATMENT OF THE NEWBORN OF A MOTHER WITH SYPHILIS

Scenario	Newborn Workup	Treatment
1. Proven or highly probable newborn disease	CSF analysis for VDRL, cell count, and protein CBC and differential and platelet counts As needed: Long-bone radiographs, chest radiograph, liver-function tests, cranial ultrasound, ophthalmologic examination, and auditory brainstem response	**Aqueous crystalline penicillin G** 100,000–150,000 units/kg/day, administered as 50,000 units/kg/dose IV every 12 hours during the first 7 days of life and every 8 hours thereafter for a total of 10 days **OR** **Procaine penicillin G** 50,000 units/kg/dose IM in a single daily dose for 10 days
2. Normal newborn examination but mother not adequately treated	CSF analysis for VDRL, cell count, and protein CBC and differential and platelet count Long-bone radiographs	If workup abnormal or not done: 10-day therapy as above. If all workup normal, may consider: **Benzathine penicillin G** 50,000 units/kg/dose IM in a single dose
3. Normal newborn examination and mother adequately treated	No evaluation	**Benzathine penicillin G** 50,000 units/kg/dose IM in a single dose
4. Normal newborn examination and mother treated prior to pregnancy	No evaluation	None needed, but some experts would give: **Benzathine penicillin G** 50,000 units/kg/dose IM in a single dose

Note: For a full description of the scenarios, see the text.
CBC count, complete blood cell count; CSF, cerebrospinal fluid; VDRL, venereal disease research laboratory.

pseudoparalysis of an extremity). Pathologic examination of the placenta or umbilical cord using specific fluorescent antitreponemal antibody staining is suggested.

Per the CDC guidelines, recommended infant workup and treatment depends on the facts of maternal treatment and on infant findings. Four scenarios are described:

(1) The infant has proven or highly probable disease.
   a. Physical examination suggestive of congenital syphilis
   or
   b. Newborn VDRL or RPR fourfold higher than that of mothers
   or
   c. Finding of spirochetes in body fluids
(2) The infant has a normal physical examination and an RPR equal to or less than fourfold the maternal titer, *but* the mother was untreated or inadequately treated, treated with a nonpenicillin regimen, or was treated <4 weeks prior to delivery.
(3) The infant has a normal physical examination and an RPR equal to or less than fourfold the maternal titer, *and* the mother was adequately treated in pregnancy >4 weeks prior to delivery.
(4) The infant has a normal physical examination and an RPR equal to or less than fourfold the maternal titer, and the mother was adequately treated prior to pregnancy without evidence of reinfection.

The infant workup and treatment of these categories of patient is outlined in Table 13.2.

SUGGESTED READINGS

CDC. Revised guidelines for HIV counseling, testing, and referral and revised recommendations for HIV screening of pregnant women. MMWR Morb Mortal Wkly Rep. 2001;50(RR-19):63–85.

CDC, Workowski KA, Berman SM. Sexually transmitted diseases treatment guidelines, 2006. MMWR Morb Mortal Wkly Rep. 2006; 55(RR-11):1–94.

Chou R, Smits AK, Huffman LH, Fu R, Korthuis PT. Prenatal screening for HIV: a review of the evidence for the U.S. Preventive Services Task Force. Ann Intern Med. 2005;143:38–54.

Geisler WM. Management of uncomplicated *Chlamydia trachomatis* infections in adolescents and adults: evidence reviewed for the 2006 Centers for Disease Control and Prevention Sexually Transmitted Diseases Guidelines. Clin Infect Dis. 2007;44(Suppl 3): S77–83.

Johnson RE, Newhall WJ, Papp JR, et al.. Screening tests to detect *Chlamydia trachomatis* and *Neisseria gonorrhoeae* infections, 2002. MMWR Morb Mortal Wkly Rep. 2002;51(RR-15):1–38.

Lyss SB, Kamb ML, Peterman TA, et al. *Chlamydia trachomatis* among patients infected with and treated for *Neisseria gonorrhoeae* in sexually transmitted disease clinics in the United States. Ann Intern Med. 2003;139:178–85.

Mast EE, Margolis HS, Fiore AE, et al. A comprehensive immunization strategy to eliminate transmission of hepatitis B virus infection in the United States. Recommendations of the Advisory Committee on Immunization Practices (ACIP) part 1: immunization of infants, children, and adolescents. MMWR Morb Mortal Wkly Rep. 2005;54(RR-16):1–31.

Newman LM, Moran JS, Workowski KA. Update on the management of gonorrhea in adults in the United States. Clin Infect Dis. 2007;44(Suppl 3):S84–101.

Romanowski B, Sutherland R, Fick GH, Mooney D, Love EJ. Serologic response to treatment of infectious syphilis. Ann Intern Med. 1991; 114:1005–9.

Stoner BP. Current controversies in the management of adult syphilis. Clin Infect Dis. 2007;44(Suppl 3):S130–46.

Wendel GO Jr, Stark BJ, Jamison RB, Melina RD, Sullivan TJ. Penicillin allergy and desensitization in serious infections during pregnancy. N Engl J Med. 1985;312:1229–32.

Thyroid Disease in Pregnancy

David E. Abel

 CASE PRESENTATION

You are about to meet your patient, Ms. Grady, for an initial visit. She is a 24-year-old primigravida who is 10 weeks pregnant by last menstrual period. Her past medical history is remarkable for a history of Graves' disease diagnosed 5 years ago. She used to take medication but doesn't remember the name. In addition, she doesn't recall when her thyroid functions were last checked. She recently moved to the area and has not established contact with an endocrinologist. When questioned about symptoms, she notes occasional sweating, palpitations, and nervousness.

On physical examination, her pulse is 105 bpm, and her weight is 140 lbs. Blood pressure is normal, and the physical examination is unremarkable, without evidence of goiter. Ultrasound confirms a viable pregnancy consistent with 10 weeks of gestation.

NEED TO KNOW

Thyroid Physiology During Pregnancy

The thyroid gland is under the influence of the hypothalamic–pituitary axis. Thyrotropin-releasing hormone, produced by the hypothalamus, induces secretion of thyroid-stimulating hormone (TSH) from the pituitary. The production of the two main thyroid hormones, thyroxine (T_4) and triiodothyronine (T_3), is induced when TSH binds to its receptors on the thyroid gland. T_3 and T_4 are mostly protein bound by thyroid-binding globulin (TBG), and only 0.04% of total T_4 (TT_4) and 0.5% of total T_3 (TT_3) are available in their free forms (FT_4, FT_3) in serum. The free hormone exerts negative feedback on the pituitary to decrease TSH production.

TT_4 and TT_3 increase early in pregnancy in association with a 200% increase in TBG. The high TBG levels plateau at 20 weeks of gestation and remain unchanged until delivery. During the first trimester, human chorionic gonadotropin (hCG) acts as a weak stimulator of the TSH receptor. This TSH-like effect by hCG leads to enhanced production of T_4 and to TSH suppression. TSH levels usually remain within the normal range, but low TSH levels may be seen in 15% of normal pregnant women in the first trimester of pregnancy, and the effect may be more pronounced in multiple gestations. Thus, a suppressed TSH in the face of a normal to high FT_4 level is consistent with normal early pregnancy and treatment is not warranted. After the first trimester, as levels of hCG decline, TSH suppression by hCG decreases and the TSH normalizes. Levels of FT_4 increase in the first trimester with hCG stimulation, then decline to levels 10% to 15% below the levels seen in nonpregnant individuals.

The effect of pregnancy on thyroid function is summarized in Figure 14.1.

? **Decision 1:** Diagnosis thyroid function tests in pregnancy

In your assessment of this patient, what laboratory tests are appropriate?

- **A.** Free thyroxine (FT_4)
- **B.** TSH
- **C.** Free triiodothyronine (FT_3)
- **D.** Thyroid-stimulating immunoglobulin (TSI)
- **E.** A and B

The correct answer is E: Both FT_4 and TSH would be appropriate. In general practice, the initial screen for thyroid dysfunction is a TSH alone. In pregnancy, however, especially in the first trimester, TSH may be misleading and the FT_4 is also of value.

FT_3 (Answer C) is not measured routinely. Although T_3 is the most active thyroid hormone, only 20% of T_3 is directly secreted from the thyroid gland. The rest is derived from peripheral conversion of T_4. However, FT_3 assessment should be considered in patients with signs of hyperthyroidism, a suppressed TSH, and a normal FT_4. In this instance, an elevated FT_3 indicates T_3 thyrotoxicosis, which may occur before increased levels of FT_4 are found.

TSIs are a feature of Graves' disease; IgG autoantibodies that directly stimulate the thyroid gland by binding to TSH receptors. The clinical utility of evaluating TSI

Mother

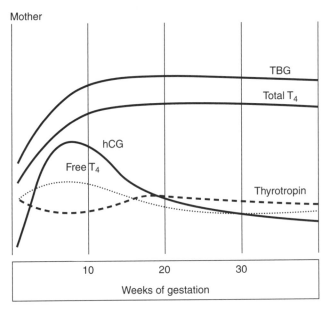

Figure 14.1 The effect of pregnancy on thyroid hormones. The rise in hCG in the first trimester is associated with an increase in free T_4 and a decrease in thyrotropin (TSH), although the levels of these hormones usually remain within the normal range. With the decrease in hCG, both TSH and free T_4 return to baseline. hCG, human chorionic gonadotropin; TBG, thyroid-binding globulin. (Adapted from Burrow GN, Fisher DA, Larsen PR. Maternal and fetal thyroid function. N Engl J Med. 1994;331(16):1072–8.)

levels (Answer D) during pregnancy is controversial. Currently, the American Congress of Obstetricians and Gynecologists (ACOG) does not endorse routine evaluation of TSI levels.

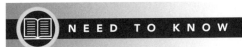

NEED TO KNOW

Thyroid Disease in Pregnancy

The diagnosis of thyroid disease in pregnancy is complicated by the fact that many of the signs and symptoms of thyroid dysfunction mimic those of pregnancy. The hypermetabolic state of pregnancy can mimic the symptoms seen in hyperthyroidism, including an increase in heart rate, fatigue, and heat intolerance. The classic symptoms of hypothyroidism include fatigue, constipation, and muscle cramps, also well-known discomforts of pregnancy. The diagnosis of thyroid disease in pregnancy, therefore, requires a high index of suspicion. A list of common signs and symptoms of hyper- and hypothyroidism is included in Table 14.1.

Hyperthyroidism

The incidence of overt hyperthyroidism in pregnancy is approximately 2 per 1,000. Most cases (95%) are due

TABLE 14.1

SIGNS/SYMPTOMS OF THYROID DISEASE

Hypothyroidism	Hyperthyroidism
■ Fatigue	■ Heat intolerance
■ Constipation	■ Nervousness
■ Somnolence	■ Weight loss
■ Cold intolerance	■ Resting tremor
■ Hair loss	■ Palpitations
■ Dry skin	■ Diaphoresis
■ Depression	■ Warm, moist skin
■ Decreased libido	■ Tachycardia
■ Weight gain despite poor appetite	■ Increased appetite
■ Periorbital puffiness	■ Exophthalmia
■ Hoarseness	

to Graves' disease, an autoimmune process characterized by the presence of autoantibodies (TSI) that stimulate the thyroid gland to release hormone. Other less common causes of hyperthyroidism include a functioning adenoma, toxic nodular goiter, and subacute thyroiditis.

Physical examination in hyperthyroidism may reveal hypertension, tachycardia, goiter, and weight loss. Symptoms specific to Graves' disease include dermopathy (localized, pretibial myxedema) and ophthalmopathy (lid lag and retraction).

Clinical hyperthyroidism is diagnosed by a suppressed TSH and elevated serum FT_4. Subclinical hyperthyroidism, defined by a suppressed TSH and normal FT_4 levels, affects 1.7% of pregnant women. This entity is not associated with adverse pregnancy outcomes, and treatment is not warranted.

Hyperthyroidism during pregnancy is associated with increased perinatal morbidity and mortality. Risks include spontaneous pregnancy loss, preterm birth, fetal growth restriction, preeclampsia, congestive heart failure, and thyroid storm. TSI can cross the placenta and cause fetal or neonatal Graves' disease (risk of 1%–5%). Fetal effects are not correlated with maternal disease status, but high levels of TSI ($\geq$200%–500%) increase the risk of fetal and neonatal hyperthyroidism. Of note, some patients with Graves' disease may produce TSH-binding inhibitory immunoglobulin (TBII) that may inhibit the fetal thyroid gland, resulting in fetal or neonatal hypothyroidism, which is usually transient. Both TSI and TBII can coexist in 30% of patients with Graves' disease. Fetal hypothyroidism can also result from transplacental passage of antithyroid medication used to treat the mother.

When hyperthyroidism is uncontrolled, excessive T_4 can lead to congestive heart failure, which has been reported to occur more commonly during pregnancy, or to thyroid storm.

Hypothyroidism

The incidence of hypothyroidism in pregnancy varies by country; in the United States, the incidence of elevated TSH in women is 2.5%. In developed countries, the most common cause of hypothyroidism is Hashimoto's thyroiditis, also known as chronic autoimmune thyroiditis. This condition is characterized by the presence of antithyroid antibodies including antimicrosomal and antithyroglobulin antibodies. Rarely, these antibodies can cause neonatal hypothyroidism, which is transient. Other causes of primary hypothyroidism include subacute viral thyroiditis, radioactive iodine treatment, thyroidectomy, and iodine deficiency. The latter is the most common cause of hypothyroidism in developing countries. Certain medications including lithium, iodine, and amiodarone are uncommon causes of hypothyroidism.

The classic symptoms of hypothyroidism include cold intolerance, dry skin, fatigue, constipation, hair loss, and muscle cramps. These may progress to weight gain, insomnia, voice changes, carpal tunnel syndrome, and intellectual slowness. Hashimoto's disease and iodine deficiency are associated with goiter. Hypothyroidism can lead to myxedema coma if left untreated. It is unusual for severe uncontrolled hypothyroidism to present during pregnancy as it is also associated with decreased fertility.

Clinical hypothyroidism is diagnosed by the finding of a high TSH and low FT_4. Well-controlled hypothyroidism has minimal impact on pregnancy. Poorly or partially controlled disease may be associated with adverse pregnancy outcomes including preeclampsia, placental abruption, preterm birth, low birth weight, and fetal death. Uncontrolled disease can also place the fetus at risk for neuropsychological deficits. The fetus does not produce thyroid hormone until approximately 12 weeks of gestation, depending on maternal FT_4 for brain development in the first trimester. Therefore, treatment should be initiated during pregnancy as early as possible.

The topic of subclinical hypothyroidism (elevated TSH and normal FT_4) has received considerable attention based on observational data suggesting a link between this entity and impaired neurocognitive development in children. These studies were retrospective and noninterventional and showed a lower intelligence quotient in children born to mothers with uncontrolled hypothyroidism (elevated TSH levels in midgestation). The results led several national endocrine authorities to recommend routine screening and treatment of subclinical hypothyroidism during pregnancy. However, the results must be interpreted with caution. To date, there have been no interventional studies to determine whether screening and treating pregnant patients for subclinical hypothyroidism will improve

TABLE 14.2

INDICATED SCREENING FOR HYPOTHYROIDISM DURING PREGNANCY: THESE RISK FACTORS MAY INDICATE A NEED FOR SCREENING

- Personal history of thyroid disease
- Symptoms of thyroid disease
- Previous treatment of hyperthyroidism
- Family history of thyroid disease
- History of high-dose neck irradiation
- Type 1 diabetes mellitus
- Goiter or palpable thyroid nodule
- Hyperlipidemia
- Medications (iodine, rifampin, amiodarone, lithium, phenytoin)

the neuropsychological performance of their offspring. Currently, ACOG does *not* recommend routine screening for subclinical hypothyroidism during pregnancy. However, it is reasonable to have a low threshold to screen patients if risk factors are present. Some risk factors that might indicate a need for screening are listed in Table 14.2.

Pregnancy-Associated Thyroid Disease

Gestational transient thyrotoxicosis is a biochemical hyperthyroidism specific to pregnancy that is associated with high hCG levels. It is commonly associated with hyperemesis gravidarum, although it can be seen in gestational trophoblastic disease. These patients are rarely symptomatic, and antithyroid treatment is not warranted. Another pregnancy-associated thyroidopathy is postpartum thyroiditis. Postpartum thyroiditis represents an autoimmune inflammation of the thyroid gland that occurs within 1 year postpartum. It is seen in 5% of normal women and can occur after pregnancy loss. The recurrence risk is 70%. The diagnosis is made by confirmation of new-onset abnormal levels of TSH, FT_4, or both. Clinically, three presentations are possible; hyperthyroidism, hyperthyroidism progressing to hypothyroidism, or hypothyroidism. Treatment of postpartum thyroiditis is controversial and is usually reserved for those with symptoms. Although usually transient, a portion of women will develop permanent hypothyroidism.

 CASE CONTINUES

On the first visit, you obtain blood for TSH and FT_4 from Ms. Grady. Her TSH is 0.1 μIU/mL, and her FT_4 is 2.8 ng/dL. The normal values for these hormones depend on the laboratory, but both of these levels are abnormal, and suggest hyperthyroidism.

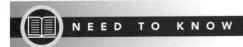

NEED TO KNOW

Management of Hyperthyroidism During Pregnancy

The treatment of hyperthyroidism during pregnancy can reduce the risk of maternal, fetal, and neonatal complications. The goal is to achieve and maintain a euthyroid state using the least possible amount of antithyroid medication. In many settings, treatment is considered for an FT_4 of >1.8 ng/dL. In the United States, the two thioamide drugs available for treatment are propylthiouracil (PTU) and methimazole (MMU). These medications decrease the synthesis of thyroid hormone by blocking the organification of iodide. PTU also inhibits peripheral conversion of T_4 to T_3. The data suggest that these medications are equally effective in achieving euthyroidism without any difference in neonatal outcomes.

PTU tends to be the preferred drug due to a possible association between MMU and fetal abnormalities, including aplasia cutis and choanal and esophageal atresia. Other proposed advantages of PTU use, including less placental transfer and an association of MMU with developmental delay, have not been confirmed in recent studies. Because of the possible association of MMU with embryopathy, many recommend avoiding the use of MMU in the first trimester if PTU is available. According to the American Academy of Pediatrics, both medications are compatible with breastfeeding.

The usual starting dose for PTU is 100 mg three times a day (range of 50–150 mg three times a day). If there is no response, the dose should be increased. On occasion, a dose as large as 600 mg/d may be necessary. MMU has a longer half-life and can be administered less frequently. A typical dose is 10 to 20 mg twice a day. Once treatment is initiated, thyroid function tests (TSH and FT_4) are obtained every 2 to 4 weeks. Improvement in the FT_4 level is usually seen within 4 weeks. TSH is not used to assess therapy as suppression may persist for months. The dose of thioamide can usually be decreased once a consistent euthyroid state is achieved. Most women will need less PTU in the third trimester, and some can discontinue treatment and remain euthyroid. Thioamides can suppress fetal thyroid function, which can lead to fetal and neonatal hypothyroidism, and possibly fetal goiter. To minimize this risk, the FT_4 is maintained in the high normal (upper third) range using the lowest thioamide dose possible.

Minor maternal side effects of thioamide treatment occurring in 5% of patients include rash, nausea, anorexia, fever, and loss of taste or smell. More serious side effects seen in 1% of patients include hepatitis, thrombocytopenia, and vasculitis. The most serious side effect is agranulocytosis, noted in 0.1% to 0.4% of women. Signs and symptoms appear acutely and include fever, sore throat, general malaise, and gingivitis. This complication is not dose related, and serial leukocyte counts are not helpful. Discontinuation of therapy and checking a complete blood cell count is warranted if a patient with hyperthyroidism receiving thioamide treatment presents with a sore throat and/or fever. Baseline white blood cell count and liver function tests are reasonable prior to the initiation of antithyroid therapy.

Beta-blockers can be used to treat symptoms of thyrotoxicosis until thioamides decrease thyroid hormone levels. Propranolol at a dose of 20 to 40 mg every 8 to 12 hours and atenolol 50 to 100 mg once a day are options.

Thyroidectomy is rarely performed during pregnancy. It is usually reserved for patients unable to tolerate thioamide therapy, those with an allergy to both thioamides, large goiters, patient preference, and the very rare case of drug resistance. Thyroid ablation with radioactive ^{131}iodine (^{131}I) is contraindicated during pregnancy.

Antepartum surveillance in the pregnant patient with hyperthyroidism includes an increased frequency of visits watching for signs and symptoms of thyrotoxicosis. Serial ultrasounds to assess fetal growth are appropriate, and weekly nonstress tests should be considered starting at 32 to 34 weeks, especially in the patient with uncontrolled symptoms. Routine ultrasound screening for fetal goiter is not recommended. However, in patients with high TSI (≥200%–500% normal), the risk of fetal goiter is increased and ultrasound assessment is reasonable. A fetal goiter may result in hyperextension of the fetal neck, creating problems at delivery and possible compromise of the airway. Ultrasound signs of fetal thyrotoxicosis include hydrops, tachycardia, and cardiomegaly. Perinatal consultation is recommended if fetal thyrotoxicosis and/or fetal goiter is identified. Because of the risk of neonatal thyroid dysfunction seen in mothers with any type of thyroid disease, the pediatrician should be made aware of the maternal diagnosis.

 ## CASE CONTINUES

Ms. Grady is started on PTU at a dose of 100 mg three times a day. She is instructed to call you if any concerns arise including sore throat or fever. A follow-up appointment to assess symptoms and obtain thyroid function tests is scheduled in 2 weeks. She misses her follow-up appointment, and calls you a few weeks later (at approximately 18 weeks of gestation) complaining of palpitations, agitation, diarrhea, and a fever of 103°F. You suspect a diagnosis of thyroid storm and instruct the patient's husband to drive her to the emergency department immediately.

Decision 2: Management

Which of the following is indicated in the treatment of thyroid storm?

- A. Admit to labor and delivery for fetal monitoring
- B. Pregnancy termination
- C. Potassium iodide
- D. Diazepam

The correct answer is C: Potassium iodide. Although iodide is required for the synthesis of thyroid hormone, it will also block the release of hormone from the gland. In contrast, fetal monitoring (Answer A) is not useful in an 18-week fetus, and very few labor and delivery units are equipped to manage a patient in thyroid storm. Pregnancy termination (Answer B) will not improve outcome in this patient and may be a risk in an unstable patient. Diazepam (Answer D) is not used specifically in thyroid storm.

Thyroid storm is a medical emergency that occurs in 1% to 2% of pregnancies complicated by hyperthyroidism. A delay in diagnosis can put the patient at risk of cardiovascular collapse and coma. It is usually seen in patients with poorly controlled disease in the setting of a precipitating factor, such as surgery, infection, labor, or preeclampsia. Signs and symptoms include fever (sometimes >103°F), palpitations, nausea, vomiting, diarrhea, mental status changes (nervousness, restlessness, confusion, rarely seizures), and cardiac arrhythmia. Tachycardia out of proportion to the fever with a pulse rate of >140 bpm is not uncommon.

In the patient with thyroid storm, the goals of treatment are to ameliorate the hyperadrenergic effects of thyroid hormone on peripheral tissues (beta-blockers), reduce the synthesis (PTU, MMU) and release (iodides) of thyroid hormone, remove thyroid hormone from the circulation (glucocorticoids, plasmapheresis, dialysis), and treat the underlying cause. Thyroid functions are obtained to confirm the diagnosis (suppressed TSH, increased FT$_4$), but treatment is initiated immediately on the basis of clinical suspicion. Table 14.3 summarizes the treatment of thyroid storm.

CASE CONTINUES

Ms. Grady recovers from her episode of thyroid storm; however, she sustains an intrauterine fetal demise at 19 weeks of gestation. She has labor induced and delivers the fetus without incident. She wants to have her thyroid treated definitively. You discuss management options and she expresses interest in a thyroid ablative procedure. She wants to know what to expect in a subsequent pregnancy if she undergoes this procedure.

TABLE 14.3
TREATMENT OF THYROID STORM DURING PREGNANCY

1. Admission to the intensive care unit for supportive therapy including fluids, correction of electrolyte abnormalities, oxygen as needed, and control of hyperpyrexia (acetaminophen).
2. Start propylthiouracil (PTU) immediately (even before any laboratory results are available), 600–800 mg, orally, followed by 150–200 mg orally every 4–6 hr. Use methimazole rectal suppositories if oral administration is not possible.
3. Start iodides 1–2 hr **after** PTU administration: Saturated solution of potassium iodide (SSKI), 2–5 drops orally every 8 hr, or sodium iodide, 0.5–1.0 g intravenously every 8 hr, or Lugol's solution, 8 drops every 6 hr, or lithium carbonate, 300 mg orally every 6 hr.
4. Dexamethasone, 2 mg intravenously or intramuscularly every 6 hr for four doses.
5. Propranolol, 20–80 mg orally every 4–6 hr, or propranolol, 1–2 mg intravenously every 5 min for a total of 6 mg, then 1–10 mg intravenously every 4 hr. If the patient has a history of severe bronchospasm, use:
   a. Reserpine, 1–5 mg intramuscularly every 4–6 hr
   b. Guanethidine, 1 mg/kg orally every 12 hr
   c. Diltiazem, 60 mg orally every 6–8 hr
6. Phenobarbital, 30–60 mg every 6–8 hr as needed to control restlessness.
7. Once clinical improvement noted, may discontinue iodides and steroids.
8. Plasmapheresis or peritoneal dialysis to remove circulating thyroid hormone is an extreme measure reserved for patients who do not respond to conventional therapy.

Adapted from ACOG Practice Bulletin, No. 37. Thyroid disease in pregnancy. Obstet Gynecol. 2002;100:387–96.

Decision 3: Counseling

In the patient contemplating a thyroid radioablation, which of the following statements is true about a subsequent pregnancy?

- A. The fetus will be at risk from the radiation when she becomes pregnant
- B. The fetus will be at risk from her medications
- C. The fetus will be at risk for hyperthyroidism
- D. The fetus will be at risk for hypothyroidism

The correct answer is C: Neonates of women who have undergone radioactive thyroid ablation prior to pregnancy and who no longer require antithyroid medication may be at greater risk for neonatal Graves' disease (Answer C) due to lack of the suppressive effect of maternal antithyroid medication. [131]I can destroy fetal thyroid tissue, thus it is contraindicated during pregnancy. Most authorities recommend that breastfeeding be discontinued for 4 months after treatment and pregnancy avoided for 4 to 6 months after radioablative therapy; however the half-life of ^{131}I is only 8 days, so no measurable maternal radioactivity will remain long before 4 months have passed. Thus, there is no risk of fetal damage from radiation if a woman becomes pregnant several months after undergoing a thyroid radioablation (Answer A). After thyroid ablation, some patients remain euthyroid without the need for thyroid replacement, whereas others become overtly hypothyroid and require medication. This medication is thyroxine (T_4), which is not teratogenic to the fetus (Answer B). Similarly, there is no risk of fetal hypothyroidism due to the maternal treatment (Answer D).

 CASE CONCLUSION

Ms. Grady elects to undergo radioablation of her thyroid. She returns 1 year later pregnant and taking 100 μg of T_4 daily. You follow her through the pregnancy with TSH levels every trimester and gradually increase her T_4 dose to 150 μg daily at term. She delivers at 38 weeks a 3,260-g male infant with an Apgar scores of 8 and 9 at one and five minutes respectively. The baby has no evidence of neonatal Graves' disease; mother and baby do well and are discharged home on the second hospital day.

SUGGESTED READINGS

ACOG Practice Bulletin, No. 37. Thyroid Disease in Pregnancy. Obstet Gynecol. 2002;100:387–96.

Alexander EK, Marquese E, Lawrence J, et al. Timing and magnitude of increases in levothyroxine requirements during pregnancy in women with hypothyroidism. N Engl J Med. 2004;351:241–9.

Ashoor G, Kametas NA, Akolekar R, Guisado J, Nicolaides KH. Maternal thyroid function at 11–13 weeks of gestation. Fetal Diagn Ther. 2010;27(3):156–63.

Burrow GN, Fisher DA, Larsen PR. Maternal and fetal thyroid function. N Engl J Med. 1994;331(16):1072–8.

Casey BM, Dashe JS, Wells CE, et al. Subclinical hyperthyroidism and pregnancy outcomes. Obstet Gynecol. 2006;107:337–41.

Casey BM, Leveno KJ. Thyroid disease in pregnancy. Obstet Gynecol. 2006;108:1283–92.

Chattaway JM, Klepser TB. Propylthiouracil versus methimazole in treatment of Graves' disease during pregnancy. Ann Pharmacother. 2007;41(6):1018–22. Epub 2007 May 15.

Gharib H, Tuttle RM, Baskin J, et al. Consensus statement #1: subclinical thyroid dysfunction: a joint statement on management from the American Association of Clinical Endocrinologists, the American Thyroid Association, and the Endocrine Society. Thyroid. 2005;15:24–8.

Goldman J, Malone FD, Lambert-Messerlian G, et al. Maternal thyroid hypofunction and pregnancy outcome. Obstet Gynecol. 2008; 112(1):85–92.

Gyamfi C, Wapner RJ, D'Alton ME. Thyroid dysfunction in pregnancy: the basic science and clinical evidence surrounding the controversy in management. Obstet Gynecol. 2009;113(3):702–7.

Haddow JE, Palomaki GE, Allan WC, et al. Maternal thyroid deficiency during pregnancy and subsequent neuropsychological development of the child. N Engl J Med. 1999;341:549–55.

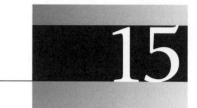

HIV in Pregnancy

Lauren Ferrara   Men-Jean Lee   Helene B. Bernstein

 ## CASE PRESENTATION

Your new patient is Ms. Anderson, a 24-year-old G3 P0020, presenting to you for her first prenatal visit. She is at 10 weeks of gestation by her last menstrual period, confirmed by ultrasound. While you are obtaining her history, she reports to you that her partner is HIV positive and she has tested negative in the past.

 ## Decision 1: Management

In a high-risk patient, what HIV testing strategy do you use?

- A. HIV enzyme-linked immunosorbent assay (ELISA) now and at term
- B. HIV ELISA and viral load now and every trimester
- C. HIV ELISA now and rapid test in labor
- D. HIV ELISA now and every trimester, rapid test in labor

The correct answer is A: HIV ELISA now and at term. In general, the Centers for Disease Control and Prevention (CDC) recommends testing all pregnant women for HIV infection as early as possible in pregnancy. The patient should be made aware that HIV screening is recommended for all women as part of routine prenatal testing; however, she may choose to opt out of the testing. Given her increased risk of seroconversion screening is highly encouraged. The CDC recommends that women like Ms Anderson who have an increased risk of HIV seroconversion should have an HIV ELISA test repeated at 36 weeks of gestation. In addition to women with an infected partner, these high-risk women include those with the factors in Table 15.1. Women who have incomplete testing (undocumented results or only one HIV test) may be screened with a rapid HIV test in labor (Answer C). If the woman is of particularly high risk or the provider suspects that she may be in the "window" period prior to seroconversion, then a plasma RNA test should be performed (Answer B). Answer D may be considered if HIV ELISA testing is inexpensive and easily accessible at your institution. If a new conversion is detected in midpregnancy, for example, at 24 weeks,

HAART (Highly Active Antiretroviral Therapy) can be initiated and cesarean delivery may be avoided if the viral load is suppressed by the end of pregnancy.

Timely identification of maternal HIV seropositivity enables early antiretroviral treatment to prevent mother-to-child transmission, allows providers to avoid obstetric practices that may increase HIV transmission, and provides an opportunity to counsel the mother against breast-feeding (also known to increase the risk for transmission). There is evidence that the adoption of "opt-out" strategies to screen pregnant women (who are informed that an HIV test will be conducted as a standard part of prenatal care unless they decline it) has resulted in higher testing rates. However, ethical and legal concerns of not obtaining specific informed consent for an HIV test using the "opt-out" strategy have been raised. While dramatic reductions in HIV transmission to neonates have been noted as a result of early prenatal detection and treatment, the extent to which detection of HIV infection and intervention during pregnancy may improve long-term maternal outcomes is unclear.

 ### NEED TO KNOW

HIV Testing Modalities

When HIV testing first became available in the mid-1980s, the primary goal was protection of the blood banking supply. When the ACTG-076 Trial demonstrated a reduction in perinatal transmission by AZT (zidovudine [ZDV]) prophylaxis during pregnancy in 1995, offering of testing to pregnant women was strongly encouraged. In 2001, the CDC recommended that offering screening for HIV should become part of routine prenatal care. Early detection and intervention with antiretroviral therapy is the best way to prevent perinatal HIV transmission. There are currently several methodologies that are available to diagnose HIV infection:

TABLE 15.1

GROUPS AT HIGH RISK OF HIV SEROCONVERSION IN PREGNANCY FOR WHOM A SECOND HIV TEST IS RECOMMENDED

1. Women who receive health care in jurisdictions with elevated incidence of HIV or AIDS among women aged 15–45 years. In 2004, these jurisdictions included

   a. Alabama
   b. Connecticut
   c. Delaware
   d. The District of Columbia
   e. Florida
   f. Georgia
   g. Illinois
   h. Louisiana
   i. Maryland
   j. Massachusetts
   k. Mississippi
   l. Nevada
   m. New Jersey
   n. New York
   o. North Carolina
   p. Pennsylvania
   q. Puerto Rico
   r. Rhode Island
   s. South Carolina
   t. Tennessee
   u. Texas
   v. Virginia.

2. Women who receive health care in facilities in which prenatal screening identifies at least one HIV-infected pregnant woman per 1,000 women screened.
3. Women who are known to be at high risk for acquiring HIV
   a. injection-drug users and their sex partners
   b. women who exchange sex for money or drugs
   c. women who are sex partners of HIV-infected persons
   d. women who have had a new or more than one sex partner during this pregnancy.
4. Women who have signs or symptoms consistent with acute HIV infection. When acute retroviral syndrome is a possibility, a plasma RNA test should be used in conjunction with an HIV antibody test to diagnose acute HIV infection.

Branson BM, Handsfield HH, Lampe MA, et al. CDC. revised recommendations for HIV testing of adults, adolescents, and pregnant women in health-care settings. MMWR Recomm Rep. 2006;55(RR-14):1–17.

1. Detecting antibodies to the virus;
2. Detecting the viral p24 antigen
3. Detecting viral nucleic acid testing
4. Culturing HIV

The standard and most commonly used tests for detecting HIV infection include the following:

1. Enzyme immunoassay (**EIA**)—This is a screening test that is widely used. It is highly sensitive for the detection of anti-HIV antibodies, but no screening test is 100% accurate. Accuracy depends on following proper procedures, as well as the person's stage of infection. Therefore, all HIV testing programs use more than one test to confirm the presence of HIV.
2. **ELISA**—Like the EIA, this very common screening test checks for the presence of antibodies to HIV; these assays do not check for the virus itself.
3. **Western blot test**, which is used to confirm the EIA/ELISA screening tests, detects the presence of antibodies to specific HIV proteins, reducing the risk of false-positive results. This confirmatory test does not detect the virus itself.
4. In general, if an ELISA screening test is positive and confirmatory test is negative, the patient is considered to have false-positive screening test. For low-risk patients, no further testing is indicated, unless a new risk factor or potential exposure develops. However, for patients who are at high risk for contracting HIV infection, the screening test should be repeated on a yearly basis.

The basis for serologic testing for HIV is the detection of IgG against HIV antigens in the serum of HIV-infected individuals. The test is based on the principle of antibody–antibody interaction. The patient's serum is placed onto an ELISA plate that is precoated with inactivated HIV antigens. If she is HIV infected (and has produced antibodies against HIV) then antibodies will be present and subsequently bind to the HIV antigen. Antihuman immunoglobulin coupled to an enzyme will detect the presence of bound antibody via a color- sensitive substrate that changes color when cleaved by the enzyme attached to the secondary antibody and results in a positive test.

Antibody response to a number of viral proteins can be detected in the serum including viral envelope (gp160, gp120, and gp41), and the translated proteins of the gag (p24, p17, p7 and p9) and pol (p32, p66, p51, and p11) genes. Gag is a polyprotein which comprises the nucleocapsid of the virus and is an acronym for Group Antigens and pol proteins include the enzymes reverse transcriptase, protease, and integrase. **Env** is the envelope glycoprotein for the virus. Antibodies to gp41, an envelope protein, and p24, a nucleocapsid protein, are the first serologically detectable markers. Gp120 is bigger and more commonly detected. Although most patients will have IgG antibodies within 6 to 12 weeks, 95% will have the antibodies by 6 months. HIV serological screening tests detect antibodies that react with the transmembrane envelope glycoproteins. These screening assays are very sensitive, but are prone to false-positivity. If two serological screening tests are positive for HIV antibodies, a confirmatory test is needed to definitively diagnose HIV infection.

Western blot is the most widely used confirmatory test for HIV infection. This test is highly specific for detecting anti-HIV antibodies recognizing specific HIV proteins. In Western blot analysis, electrophoresis is performed on a panel of HIV proteins to separate the proteins followed by protein transfer onto a solid membrane. The patient's serum is incubated with the membrane containing the separated HIV proteins. If the patient has antibodies against any of the proteins in this HIV protein panel, enzyme-labeled antibodies recognizing human IgG will permit delineation of how many and which HIV-specific proteins are recognized by the patient's serum. Worldwide, different organizations use slightly different criteria for the interpretation of Western blots. The CDC requires detection of antibodies to at least two of the following antigens: p24, gp41, and gp120 to diagnose HIV infection. The American Red Cross criteria requires the detection of anti-HIV antibodies against at least one HIV protein derived from each env, gag, and pol gene to confirm the diagnosis of HIV infection.

Rapid HIV antibody testing is also highly accurate and can be performed in 10 to 30 minutes. When offered at the point of care, the rapid HIV test is useful for screening high-risk patients who do not receive regular medical care (e.g., those seen in emergency departments), as well as women with unknown HIV status who present in active labor.

Confirmation of positive or indeterminate serological screen for HIV infection can also be done by indirect immunofluorescence assay (IFA). IFA is less commonly used in the United States but is a valid confirmatory test. IFA is performed by incubating the patient's serum on a slide containing human T-cells that express HIV antigens on their surface. HIV-specific antibodies present within serum bind HIV antigens expressed by the human T-cells and are detected by a fluorescein-labeled secondary antibody to human immunoglobulin. The presence of fluoresceinated cells on the microscope slide in this test is indicative of HIV infection.

A two-step protocol to diagnose HIV infection, the repeatedly reactive EIA (or ELISA) followed by confirmatory Western blot or immunofluorescent assay, is highly accurate at detecting HIV infection. According to a survey done by the CDC, the Western blot has been shown to be 99.3% sensitive and 99.7% specific. Serologic screening by ELISA and Western blot confirmation represents a highly sensitive, inexpensive, and rapid method to diagnose HIV infection. However, some patients who are suspected of having an acute infection may have not yet seroconverted, so the antibody testing will be negative. In these patients, HIV nucleic acid quantification (viral DNA or RNA), p24 antigen detection, or isolation via culture should be used for diagnosis.

The p24 antigen is one of the gag-encoded viral core proteins that can be detected in the serum during the "window period" of primary HIV infection. Levels of p24 antigen can be measured by anti–p24-specific monoclonal antibodies coated to a solid support and detected with another p24-specific detection antibody. This test is 50% to 75% sensitive, and is >95% specific for the detection of HIV infection. HIV can be isolated by culturing peripheral mononuclear cells. The presence of the virus is detected by the demonstration of the presence of p24 antigen, reverse transcriptase, or HIV RNA. Isolation of HIV is a time-consuming and expensive process, and therefore used primarily for only research purposes. These tests are not the primary means to diag-

nose HIV infection and should be reserved for special situations.

An RNA viral load test measures the quantity of viral RNA in the blood. This test is often used to measure the effectiveness of drugs used to treat HIV-infected patients. HIV-1 RNA quantification from plasma to determine viral load is considered the best method for monitoring disease progression and response to antiretroviral therapy. There are three molecular amplification methods to determine HIV-1 viral load. One is based on the use of polymerized chain reaction (PCR) to detect the nucleic acid sequence of HIV-1, one uses nucleic acid sequence–based amplification, and the other is based on branched-chain DNA hybridization signal amplification (bDNA assay). These nucleic acid–based protocols are capable of detecting HIV-1 RNA down to 20 to 50 copies/mL. PCR-based assays are so sensitive that they may yield false-positive results, thus these tests should not be used for diagnosis.

As of February 2008, six rapid tests have received FDA approval. These tests are rapid primarily serological screening tests based on ELISA technology that have become standard in many parts of the world because of quick availability of results, high diagnostic accuracy, and low cost. Generally, the results are available within 5 to 40 minutes. The sensitivity of these results is >99%. Positive and negative predictive values vary with the prevalence of HIV infection in a specific population. As a result of this, the CDC recommends that a positive screening result should be considered preliminary and should be followed by standard serology testing including the Western blot. No further testing is needed if the rapid test is negative, unless the test was performed because of a recent exposure. Then the patient may be in the "window period" of an acute infection and should have follow-up testing. In the labor and delivery setting, if the rapid test is positive the patient should be offered antiretroviral therapy while her confirmatory tests are being undertaken to protect the fetus from intrapartum perinatal HIV transmission. Risk of drug exposure is minimal to the mother and fetus.

Consumer-controlled test kits (popularly known as "home test kits") were first licensed in 1997. The Home Access Express HIV-1 Test System manufactured by Home Access Health Corporation is approved by the U.S. Food and Drug Administration (FDA) and can be purchased at most local drug stores. This testing procedure involves a finger prick and placing drops of blood on a specially treated card that is mailed in to be tested at a licensed laboratory. Customers then call the laboratory to obtain the test results. The accuracy of home test kits other than the Home Access kit cannot be verified.

Oral tests for HIV infection can also be performed in a doctor's office or clinic. To use an oral HIV test, the inside of the mouth is gently scraped and the saliva is tested for the presence of HIV antibodies. The result is as accurate as the blood tests because the saliva is tested using an EIA test and then a Western blot test if necessary. Urine-based tests are also available for HIV screening in a doctor's office or clinic. However, it is somewhat less accurate than the blood- or saliva-based tests. Like other tests, positive results must be confirmed with the Western blot test.

 CASE CONTINUES

The patient's ELISA and Western blot come back as positive for HIV infection. Routine baseline labs are sent. Her viral load is 100,000 copies, and her CD4 count is 400.

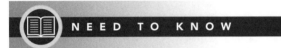 **N E E D   T O   K N O W**

Additional Workup of HIV-Infected Women

In addition to her routine prenatal labs (complete blood cell [CBC] count, type and screen, rubella antibody screen, hepatitis B antigen screen, purified protein derivative (PPD), GC culture, chlamydia DNA screen, and Papanicolaou test), an HIV-infected woman should have additional laboratory work performed to optimize her health for the pregnancy and beyond. A baseline viral load, genotype, phenotype, resistance panel, and CD4 count should be sent. The patient should have additional serology evaluation including hepatitis C virus antibody and antibodies to both cytomegalovirus and *Toxoplasma gondii*. A baseline CBC count, SMA-7 (chemistry panel), liver function tests (LFTs), and cholesterol/lipid panel should be sent because of potential toxic effects of some antiretroviral medications.

Although not considered part of a workup in an HIV-infected patient, it is important to recommend both influenza and pneumococcal vaccines at the appropriate seasons and times. The pneumococcal vaccine is recommended for all HIV-infected patients with revaccination being considered every 5 years. It is should be noted that if the patient's CD4 count is <200, the vaccine may not be as effective and the patient should be revaccinated if the CD4 count improves after HAART. The influenza vaccine should be given annually in the fall and winter months. It is most effective among persons with CD4 count >100 and viral load <30,000 copies. Hepatitis B vaccination is not contraindicated in pregnancy. PPD testing for tuberculosis screening is also recommended for pregnant women who are HIV positive. Chest x-ray

with shielding after the first trimester of pregnancy is recommended for those women with positive PPD testing. Isoniazid prophylaxis is well tolerated during pregnancy in women who are PPD positive (latent tuberculosis). For those HIV-positive women with a high index of suspicion for active tuberculosis during pregnancy, chest x-ray, induced sputum for culture, and optimal, multidrug antituberculosis treatment, regardless of the trimester, must be initiated immediately. Isoniazid, rifampin, and ethambutol are the first-line multidrug antituberculosis regimen during pregnancy. Pyrazinamide is usually a part of the four-drug regimen in nonpregnant patients, but during pregnancy, pyrazinamide is not included in the initial therapy because of the lack of pregnancy safety data.

Pneumocystis jiroveci pneumonia (PCP) remains one of the most common life-threatening opportunistic infections in patients with advanced HIV disease. This fungus can affect many organ systems but pneumonia is the most common. A patient with CD4 count <200, a previous history of PCP, or a history of oral thrush should be started on prophylaxis. PCP prophylaxis may also be considered in patients already affected by other opportunistic infections or with persistent fever. If a patient's CD4 count is declining, it should be watched very closely. The typical regimen is Bactrim DS, one tab every day, although three times a week is also effective and may improve compliance. The single-strength dose may be used but may not be as effective. If the patient is allergic to or cannot tolerate sulfa drugs, then alternative regimens may be used. In patients with a mild allergic reaction, desensitization may be considered.

If a patient's Papanicolaou test is abnormal, human papillomavirus (HPV) testing is automatically done. If her HPV-PCR is positive for high-risk serotypes, a screening colposcopy is typically done. Very suspicious areas may be biopsied; however, in the absence of malignant appearing lesions, biopsy is typically deferred until the postpartum period. Recent evidence suggests that Papanicolaou test abnormalities are common but high-grade lesions are not.

There are no recommendations regarding antepartum testing in HIV patients. Antenatal fetal surveillance is reserved for routine obstetrical indications.

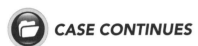 **Decision 2:** Patient counseling

What is the risk of perinatal (infant) HIV infection with and without treatment?

   A. 0% with/10% without

   B. 2% with/30% without

   C. 10% with/20% without

   D. 20% with/60% without

The correct answer is B. The risk of transmission with antiretroviral therapy is <2% and 15% to 40% without treatment.

In 1994, the PACTG 076, a randomized, double-blinded, placebo controlled trial conducted in the United States and France, found that administration of antiretroviral therapy in the form of ZDV could reduce the risk of perinatal transmission by up to 70%. This trial enrolled HIV-infected women between 14 and 34 weeks of gestation, who were not on antiretroviral medication and had CD4 counts >200. The goal was preventing HIV transmission. The study included three treatment components: antepartum, intrapartum, and neonatal. Antepartum treatment consisted of 100 mg of ZDV five times/day starting at enrollment. Since prior studies had shown that ZDV crosses the placenta, one goal of this treatment was to decrease *in utero* transmission. Intrapartum therapy consisted of intravenous ZDV, with a loading dose of 2 mg/kg over the first hour followed by 1 mg/kg/hr until delivery. This component was intended to provide prophylaxis against potential exposure during delivery through the birth canal. Postpartum the neonate also received prophylactic ZDV treatment, 2 mg/kg four times a day, for the first 6 weeks of life. Using this protocol, the perinatal transmission of HIV infection was reduced from 22.5% down to 7.6%.

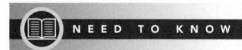

HAART Treatment and Risks to the Fetus

The overall goals of HAART during pregnancy are the same as in the nonpregnant state: to suppress the viral load to as low as possible for as long as possible, to preserve/restore immune function, and to prolong life. During pregnancy, there is the additional goal of reducing the risk of perinatal HIV transmission. The initiation of therapy should be discussed with the patient and special consideration should be made when choosing a treatment regimen. Factors impacting therapy include safety and potential toxicity to both the mother and fetus, and potential changes in dose requirements due to the normal physiologic changes in pregnancy. There is limited data available on the safety of antiretrovirals; however, there have been no reported long-term effects of antiretroviral exposure on HIV-exposed neonates and children. In terms of teratogenesis, there is minimal fetal risk with most medications. The exception to this is Sustiva (efavirenz). Exposure to efavirenz, particularly in the first trimester, has been associated with neural tube defects.

Agenerase (amprenavir) is contraindicated because it may not be properly metabolized during pregnancy.

There is maternal risk of hepatotoxicity from nevirapine started in women with CD4 counts >250 cells/μL. It should be started in these women only if the benefits outweigh the risk. Abacavir is also associated with a maternal hypersensitivity reaction and lopinavir/ritonavir (Kaletra) levels can be subtherapeutic late in pregnancy. Antiretroviral management during pregnancy should be performed by a provider knowledgeable about the risks, benefits, and limitations of the available drugs. It is important to remember that the goal of treatment during pregnancy is not only maintenance of maternal wellbeing but also prevention of perinatal transmission. The HIV viral load is strongly predictive of risk for transmission, therefore, the goal is to suppress viral load to very low levels and if possible to undetectable.

For prevention of perinatal HIV transmission, combination drug therapy has become the standard of care in the United States. If HIV RNA is detectable, resistance testing should be sent to tailor therapy appropriately. If the patient presents in advanced gestation, therapy should be initiated while awaiting the results of this testing. The therapy that is initiated will depend on whether or not she is already on therapy, what medications the patient has been exposed to in the past, and resistance testing.

Typically HAART regimens should include three drugs from at least two different classes of antiretroviral medications. The most common antiretroviral drug classes are nucleoside reverse transcriptase inhibitors (NRTIs), nonnucleoside reverse transcriptase inhibitors (NNRTIs), and protease inhibitors (PIs). Other classes of drugs such as entry inhibitors, CCR5 antagonists, or integrase inhibitors are not used as first-line therapy. When talking about antiretroviral therapy many authors classify the drugs as either a "base" or a "backbone." The most widely utilized regimen is composed of a Combivir (ZDV 300 mg/lamivudine 150 mg) backbone in conjunction with a PI. There is extensive experience as well as efficacy studies with these drugs. Some form of ZDV should be used unless there is evidence of toxicity or resistance. Kaletra (lopinavir/ritonavir) is the PI that is recommended for use in pregnancy (In the past, nelfinavir was the pregnancy-recommended PI). When using Kaletra in pregnancy, the provider should remember to check the drug level or increase the dosage in the third trimester because of the increased volume of distribution in pregnancy.

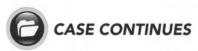

CASE CONTINUES

This patient is started on Combivir and Kaletra as a part of her first-line HAART regimen and is compliant with her treatment. She undergoes QUAD serum marker screening at 16 weeks of gestation, which reveals a 1/200 risk for Down's syndrome. This is followed by a level II ultrasound, which is normal, and a genetic counseling consultation to discuss the risks and benefits of amniocentesis, an invasive procedure to obtain fetal amniocytes for karyotyping. After consideration of the potential increased risk for vertical HIV transmission with amniocentesis, the slightly increased risk for Down's syndrome based on serum screening, and the risk of pregnancy loss following invasive testing, the patient declines amniocentesis. Recent studies have shown that there is not a statistically significant increased risk of HIV transmission following invasive prenatal karyotype determination. Her glucose challenge test and repeat VDRL are both negative at 28 weeks of gestation. At 37 weeks the patient's viral load remains detectable at 5,000 copies.

Decision 3: Delivery

How should the patient be delivered?

A. Cesarean section at 38 weeks on current meds
B. Cesarean delivery at 38 weeks after 3 hours of IV AZT
C. Vaginal delivery on current meds
D. Vaginal delivery on IV AZT

The correct answer is B: Cesarean delivery at 38 weeks after 3 hours of IV AZT. The American College of Obstetrics and Gynecology recommends consideration of elective cesarean delivery at 38 weeks of gestation for HIV-infected women with a viral load of >1,000 copies/mL near the time of delivery. Elective cesarean delivery is not mandatory but should be carefully considered after a detailed discussion with the patient regarding her disease state, viral load, compliance with HAART, and risks of postoperative complications. A planned cesarean should be scheduled at 38 weeks, as there is minimal benefit of elective cesarean delivery following spontaneous rupture of membranes or when labor has ensued. Intravenous ZDV should be started at least 3 hours prior to elective cesarean delivery. When a vaginal delivery is planned, women should be advised to proceed to the hospital at the first signs of labor. IV ZDV should be administered upon presentation. A loading dose of 2 mg/kg is given over the first hour followed by a maintenance dose of 1 mg/kg/hr. If membranes rupture early, oxytocin (Pitocin) augmentation should be considered to decrease the interval to delivery. Fetal scalp electrode placement, episiotomy, and any other procedures, which could result in additional exposure to maternal blood should be avoided when possible, secondary to a likely increased risk of perinatal HIV transmission.

In the case of preterm, premature rupture of membranes, one must weigh the risk of prematurity against the potential risk for vertical transmission of HIV infection. This patient's case was significant for suboptimal viral load suppression. Viral loads are usually monitored 2 to 6 weeks

after initiation or change in therapy. 1 $\log_{10}$ copies/mL decrease within 1 month following initiation of drug therapy denotes an adequate response. Viral load and CD4 counts should be checked every trimester in aviremic patients on a stable therapeutic regimen. Patients on a new therapeutic regimen, women with compliance issues and viremic patients require closer monitoring. The patient should also be monitored for potential complications of therapy; that is, hepatic and hematologic dysfunction.

If there is not continuing appropriate decreases in viral load and/or the viral load does not become completely suppressed, the patient should be evaluated for viral resistance, adherence to the regimen, medication dosing, as well as tolerance. In this patient, B is the most appropriate answer.

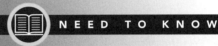

Delivery with HIV Infection—Options in Untreated and Treated Patients

There are several scenarios involving HIV-infected pregnant women in which cesarean delivery for obstetric indications is the best choice. In treated women, there is no evidence that elective cesarean delivery benefits women with undetectable viral loads. Furthermore, HIV-infected women have higher morbidity following cesarean delivery.

If there is a detectable viral load at term and the patient is not in labor and has intact membranes, an elective cesarean delivery at 38 weeks may limit HIV transmission. However, multiple studies have shown that there is little benefit to cesarean delivery following the initiation of labor or spontaneous rupture of membranes, thus delivery for obstetrical indications is most appropriate in this patient group.

In women who decline treatment of their HIV infection during pregnancy, one should consider an elective cesarean delivery at 38 weeks to limit perinatal HIV transmission. Studies demonstrate that within this population, elective cesarean delivery limits perinatal HIV transmission compared to untreated and AZT monotherapy-treated women. As HIV-infected women have a higher risk of preterm delivery and preterm premature rupture of membranes, we recommend antiretroviral therapy in all patients.

CASE CONCLUSION

The patient is admitted to labor and delivery at 38 weeks. Intravenous AZT is started and running 3 hours prior to delivery. She undergoes an uncomplicated primary elective cesarean section. She has a healthy female infant weighing 3,000 g, with Apgar scores of 9 and 9 and one and five minutes. The patient and her baby go home on postpartum day 4. The initial HIV DNA PCR and the 1- and 6-month HIV-PCR test results are negative on the infant.

All HIV-exposed neonates should receive therapy for the first 6 weeks of life. The standard therapy is ZDV 2 mg/kg orally or 1.5 mg/kg intravenously. HIV infection in the neonate is diagnosed via HIV DNA PCR or RNA assays. Maternal IgG antibodies cross the placenta and will be detectable in these infants for up to 18 months of life, so serologic assays should not be used for diagnosis. HIV PCR should be done at first week of life, 1 month, and 6 months of age. If a positive result is encountered, the test should be repeated. Two positives confirm infection. There is no evidence to suggest that the standard ZDV therapy in the neonatal period delays the diagnosis.

SUGGESTED READINGS

Allain JP, Laurian Y, Paul DA, Senn D. Serological markers in early stages of human immunodeficiency virus infection in haemophiliacs. Lancet. 1986;2(8518):1233–6.

Benson CA, Kaplan JE, Masur H, et al. Treating opportunistic infections among HIV-infected adults and adolescents: recommendations from CDC, the National Institutes of Health, and the Infectious Diseases Society of America. MMWR Recomm Rep. 2004;53(RR-15):1–112.

Bernstein HB. In: Gabbe SG, Niebyl JR, Simpson JL, editors. Maternal and Perinatal Infection—Viral In: Gabbe SG, Niebyl JR, Simpson JL, editors Obstetrics: Normal and Problem Pregnancies. 5th ed. Philadelphia, PA: Elsevier; 2007, pp. 1203–1232.

Branson BM, Handsfield HH, Lampe MA, et al. Revised recommendations for HIV testing of adults, adolescents, and pregnant women in health-care settings. MMWR Recomm Rep. 2006;55(RR-14):1–17.

CDC issues updated TB prevention guidelines. Healthcare Benchmarks Qual Improv. 2006;13(3):34–5.

Centers for Disease Control and Prevention. Guidelines for laboratory test result reporting of human immunodeficiency virus type 1 ribonucleic acid determination. Recommendations from a CDC working group. MMWR Recomm Rep. 2001;50(RR-20): 1–12.

Centers for Disease Control and Prevention. HIV infection reporting—United States. MMWR Morb Mortal Wkly Rep. 1989;38(28): 496–9.

Connor EM, Sperling RS, Gelber R, et al. Reduction of maternal-infant transmission of human immunodeficiency virus type 1 with zidovudine treatment. Pediatric AIDS Clinical Trials Group Protocol 076 Study Group. N Engl J Med. 1994;331(18):1173–80.

Ekoukou D, Khuong-Josses MA, Ghibaudo N, Mechali D, Rotten D. Amniocentesis in pregnant HIV-infected patients. Absence of mother-to-child viral transmission in a series of selected patients. Eur J Obstet Gynecol Reprod Biol. 2008;140(2):212–7.

Horsburgh CR Jr, Ou CY, Jason J, et al. Duration of human immunodeficiency virus infection before detection of antibody. Lancet. 1989;2(8664):637–40.

Luciw PA. Human immunodeficiency viruses and their replication. In: Fields B, Knipe P, Howley P, et al., editors. Fields Virology. 3rd ed. Philadelphia, PA: Lippincott-Raven; 1996. pp. 1881–952.

Mandelbrot L, Jasseron C, Ekoukou D, et al. Amniocentesis and mother-to-child human immunodeficiency virus transmission in the Agence Nationale de Recherches sur le SIDA et les Hepatites Virales French Perinatal Cohort. Am J Obstet Gynecol. 2009; 200(2):160.e1–9.

Massad LS, Seaberg EC, Wright RL, et al. Squamous cervical lesions in women with human immunodeficiency virus: long-term follow-up. Obstet Gynecol. 2008;111(6):1388–93.

Shapiro DE, Sperling RS, Coombs RW. Effect of zidovudine on perinatal HIV-1 transmission and maternal viral load. Pediatric AIDS Clinical Trials Group 076 Study Group. Lancet. 1999;354(9173): 156.

Somigliana E, Bucceri AM, Tibaldi C, et al. Early invasive diagnostic techniques in pregnant women who are infected with the HIV: a multicenter case series. Am J Obstet Gynecol. 2005;193(2): 437–42.

US Preventive Services Task Force. Screening for HIV: recommendation statement. Ann Intern Med. 2005;143(1):32–7.

Acute Abdominal Pain in Pregnancy

16

Ramy Eskander

 CASE PRESENTATION

Ms. Ruiz, a 16-year-old G1 P0 at 34 weeks 3 days of gestation presents to labor and delivery with a 2-day history of abdominal pain, fever, chills, nausea, vomiting, and decreased appetite. She states that the pain started around her umbilicus but has moved to her lower right side since this morning. She describes the automobile ride to the hospital as "horrible" with severe abdominal pains every time the car went over a bump. She currently denies vaginal bleeding, loss of fluid, or dysuria. There are no sick relatives at home.

Initial vitals signs reveal a temperature of 102.7°F, heart rate of 107 bpm, respiratory rate of 23/min, blood pressure of 127/78 mm Hg, and 100% O₂ saturation on room air. She rates her pain as 7/10. A bedside ultrasound confirms the patient's dating with a fetal heart rate of 175 bpm and a vertex presentation. Estimated fetal weight is 2,365 g with an amniotic fluid index of 17 cm. A vaginal examination demonstrates a cervix that is <1 cm dilated, 20% effaced, and −3 station. You place the patient on continuous external fetal heart rate monitoring with tocodynamometry that shows the tracing seen in Figure 16.1.

 N E E D T O K N O W

Differential Diagnosis of Acute Abdominal Pain in Pregnancy

Abdominal pain in pregnancy can pose a diagnostic dilemma to even the seasoned obstetrician, as the differential diagnosis is vast and covers multiple organ systems with diverse treatments. Delay in diagnosis and treatment may result in increasing morbidities to both the mother and the fetus, though unnecessary surgical intervention also has significant pregnancy risks.

Gallbladder disease in the form of biliary sludge and stone formation complicates up to 31% and 2% of

pregnancies, respectively. Most cases are entirely asymptomatic, with only 28% of women reporting pain symptoms. The rate of acute cholecystitis remains unchanged during pregnancy. Presenting symptoms, which include right upper quadrant pain, anorexia, nausea, vomiting, and fever are quite nonspecific. Appendicitis, hepatitis, pancreatitis, abscess, and right-sided pneumonia are the most common conditions that overlap symptomatically with gall bladder disease during pregnancy.

Pancreatitis, which occurs in roughly 1/3,000 pregnancies is commonly due to cholelithiasis with passage of obstructing stones into the common bile duct that either block or compress the pancreatic duct. Most cases occur in the third trimester and are usually mild. Conservative medical treatment is usually successful and should be the initial approach. Bowel rest, hydration, nasogastric suction, and electrolyte repletion are often sufficient for symptom resolution.

Acute appendicitis, a common medical and surgical problem encountered in the young population, complicates approximately 1/1,500 pregnancies. Symptoms of anorexia, nausea, vomiting, and abdominal pain are similar to the symptoms of appendicitis in a nongravid female. The *location* of the appendiceal pain may be altered by the physical relocation of the appendix with increasing uterine size. Figure 16.2 demonstrates the most common locations for appendiceal pain by gestational age. In pregnancy, fever and leukocytosis are not helpful, being similar for women found to have appendicitis compared with women with a negative appendix at laparotomy. A high index of suspicion is crucial since a delay in diagnosis can lead to rupture of an inflamed appendix. Rupture dramatically increases the rate of fetal loss from 3% to 5% to 20% to 25%.

Rarer causes of acute, severe third trimester abdominal pain may include small bowel obstruction (1/3,000), acute hepatitis, intra-abdominal abscesses, degenerating leiomyomata, ovarian neoplasms, and torsion, but the scarcity of such cases should steer the clinician to rule out the more common causes before entertaining these "zebras."

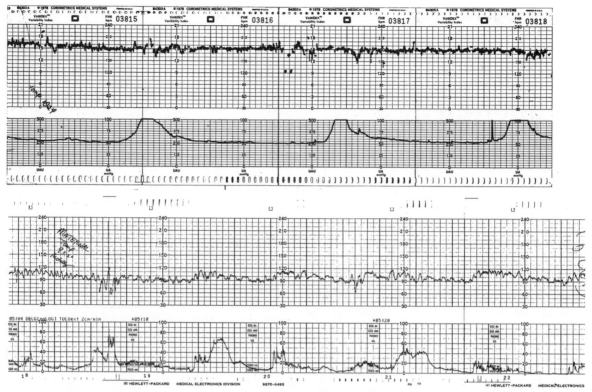

Figure 16.1 Fetal heart rate tracing on admission. The baseline heart rate is 180 bpm, with decreased variability and one suspicious deceleration (arrow). Used with permission from Cabaniss and Ross. Fetal Monitoring Interpretation, second edition. Wolters Kluwer, Philadelphia, 2010 p. 292.

? Decision 1: Management

What should be done immediately?

A. Delivery
B. Antibiotics and labor induction
C. Hydration and fetal monitoring
D. Hydration and abdominal imaging

The correct answer is D: Hydration and abdominal imaging. At this point in time, there is no indication for delivery of this preterm fetus, whether by cesarean delivery or by induction of labor. Given the severity of maternal

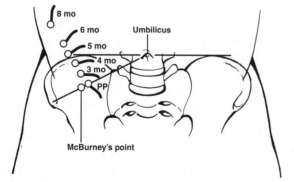

Figure 16.2 Location of appendiceal pain with increasing gestational age. The appendix rises from McBurney's point to well above the umbilicus in a term pregnancy.

fever and fetal tachycardia, this patient does require vigorous hydration with IV fluids. Furthermore, her presenting symptoms, history, and physical examination raise suspicion for a possible intra-abdominal infection, and thus, further testing in the form of abdominal imaging is indicated.

Medical imaging and pregnancy have often been problematic, with many clinicians hesitant to order proper studies for fear of fetal radiation exposure. A pregnant woman should not be penalized for being pregnant. Unrealistically high fears of fetal harm continue to be reported by many obstetricians despite numerous articles, bulletins, and publications documenting no evidence of fetal harm with judicious use of ionizing radiation studies (e.g., computed tomography [CT] scan). In fact, exposure to <5 rad has not been associated with an increase in any fetal anomaly or pregnancy loss (Table 16.1).

Initial screening with an abdominal ultrasound to evaluate the gallbladder, appendix, and adnexa is acceptable, but is often limited by the obscuring, gravid uterus. Although several studies show equal efficacy between helical CT and compression ultrasonography in the diagnosis of diseases like acute appendicitis, the most commonly studied and most available imaging modality is CT.

Expedient hydration and imaging will aide in the accurate diagnosis and treatment of this patient. Depending on the radiologic findings, the patient may be started on the appropriate antibiotics, counseled on her pregnancy risks, and prepared for exploratory surgery if necessary.

TABLE 16.1

FETAL EXPOSURE FROM COMMON RADIOLOGIC PROCEDURES

Procedure	Fetal Exposure
Chest X-ray (2 views)	0.02–0.07 mrad
Abdominal film (single view)	100 mrad
Intravenous pyelography	≥1 rad
Hip film (single view)	200 mrad
Barium enema or small bowel series	2–4 rad
CT scan of head or chest	<1 rad
CT scan of abdomen and lumbar spine	3.5 rad
CT pelvimetry	250 mrad

Modified from: ACOG Committee on Obstetric Practice. ACOG Committee Opinion. Number 299, September 2004. Guidelines for diagnostic imaging during pregnancy. Obstet Gynecol. 2004 Sep;104(3):647–51.

As previously described, the diagnosis of appendicitis in a pregnant woman requires a high level of suspicion. As with this patient, most will present with vague abdominal pain originating in the mid abdomen, but later localizing to the right side as the inflamed appendix continues to irritate the parietal peritoneum. Nausea, vomiting, and anorexia, although quite common in appendicitis, are also common in pregnancy. They cannot be used independent of other findings to include or exclude the diagnosis of appendicitis. The mild to moderate leukocytosis common in pregnancy is not helpful in diagnosis, but there is often a bandemia indicating an acute infectious process that is significant.

 CASE CONTINUES

A complete blood cell (CBC) count, chemistry panel, liver function tests, amylase, and lipase are drawn. You begin aggressive hydration providing a liter of normal saline over 30 minutes, then run a maintenance rate of 150 mL/hr. You start Ms. Ruiz on cooling measures and administer acetaminophen for her fever.

Your suspicion for appendicitis is high, and after counseling, Ms. Ruiz consents to a CT scan of the abdomen and pelvis with PO and IV contrast. You receive a call from the on-call radiologist who tells you that the appendix does not fill with contrast, appears thickened, and has surrounding fat stranding; all of these signs are consistent with a diagnosis of nonperforated, acute appendicitis.

The results of Ms. Ruiz' labs are now available. She has a white blood cell count of 17.9 with 88% neutrophils, 6% lymphocytes, and 6% bands. Her other test results are unremarkable.

The surgeon is consulted and she agrees with the diagnosis of appendicitis. She recommends immediate appendectomy via an open incision, as the 34-week gravid uterus makes laparoscopic surgery difficult.

After explaining the above risks and benefits of surgery, the patient consents and agrees to proceed. **Informed consent is obtained by the treating obstetrician in conjunction with the general surgeon.**

 Decision 2: Management

What is the most appropriate management of this pregnancy during surgery?

A. Tocolysis with magnesium sulfate during surgery
B. Continuous fetal monitoring during the procedure
C. Pregnancy termination at the time of surgery
D. Indomethacin tocolysis after the procedure

The correct answer is B: Continuous fetal monitoring during the procedure. In regards to fetal monitoring during the procedure, there is no evidence to support or refute its use. No comparative studies exist suggesting that this improves fetal outcome. According to the American College of Obstetricians and Gynecologists, "··· this decision should be individualized, and, if used may be based on gestational age, type of surgery, and facilities available." In the example of this patient, given a viable fetus and facilities capable of supporting immediate delivery, intraoperative fetal monitoring will most often be considered as a part of routine operative care.

The decision to prophylactically tocolyze the patient can be a difficult one to make. Although many perceive the risks of tocolysis to be low, they are real. Tocolytics used in conjunction with sedatives and paralytics intraoperatively, as in answer A, can pose unnecessary risks to both mother and fetus. Although the current body of literature is equivocal, many papers fail to show any benefit of prophylactic tocolysis. Postoperative tocolysis is often used to "prevent" contractions and possible preterm labor without evidence to support its use. Tocolysis is indicated for cases with documented uterine contractions, but no data support prophylactic tocolytics. Despite this lack of evidence, most centers will treat with a tocolytic to reduce the risk of premature delivery. Answer D is, however, incorrect as indomethacin tocolysis would be relatively contraindicated in a pregnancy of this gestational age due to the risk of oligohydramnios and ductal closure.

The ultimate decision to terminate the pregnancy and deliver the fetus prematurely, or answer C, must be heavily weighed. The fetal tachycardia and uterine activity can be attributed to maternal fever and infection. It is reasonable to expect that expedient surgery, hydration, and treatment with antibiotics will normalize the fetal heart rate and reduce the uterine contractions. There is little to be gained by abdominal delivery prior to therapy since the short-term anesthetic exposure at this gestational age has not been associated with any teratogenic risks. The risk of premature delivery following surgery is quite low and would only increase with time since delay would increase the risk of appendiceal rupture.

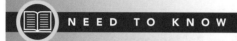

NEED TO KNOW

Anesthesia in Pregnancy

The issues to consider regarding anesthesia for the pregnant patient undergoing nonobstetric surgery are similar to those in cesarean delivery. Anesthesia in pregnancy is complicated by the need to consider the unique physiologic state of the pregnant woman, as well as the status of the fetus. One option is the use of regional anesthesia when possible, due to the reduction in maternal risk associated with this modality. When general anesthesia is needed, pregnancy is associated with changes in cardiopulmonary physiology, affecting anesthesia. The normal pregnant woman demonstrates increased oxygen consumption and decreased functional residual capacity, making her more prone to becoming hypoxemic with apnea. Anatomic changes in the pregnant woman may make intubation more difficult and the increased vascularization may lead to bleeding when intubation is attempted. Venous return from the lower body may be obstructed by the pregnant uterus when the patient is supine, leading to maternal hypotension. The pregnant woman is usually positioned with a wedge under the right hip to avoid the supine position. Gastric aspiration is a concern in pregnancy, due to relaxation of the gastroesophageal sphincter and to the anatomic distortion associated with the pregnant uterus. Pregnant women are treated as having a full stomach during induction of anesthesia due to their increased risk of aspiration. Finally, maternal anesthesia requirements may be reduced in pregnancy for both inhaled and intravenous anesthetics.

Proper informed consent for the patient requires an explanation of the risks to her and her fetus. Managing two patients (mother and fetus) requires certain compromises for each to maximize the outcome.

Nontreatment and delayed surgery exposes the mother to the risk of appendiceal rupture and ensuing sepsis, infection, preterm delivery, fetal death, and maternal death. Proceeding to surgery poses unique risks including preterm labor, preterm delivery, fear of drug exposure, limitation of certain anesthetics due to concern of fetal effects, and the risk of fetal hypoperfusion. Most of the surgical

risks are justified if the diagnosis is correct. However, there is always some chance of a negative laparotomy.

Fetal risks include preterm delivery and drug effects. The rate of preterm labor after nonobstetric surgery during pregnancy tends to increase with increasing gestational age and depends on the type and duration of the procedure performed. Furthermore, the safety of the anesthetics used should be considered, though there is little evidence that any drug used during general anesthesia is teratogenic in humans.

Finally, adequate fetal perfusion must be maintained throughout the entire procedure. Maternal hypotension, hypoxia, or obstruction of vena caval blood return may compromise the fetus. This can be avoided by strict monitoring of maternal vital signs and tilting or placing a wedge under the patient to avoid a completely supine position. Intraoperative fetal monitoring may aide in evaluating fetal perfusion.

 CASE CONTINUES

Ms. Ruiz undergoes an uncomplicated open appendectomy through a 5-cm transverse incision in the right lower quadrant over the point of maximal tenderness. Fetal heart tones are documented to be in the range of 170–175 bpm during and after the procedure. Following surgery, the patient is placed on continuous fetal monitoring and tocodynamometry. You are called by the nurse to evaluate the fetal heart rate tracing that shows variable decelerations with increasingly frequent and forceful contractions that are confirmed by palpation. A vaginal examination demonstrates a cervix that is 4 cm dilated, 70% effaced with the vertex at 0 station.

 Decision 3: Management

How should this delivery be managed?

A. Immediate cesarean due to the risk of wound dehiscence
B. Immediate cesarean due to the risk of fetal infection
C. Vaginal delivery in the intensive care unit (ICU)
D. Vaginal delivery in labor and delivery

The correct answer is D: Vaginal delivery in labor and delivery. Decision making regarding delivery of a patient in the immediate postoperative period differs little from normal considerations.

In the case of this patient who is immediately postoperative, cesarean delivery is reserved for obstetric indications. In the event of fetal distress or an arrest of labor, a cesarean may be performed. Otherwise, a vaginal route is preferred. There is no evidence that an immediate cesarean delivery offers any protection for the mother or fetus. Labor and a vaginal delivery do not increase the chances of a wound dehiscence (answer A).

A vaginal delivery in the ICU is an uncommon event and often makes the patient, the nurses, and the physicians uncomfortable. If a patient is hemodynamically unstable, or if there is a likelihood of hemodynamic instability in the peripartum period, then an ICU delivery may be indicated. There is no evidence of instability in this case so there is no need for a delivery in the ICU setting.

The best option for this patient is a vaginal delivery in labor and delivery where she and the fetus will be closely monitored. Should obstetric indications arise, cesarean delivery may be performed.

 ## CASE CONCLUSION

Ms. Ruiz progresses rapidly in labor to complete cervical dilatation. After 1 hour of pushing, she experiences fatigue and pain, and refuses further pushing efforts. With the fetal head at +3 station, a forceps delivery is performed, with delivery of a 2,340-g female infant, Apgar scores of 7 and 8 at 1 and 5 minutes. Recovery for both mother and infant is unremarkable, and the infant is discharged home on day of life 14.

SUGGESTED READINGS

ACOG Committee on Obstetric Practice. ACOG Committee Opinion Number 284, August 2003: Nonobstetric surgery in pregnancy. Obstet Gynecol. 2003 Aug;102(2):431.

ACOG Committee on Obstetric Practice. ACOG Committee Opinion. Number 299, September 2004. Guidelines for diagnostic imaging during pregnancy. Obstet Gynecol. 2004 Sep;104(3):647–51.

ACOG Committee Opinion. Guidelines for diagnostic imaging during pregnancy. Number 299. September 2004.

Dietrich CS, Hill CC, Hueman M. Surgical diseases presenting in pregnancy. Surg Clin North Am. 2008;88(2):403–19.

Kilpatrick C, Monga M. Approach to the acute abdomen in pregnancy. Obstet Gynecol Clin N Am. 2007;34:389–402.

Van De Velde M, De Buck F. Anesthesia for non-obstetric surgery in the pregnant patient. Minerva Anesthesiol. 2007;73(4):235–40.

Young BC, Hamar BD, Levine D, Roqué H. Medical management of ruptured appendicitis in pregnancy. Obstet Gynecol. 2009;114(2 Pt 2):453–6.

Ultrasound Diagnosis of a Congenital Anomaly

17

Aisling Murphy   Lawrence D. Platt

 CASE PRESENTATION

Ms. Robinson, a 25-year-old G2 P1001, has been attending prenatal care at your outpatient department since 15 weeks of gestation. She has had an uncomplicated early antenatal course and is dated by a certain last menstrual period. She returns today at 19 weeks of gestation to discuss the results of her recent second trimester serum analyte screen (quadruple test), which includes a markedly elevated maternal serum (MS) alpha fetoprotein (AFP) (Table 17.1).

 Decision 1: Workup

What testing may help eliminate a false-positive MSAFP?

 A. Maternal estriol and human chorionic gonadotropin (hCG)
 B. Ultrasound for dating
 C. MS acetylcholinesterase
 D. Repeat MSAFP

The correct answer is B: Ultrasound for dating. AFP is a fetal glycoprotein that is produced by the yolk sac in early pregnancy and thereafter by the fetal liver and gastrointestinal tract. Levels of MSAFP start to rise after approximately 10 weeks of gestation. In the second trimester, levels rise rapidly to reach a maximum at about 30 to 32 weeks of gestation.

Screening for open neural tube defects (NTDs) using measurement of MSAFP is offered to all pregnant women between 15 and 20 weeks of gestation. MSAFP results are reported as multiples of the median (MoM) for the week of gestation.

Values above either 2.0 MoM or 2.5 MoM are considered to be positive, depending on the reporting laboratory. The interpretation of results is based on the precise gestational age, and a false-positive or false-negative result is most commonly due to incorrect dating. For this reason, an ultrasound assessment of gestational age may be helpful in

eliminating a false positive. In addition, an ultrasound may detect a previously unsuspected twin gestation or fetal demise, other potential causes of a false-positive result.

Answer A, maternal estriol and hCG is incorrect because both are not useful in the diagnosis of open NTDs. These MS analytes are used in conjunction with MSAFP and inhibin in the second trimester to screen for fetal trisomy 21 and trisomy 18. In both of these conditions, MSAFP levels are typically reduced.

Answer D, repeating the test, is incorrect. In cases where there is a positive MSAFP, there is little benefit in repeating the test, and most authorities recommend proceeding to a detailed anatomic ultrasound as the next step in evaluation. At the time of the ultrasound, gestational age can be confirmed, and the majority of anatomic anomalies associated with an elevation in MSAFP can be readily identified.

Answer C, MS acetylcholinesterase, is incorrect because MS acetylcholinesterase is not useful in eliminating a false-positive MSAFP. Acetylcholinesterase is an enzyme that is produced by neural tissue. In cases where, following a positive MSAFP, a detailed fetal ultrasound is nondiagnostic, further evaluation via amniocentesis may be offered. A sample of amniotic fluid is sent for AFP and acetylcholinesterase determination. An elevated level of both amniotic fluid AFP and acetylcholinesterase has a detection rate for an open NTD of 96%. The false-positive rate is 0.14% overall, and only 0.06% in samples that were not blood stained.

 NEED TO KNOW

Differential Diagnosis of an Elevated MSAFP

As described above, an accurate determination of gestational age is essential to avoid a false-positive or false-negative screening test result. Likewise, there are a number of other factors that may affect the measurement of MSAFP. These include maternal weight, ethnicity, the presence of twins, and the presence of insulin-dependent

TABLE 17.1

RESULTS OF PATIENT QUADRUPLE SCREEN PERFORMED AT 17 WEEKS AND 3 DAYS OF GESTATION

AFP MoM:	6.38
hCG MoM:	1.23
uE3 MoM:	0.78
Inhibin MoM:	0.85

Test interpretation:
Down syndrome risk assessment – SCREEN NEGATIVE
Trisomy 18 risk assessment – SCREEN NEGATIVE
Risk assessment for Smith-Lemli-Optiz syndrome – SCREEN NEGATIVE
Open neural tube defect risk assessment – SCREEN POSITIVE – INCREASED RISK

AFP, alpha fetoprotein; hCG, human chorionic gonadotropin; MoM, multiples of the median; uE3, unconjugated estriol.

maternal diabetes. The reporting laboratory makes adjustments based on these variables to provide the most accurate MSAFP result.

A list of the most common causes for an elevated MSAFP screen is given in Table 17.2. Even in the absence of any known cause, an elevated MSAFP remains a risk factor for perinatal complications including intrauterine growth restriction, preterm delivery, and fetal demise. It has been proposed that elevation of MSAFP in such cases is a result of placental injury, resulting in increased transfer of AFP from the fetal compartment to the maternal circulation.

 CASE CONTINUES

In light of Ms. Robinson's markedly elevated MSAFP, you refer her for detailed anatomic ultrasound, as well as genetic counseling. At the time of the sonogram, an abdominal wall defect is identified to the right of the umbilical cord insertion, with herniation of the bowel through this defect. The intestine outside the abdomen is not surrounded by a membrane. A diagnosis of gastroschisis is made.

 NEED TO KNOW

Prognosis of a Fetus with Gastroschisis

In contrast to omphalocele, where more than 50% of cases are associated with an abnormal karyotype, and other major malformations occur in as many as 40% of cases, the karyotype in gastroschisis is typically normal and extraintestinal malformations are uncommon. There is, however, an association with amyoplasia, a form of arthrogryposis, and a possible increased risk for congenital cardiac disease.

Associated intestinal malformations occur with a frequency of 10% to 15% in patients with gastroschisis. Most common are intestinal atresia or stenosis, which may be related to the primary vascular event implicated in the development of the gastroschisis itself. Alternatively, they

TABLE 17.2

DIFFERENTIAL DIAGNOSIS OF AN ELEVATED MSAFP

Fetal Causes
1. Multiple gestation
2. Fetomaternal hemorrhage
3. Fetal demise
4. Open NTDs. The sensitivity of MSAFP for detection of an open NTD depends on gestational age at the time of screening and the cutoff used in terms of MoMs. Overall it is between 75% and 85%. The detection rate of an anencephaly is higher, usually on the order of >90%, whereas in the case of encephalocele it is lower, as there is skin overlying the defect. The optimum time for screening is 16 to 18 weeks.
5. Fetal abdominal wall defects, such as omphalocele and gastroschisis. MSAFP is elevated in almost all cases of gastroschisis and in most cases of omphalocele. Levels in pregnancies affected by omphalocele tend to be lower, due to the presence of a membrane overlying the defect. In one study of 72,782 women who underwent second trimester screening between 1979 and 1987, the median values for the two lesions were 4.1 MoM for omphalocele and 7.0 MoM for gastroschisis.
6. Skin defects of the fetus, such as epidermolysis bullosa or aplasia cutis
7. Congenital nephrosis (Finnish type)
8. Sacrococcygeal teratoma
9. Other fetal anomalies including duodenal and esophageal atresias

Maternal Causes
10. Maternal tumors, e.g., hepatocellular carcinoma and endodermal sinus tumors (yolk sac tumors) of the ovary
11. Hereditary persistence of AFP production. This is a rare autosomal dominant condition

Placental Causes
12. Placental abnormalities such as placenta accrete

MoM, multiples of the median; NTD, neural tube defect.

may result at a later stage from volvulus or compression of the mesenteric vascular pedicle by a narrowing abdominal ring. Patients with associated intestinal anomalies face a more difficult operative course and are at more risk for long-term complications.

Overall the prognosis in gastroschisis is favorable, with survival rates of 90% to 95% reported. However, there is an increased incidence of intrauterine growth restriction, which may occur in up to 61% of fetuses. One theory suggests that this is the result of loss of protein across the exposed bowel. The diagnosis of intrauterine growth restriction may be complicated by the fact that the abdominal circumference is already smaller than expected, and in fact, some authors have proposed a specific ultrasonographic weight estimation formula for these infants, which excludes the abdominal measurement, and may be more accurate than commonly used formulae.

Rates of intrauterine demise are also increased in gastroschisis and have been reported to occur even in normally grown fetuses. For this reason, antenatal testing is usually instituted in pregnancies complicated by gastroschisis. In addition, while most fetuses with gastroschisis are delivered at full term, there is an increased rate of spontaneous preterm birth with this condition. Immediate postnatal complications include heat and fluid loss from the exposed bowel and also electrolyte disturbances. Surgical complications include infection, postoperative respiratory distress due to raised abdominal pressure, and bowel ischemia due to replacement of volved bowel. Other important complications include necrotizing enterocolitis, which has an incidence of up to 20%, central venous line infection and gastrointestinal dysmotility, which may delay enteral feeding and result in prolonged need for total parenteral nutrition (TPN). In patients exposed to TPN for prolonged periods, liver damage is a significant risk.

? Decision 2: Follow-up

What additional studies might be helpful?

A. Paternal karyotype
B. Umbilical artery Doppler assessment
C. Amniocentesis
D. Fetal blood sampling

The both B and C are correct. The best answer is B: Umbilical artery Doppler assessment. As discussed above, fetuses with gastroschisis are at increased risk of growth disturbances. In addition, abnormalities of amniotic fluid volume, most commonly oligohydramnios may develop.

Since intrauterine fetal demise occurs in as many as 10% of these infants, most authors recommend serial assessment of fetal growth and amniotic fluid volume to identify pregnancies at risk. Assessment of the umbilical artery Doppler is useful as a tool for surveillance of fetuses affected by growth restriction, as it has been shown to significantly reduce the risk of perinatal death in that setting. A normal Doppler is a reassuring finding and has also been shown to reduce unnecessary iatrogenic preterm delivery in numerous randomized controlled trials.

Amniocentesis (Answer C) is controversial. Since the risk of aneuploidy is not increased above background levels in cases of fetal gastroschisis, many authorities believe that a genetic amniocentesis or chorionic villus sampling procedure is not warranted except for an additional indication, such as the identification of an additional malformation on ultrasound. A discussion of the relative risks and benefits of invasive testing should be had with the patient when the diagnosis of gastroschisis is made. Later in gestation, however, amniocentesis for determination of fetal lung maturity may prove useful in timing delivery in certain cases.

Answer A (paternal karyotype) and answer D (fetal blood sampling) are incorrect. There is no indication for paternal karyotype or fetal blood sampling.

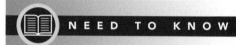 **NEED TO KNOW**

Risk Factors for Gastroschisis

Gastroschisis is believed to result from a vascular insult to the developing anterior abdominal wall resulting in ischemia with consequent breakdown of tissue leading to a defect. It is thought that the right paraumbilical area might be at particular risk of this complication because it is supplied by the right umbilical vein and right omphalomesenteric artery until they involute. If involution is disturbed in degree or timing, gastroschisis may result.

Reported risk factors for this malformation that tend to lend credence to the vascular theory of pathogenesis include maternal use of vasoactive medications such as pseudoephedrine and phenylpropanolamine, maternal smoking, and alcohol and illicit drug use. In addition, use of cyclooxygenase inhibitors such as aspirin and ibuprofen has been associated with an increased risk of gastroschisis in some studies.

Young maternal age is a risk factor that is reported by the vast majority of studies, with mothers younger than 20 years having a relative risk of 7.0. The reason for this is unclear. Interestingly, young maternal age is also reported as a risk factor for several other malformations that are thought to have a vascular etiology, including hydranencephaly and porencephaly, as well as some cases of oculoauriculovertebral syndrome and septo-optic dysplasia.

Other reported risk factors include primiparity, low maternal body mass index, poor maternal diet, and low socioeconomic status. In addition, a genetic component is likely to be involved, at least in some cases. There are cases of familial occurrence of the disorder, and the recurrence rate is estimated to be in the order of 3.5%.

 CASE CONTINUES

Ms. Robinson continues to see you in your office for the remainder of her pregnancy. She undergoes regular ultrasounds for follow-up of fetal growth and amniotic fluid volume. In addition, antenatal testing is commenced at 32 weeks of gestation. There is no evidence of fetal growth restriction or compromise. At 37 weeks, she presents to the hospital complaining of regular painful contractions and a bloody show. She is examined and found to be 4 cm dilated and is admitted to labor and delivery. She has an uncomplicated labor course and delivers a vigorous female infant.

At the time of delivery, a right paraumbilical defect can be seen with herniation of small bowel. In the delivery room the neonatal intensive care unit (NICU) team wraps the bowel in with plastic wrap and places an orogastric tube. The baby is brought to the NICU where she is assessed by the pediatric surgeon on call.

In this case, a decision is taken to proceed to the OR for primary closure of the defect under general anesthesia. At the time of the procedure, primary closure is not possible, and a silastic silo is placed. The patient is brought back to the NICU and daily reduction of the silo is carried out until the fascial defect can be closed after 6 days.

 N E E D   T O   K N O W

Perinatal/Neonatal Management of Gastroschisis

Timing of Delivery

Timing of delivery in gastroschisis involves consideration of several variables including fetal growth, amniotic fluid volume, and the results of antenatal testing. In the absence of fetal growth restriction or nonreassuring fetal

testing, the optimal age for delivery has yet to be determined. In such cases, there appears to be no benefit to elective delivery prior to 37 weeks.

Mode of Delivery

The optimal mode of delivery has been another area of controversy in the management of pregnancies affected by gastroschisis. Available data suggest no clear advantage to elective caesarean delivery and therefore vaginal delivery can be safely undertaken.

Immediate Postnatal Management

Early neonatal management of gastroschisis involves stabilization of the bowel and prevention of heat and fluid loss. Stabilization of bowel in the midline prevents twisting of the mesentery and constriction of blood supply at the edge of the defect. The bowel is then regularly observed to ensure adequate perfusion. Generally the bowel is immediately wrapped in plastic wrap to minimize heat and fluid loss and an orogastric tube is placed to decompress the stomach. IV access is obtained and fluid resuscitation is instituted. Any electrolyte abnormalities are corrected as needed.

Surgical Closure

The optimum method and timing of surgical repair are controversial.

Traditionally, repair is carried out via primary closure of the defect under general anesthetic within hours of delivery. This may involve enlarging the defect to facilitate reduction of the bowel into the abdominal cavity. If the bowel cannot be reduced in this way, or if the reduced gastroschisis is too tight to allow adequate ventilation, a silo may be used to facilitate staged reduction. The silo is a pouch or bag, usually made of silastic sheeting, which is sutured to the abdominal wall around the defect to contain the bowel. The silo is gradually reduced in size over a period of days until secondary closure of the fascia may be carried out. This staged closure was undertaken in our case as described above.

Alternatively, several studies have investigated other surgical approaches. These include primary reduction of the bowel at the bedside or staged reduction at the bedside using a preformed silo, followed by secondary closure in the OR. Some studies have reported that a staged bedside reduction may be associated with better outcomes than the traditional approach; however, a recent randomized controlled trial failed to show any clear advantages.

Long-Term Management

Long-term feeding difficulties due to gastrointestinal dysmotility are not uncommon in gastroschisis, and regular follow-up is needed for all infants after leaving the hospital so that these problems can be identified and corrected.

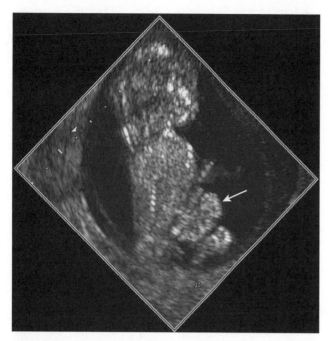

Figure 17.1 An example of a 13-week fetus with gastroschisis (arrow). The herniated bowel has a cauliflower-like appearance and is not covered by a membrane.

 Decision 3: Counseling

What options are available for this patient in the next pregnancy?

A. Early ultrasound screening (13 weeks)
B. First trimester serum testing
C. Second trimester serum testing
D. DNA (genetic) testing

The best answers are A and C. Answer A (early ultrasound) is correct. A recurrence of gastroschisis would be a concern in a future pregnancy. Physiologic herniation of the fetal bowel has resolved by 12 weeks, and late first trimester sonographic diagnosis of gastroschisis is possible (Fig. 17.1). An early ultrasound would be valuable in excluding a recurrence of this anomaly.

Answer C (second trimester serum screening) is also correct. The MSAFP component of the second trimester analyte screen would be valuable in excluding a recurrence of gastroschisis, as almost all cases of fetal gastroschisis are associated with an elevation on MSAFP.

First trimester screening (Answer B) is a part of routine prenatal care, but is not effective in the diagnosis of gastroschisis.

Answer D (DNA testing) is incorrect as DNA (genetic) testing of the mother or fetus is not useful in the diagnosis of gastroschisis.

In addition to the options mentioned above, it would be prudent to advise a reduction in any modifiable risk factors that the mother may have such as smoking and the use of vasoactive medications or illicit drugs.

 CASE CONCLUSION

Following a successful second surgery for closure of the defect, the infant is continued on TPN. Enteral feeds with maternal breastmilk are gradually introduced, but the baby makes slow progress. When you see Ms. Robinson again at her postpartum visit, she is happy to tell you that her baby is now taking full enteral feeds and is due to be discharged soon.

SUGGESTED READINGS

Boutros J, Regier M, Skarsgard ED. Canadian Pediatric Surgery Network. Is timing everything? The influence of gestational age, birth weight, route, and intent of delivery on outcome in gastroschisis. J Pediatr Surg. 2009;44(5):912–7.

Dugoff L, Hobbins JC, Malone FD, et al. Quad screen as a predictor of adverse pregnancy outcome. Obstet Gynecol. 2005;106(2):260–7.

Gilbert WM, Nicolaides KH. Fetal omphalocele: associated malformations and chromosomal defects. Obstet Gynecol. 1987;70(4):633–5.

Hunter AG, Stevenson RE. Gastroschisis: clinical presentation and associations. Am J Med Genet C Semin Med Genet. 2008;148C(3):219–30.

Jones KL, Benirschke K, Chambers CD. Gastroschisis: etiology and developmental pathogenesis Clin Genet. 2009;75(4):322–5.

Kunz LH, Gilbert WM, Towner DR. Increased incidence of cardiac anomalies in pregnancies complicated by gastroschisis. Am J Obstet Gynecol. 2005;193(3 Pt 2):1248–52.

Ledbetter DJ. Gastroschisis and omphalocele. Surg Clin North Am. 2006;86(2):249–60, vi.

Marven S, Owen A. Contemporary postnatal surgical management strategies for congenital abdominal wall defects. Semin Pediatr Surg. 2008;17(4):222–35.

Neilson JP, Alfirevic Z. Doppler ultrasound for fetal assessment in high risk pregnancies. Cochrane Database Syst Rev. 2000;(2):CD000073.

Netta DA, Wilson RD, Visintainer P, et al. Gastroschisis: growth patterns and a proposed prenatal surveillance protocol. Fetal Diagn Ther. 2007;22(5):352–7. Epub 2007 Jun 5.

Palomaki GE, Hill LE, Knight GJ, Haddow JE, Carpenter M. Second-trimester maternal serum alpha-fetoprotein levels in pregnancies associated with gastroschisis and omphalocele. Obstet Gynecol. 1988;71(6 Pt 1):906–9.

Pastor AC, Phillips JD, Fenton SJ, et al. Routine use of a SILASTIC spring-loaded silo for infants with gastroschisis: a multicenter randomized controlled trial. J Pediatr Surg. 2008;43(10):1807–12.

Rasmussen SA, Frías JL. Non-genetic risk factors for gastroschisis. Am J Med Genet C Semin Med Genet. 2008;148C(3):199–212.

Santiago-Munoz PC, McIntire DD, Barber RB, Megison SM, Twickler DM, Dashe JS. Outcomes of pregnancies with fetal gastroschisis. Obstet Gynecol. 2007;110(3):663–8.

Segel SY, Marder SJ, Parry S, Macones GA. Fetal abdominal wall defects and mode of delivery: a systematic review. Obstet Gynecol. 2001; 98 (5 Pt 1):867–73.

Siemer J, Hilbert A, Hart N, et al. Specific weight formula for fetuses with abdominal wall defects. Ultrasound Obstet Gynecol. 2008; 31(4):397–400.

Snyder CL, Miller KA, Sharp RJ, et al. Management of intestinal atresia in patients with gastroschisis. J Pediatr Surg. 2001;36(10):1542–5.

Waller DK, Lustig LS, Cunningham GC, Feuchtbaum LB, Hook EB. The association between maternal serum alpha-fetoprotein and preterm birth, small for gestational age infants, preeclampsia, and placental complications. Obstet Gynecol. 1996;88(5):816–22.

Fetal Chromosomal Anomaly

Marie H. Beall

 CLINICAL CASE

Your next office patient is Mrs. Johnson, a 35-year-old G3 P0 currently at 10 weeks and 3 days of gestation by last menstrual period, presenting for her initial prenatal care visit. You cared for her in her last pregnancy, which ended in a spontaneous abortion 8 months ago. She also has a history of an early therapeutic abortion 12 years ago with a different partner. The remainder of her medical history is unremarkable. Her family history is remarkable, as she has both a brother and a maternal uncle with Down syndrome. She is quite clear about the diagnosis and insists that it "runs in her family." Her uncle is deceased, but her brother is still living. She shows you photographs of her brother, who appears to have the typical stigmata of Down syndrome (Fig. 18.1). She would not terminate a fetus with Down syndrome, but states that she wants to know her risk so that she can be prepared.

Physical examination reveals a 10-week–sized uterus. A brief ultrasound confirms gestational age and documents fetal heart motion. Routine prenatal labs are sent and are later found to be normal.

 Decision 1: Risk

What is the Down syndrome risk for this patient?

A. 1/270
B. 5%
C. 25%
D. Depends on maternal karyotype

The correct answer is D: Depends on the maternal karyotype. Down syndrome risk is typically quoted as the risk of Down syndrome in the fetus at mid trimester. This risk of fetal Down syndrome is higher than the risk of a liveborn Down syndrome child at term, as there is excess mortality in Down syndrome pregnancies in the second half of gestation. Answer A (1/270) is the Down syndrome risk at mid trimester based on a maternal age of 35 years

at delivery; the risk of a liveborn Down syndrome newborn is 1/350 at this maternal age. A family history of Down syndrome, such as was found in this family, might indicate the presence of familial Down syndrome due to a chromosomal rearrangement. This would increase the risk of a Down syndrome pregnancy (see below).

NEED TO KNOW

Chromosomal Rearrangements

Most often, Down syndrome is a consequence of having an extra chromosome 21, with a total chromosome number of 47. This is often reported as 47, XY, +21 (for a male), indicating 47 total chromosomes, XY sex chromosome complement, and an extra chromosome 21. Chromosomal trisomies (a single extra chromosome) are most often a result of an error in chromosome separation (nondisjunction) at meiosis. Although some families appear to have an increased risk of nondisjunction, chromosomal trisomies are not themselves inherited from normal parents.

Inherited or familial Down syndrome is typically not due to a chromosomal trisomy. Familial Down syndrome may result from a chromosomal rearrangement that leads to the fetus getting three copies of all or part of chromosome 21. In such cases, the total number of chromosomes may be normal. A Robertsonian translocation (also called a centric fusion) is the most common chromosomal rearrangement leading to familial Down syndrome. In such translocations, two acrocentric (with the centromere very near one end) chromosomes fuse at the centromere. The most common such translocation is 14:21; however, chromosomes 13 and 15 may also be involved, and it is also possible to have a 21:21 translocation (Fig. 18.2). In such cases, the carrier is generally phenotypically normal, but has 45 chromosomes. The carrier can form gametes with normal, balanced, or unbalanced karyotypes (Fig 18.3),

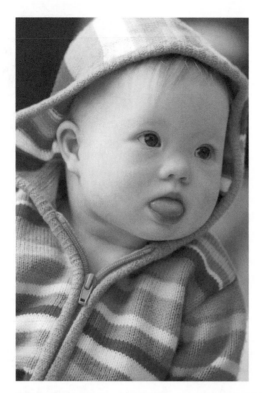

Figure 18.1   Down syndrome child. Note the epicanthal folds of the eye, round face, and depressed nasal bridge; all typical features of Down syndrome.

leading to normal, carrier, or trisomic offspring, except in the case of a 21:21 translocation carrier, when only unbalanced forms are possible. Because of increased intrauterine mortality in pregnancies with unbalanced karyotypes, the risk of a liveborn Down syndrome offspring is less than the proportion of unbalanced gametes; also the risk of an unbalanced offspring is greater when the carrier is the mother. Therefore, the risk of a Down syndrome child is empirical but is usually between 5% and 25%.

 CASE CONTINUES

You obtain blood for karyotype from the mother, with the plan that you may test her partner later, as he is not present. Five days later, the nurse calls you from the clinic as the patient's karyotype has returned, and is 45, XX t13:21, meaning that she is a balanced translocation carrier for a 13:21 translocation. You inform the patient that she is at increased risk for fetal Down syndrome, and also for trisomy 13, and offer her prenatal diagnosis with chorionic villus sampling (CVS). She declines CVS as she has been told that there is an increased risk of fetal loss

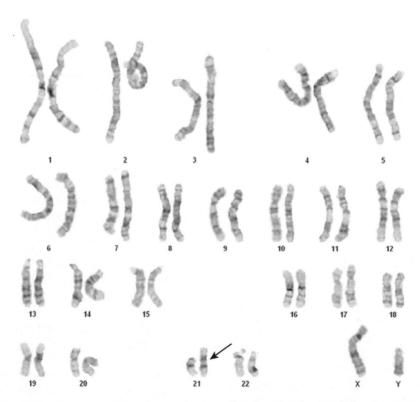

Figure 18.2   Karyotype of a female with translocation Down syndrome. Note the 21:21 translocation (arrow), giving three copies of chromosome 21, although there are only 46 chromosomes. (Picture courtesy of Rezaur Rahman, PhD.)

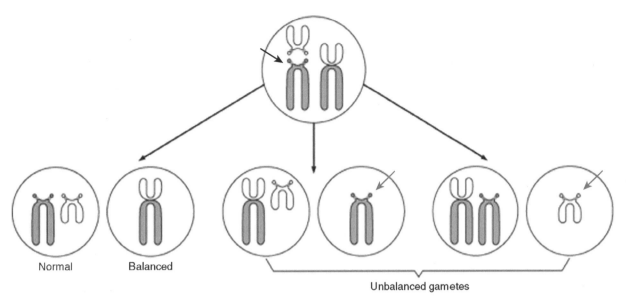

Figure 18.3   A mother with a 13:21 or 14:21 translocation (black arrow) can produce gametes with one copy of each chromosome (balanced), or with extra or missing chromosomes (unbalanced). Zygotes missing a chromosome, produced by gametes indicated by gray arrows, do not survive.

after the procedure compared with amniocentesis. However, she states that she wants to have an amniocentesis at 16 weeks.

At 16 weeks of gestation, Mrs. Johnson returns for a genetic amniocentesis. The fetal anatomy survey is suboptimal due to gestational age and maternal body habitus; however, there are no fetal anomalies apparent. Amniocentesis results show the fetus with an unbalanced karyotype suggestive of fetal Down syndrome. The mother again states that she does not want to consider pregnancy termination. However, her brother has recently been diagnosed with leukemia, and she wants to know what the risks are that her baby will have this or other problems associated with Down syndrome.

 Decision 2: Workup

What additional workup might be helpful?

A. Paternal karyotype
B. Umbilical artery (UA) Doppler
C. Fetal echocardiogram
D. Fetal blood sampling

The correct answer is C: Fetal echocardiogram. Individuals with Down syndrome have an up to 50% risk of congenital heart disease. Although the mother has stated that she would not terminate, a fetus with congenital heart disease may require a higher level of care at delivery, depending on the specific lesion. The heart lesion most typical of

Down syndrome is an endocardial cushion defect (see below). The paternal karyotype is not an issue at this point as the fetal karyotype is known. UA Doppler at 16 weeks and fetal blood sampling would not be helpful at this time in this pregnancy.

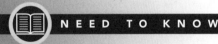 **NEED TO KNOW**

Prognosis of a Child with Down Syndrome

The individual with Down syndrome is at higher risk of a number of health problems. A number of serious congenital anomalies are more prevalent in Down syndrome, and identification of one of these anomalies is often the initial clue to the diagnosis. In particular, cardiac anomalies occur in 25% to 50% of individuals with Down syndrome, as compared with 0.9% of the general population. During the course of pregnancy, the Down syndrome pregnancy is more likely to be complicated by polyhydramnios or fetal growth restriction, and additional pregnancy monitoring for fetal growth may be prudent.

In childhood, Down syndrome individuals demonstrate slow body growth. They are at a 10-fold higher risk for leukemia, as well as at increased risk for infectious diseases. About 15% to 40% of individuals with Down syndrome have abnormalities of the cervical spine and may be at risk for odontal-axial subluxation and spinal

TABLE 18.1

PHYSICAL AND MENTAL DISORDERS WITH INCREASED PREVALENCE IN ADULTS WITH DOWN SYNDROME[a]

Selected Medical Conditions with a Higher Prevalence in Adults with Down Syndrome[a]

Endocrine
  Thyroid disease—hypothyroidism
    and hyperthyroidism
  Diabetes mellitus
Mental health
  Depression
  Obsessive-compulsive disorder
  Abuse (physical or sexual)
  Conduct disorder

Otolaryngology
  Obstructive sleep apnea
  Hearing loss
Musculoskeletal
  Spinal cord compression
  Atlantoaxial subluxation
Periodontal disease
Alzheimer's disease

Cataracts, refractive errors and keratoconus
Seizures
Testicular cancer
Xerodermatitis
Acquired valvular heart disease, including
  mitral valve prolapse

[a]Listed in approximate order of clinical importance.
Adapted from Smith DS. Health care management of adults with Down syndrome. Am Fam Physician. 2001;64(6): 1031–8.

cord injury. Down syndrome individuals also typically demonstrate developmental delay, although this can be very variable. Although most individuals with Down syndrome have intelligence quotients (IQs) in the mild (50–69) or moderate (35–49) mental retardation range, some individuals may have near normal intelligence, and others may be profoundly impaired.

The average life expectancy of a child with Down syndrome is about 50 years, and most children without life-threatening physical abnormalities will achieve adulthood. In adolescence, individuals with Down syndrome become sexually mature. Men with Down syndrome are usually subfertile, but women can become pregnant and carry pregnancies to term. Down syndrome adults continue to have an increased risk of health problems (Table 18.1). In particular, they tend to experience premature aging, and early Alzheimer's disease.

All states in the United States offer educational services for individuals with intellectual handicaps, and parents should be assisted to access these services. Parents may also benefit from referral to local parents support groups. As with any special-needs child, parents should be encouraged to make plans for both financial and social support if or when the parents can no longer provide a home to their adult child.

 NEED TO KNOW

Prognosis of Other Chromosomal Abnormalities

In addition to Down syndrome, this patient was at risk for another chromosomal trisomy. In fact, there

are two other chromosomal trisomies that are commonly seen at delivery. These are trisomy 13 and trisomy 18, also called Patau syndrome and Edwards syndrome, respectively. Infants with these conditions are much more severely affected than those with Down syndrome, with some studies quoting a 100% risk of congenital anomalies, and a very high risk of death in the first year of life (Table 18.2). In surviving individuals, IQ has seldom been recorded and may not be possible to assess due to the lack of language skills in these individuals. The developmental quotient (developmental age divided by actual age) has been reported to be between 0.2 and 0.3 for trisomy 13 and between 0.1 and 0.2 for trisomy 18 in children older than 1 year.

 CASE CONTINUES

This patient is referred for a high-resolution ultrasound and fetal echocardiogram, which are reported to be normal. Because of the risk for fetal growth restriction, she has ultrasound performed for fetal growth at 28, 33, and 36 weeks. On each of the ultrasounds, the fetus appears to be growing at the 20th percentile.

Decision 3: Labor management

How should labor and delivery be managed with a Down syndrome fetus?

  A. Elective cesarean prior to labor
  B. Early maternal epidural

TABLE 18.2

OUTCOME OF FETUSES WITH TRISOMY 13 AND 18 (IN A POPULATION WITH NO ELECTIVE PREGNANCY TERMINATIONS)

	Trisomy 18 (%)	Trisomy 13 (%)
Antepartum stillbirth	12.5	33
Intrapartum stillbirth	6	17
Born alive Death <24 hours	23	No information
Born alive Death <14 days	69	44–100
Total perinatal mortality	94	77–100
Survival >1 year	6	0–7
Major anomalies	100	100

C. Using regular L&D protocols
D. Forceps delivery to shorten the second stage

The correct answer is C: Using regular L&D protocols. Fetuses with Down syndrome do not have an increased risk of cesarean section for fetal compromise, or an increased risk of stillbirth intrapartum, and no special interventions are recommended. Although individuals with Down syndrome do demonstrate an increased risk of instability of the high cervical spine, there is no evidence of an increase in birth injures referable to this, and elective cesarean is not recommended.

 ## CASE CONTINUES

At 39 weeks of gestation, the patient goes into spontaneous labor and delivers a 2,970-g female infant without incident. The infant is noted to be hypotonic at birth, and for this reason the 5-minute Apgar score is 6, although the cord blood pH is normal. The infant initially is sent to room in with her mother, but she is then taken to the nursery for poor feeding effort. After attempting to breast-feed for 2 days, Mrs. Johnson becomes discouraged and begins to supplement with a bottle. Postnatal cardiac examination reveals no heart lesion. On day of life 3, the infant is discharged home with her mother.

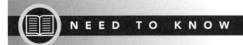 **NEED TO KNOW**

Appearance of the Newborn with Down Syndrome

After delivery, the newborn is typically hypotonic, and the tongue may be enlarged and protruding. These symptoms may impair feeding, and Down syndrome infants feed slowly and may not be successful breast-feeders. The newborn may also demonstrate hypothyroidism or hearing loss, in addition to congenital heart disease that may not have been identified prenatally. Prudent management of any newborn with Down syndrome includes assessment for congenital heart disease. Newborn testing for hypothyroidism and hearing loss should be considered if they are not part of the normal newborn screening protocol. Finally, the newborn should be carefully followed for growth and weight gain; normal standards for Down syndrome infants have been developed and may be more appropriate to assess growth.

 ### Decision 4: Infant workup

What special interventions are recommended in this baby?

A. Complete blood cell count
B. X-ray examination of the spine and possible spinal fusion
C. Administration of neuroprotective peptides
D. Screening for celiac disease

The correct answer is A: Complete blood cell count. Newborns with Down syndrome have a small risk for leukemia, and a much higher risk for polycythemia and a leukemoid reaction. For these reasons, the American Academy of Pediatrics recommends a blood count on the Down syndrome newborn. X-ray examination of the spine is recommended, but only later in childhood, and the usefulness of this in asymptomatic children has been questioned. Neuroprotective peptides administered during pregnancy have been shown to reduce the developmental delay associated with Down syndrome in a mouse model, but this intervention has not been tried in humans. Celiac disease is increased in Down syndrome, but there is no evidence that identifying it presymptomatically is of benefit.

 ## CASE CONCLUSION

Mrs. Johnson takes her baby home. One year later she returns to your office to plan another pregnancy. She is still unwilling to consider a pregnancy termination, but she has discovered that her sister is not a translocation carrier. She wants to discuss with you having ovum donation from her sister so as to avoid the risk of fetal chromosomal anomalies.

SUGGESTED READINGS

American Academy of Pediatrics. Committee on Genetics. Health supervision for children with Down syndrome. Pediatrics. 2001;107(2): 442-9.

Baty BJ, Blackburn BL, Carey JC. Natural history of trisomy 18 and trisomy 13: I. Growth, physical assessment, medical histories, survival, and recurrence risk. Am J Med Genet. 1994;49(2):175-88.

Baty BJ, Jorde LB, Blackburn BL, Carey JC. Natural history of trisomy 18 and trisomy 13: II. Psychomotor development. Am J Med Genet. 1994;49(2):189-94.

Hill LM. The sonographic detection of trisomies 13, 18, and 21. Clin Obstet Gynecol. 1996;39(4):831-50.

Moran CJ, Tay JB, Morrison JJ. Ultrasound detection and perinatal outcome of fetal trisomies 21, 18 and 13 in the absence of a routine fetal anomaly scan or biochemical screening. Ultrasound Obstet Gynecol. 2002;20(5):482-5.

NIH NICHHD. Facts about Down syndrome. http://www.nichd.nih.gov/publications/pubs/downsyndrome.cfm accessed 11/1/2009.

Smith DS. Health care management of adults with Down syndrome. Am Fam Physician. 2001;64(6):1031-8.

Multiple Gestation

Julie Boles

19

 ## CASE PRESENTATION

Ms. Jason, a 31-year-old G2 P1 patient presents to your office seeking prenatal care. She is unsure of her last menstrual period due to a history of irregular menses. On physical examination, her uterus is noted to be approximately 12-week size. You perform an abdominal ultrasound to establish an estimated due date. You see the following image (Fig. 19.1).

You give the shocked patient the news that she is pregnant with monochorionic/diamniotic twins.

 ## Decision 1: Diagnosis

How is the diagnosis of zygosity made on this ultrasound?

A. By the presence of a "T" sign
B. By the presence of a "lambda" sign
C. By the presence of a single placenta
D. By the presence of a common extraamniotic fluid space

The correct answer is D: Monochorionic twinning is established in this case by the presence of a common extraamniotic space. At this early gestation, the amnion is not fused to the chorion, and there is a relatively large amount of extraamniotic fluid (extraamniotic coelom). The fact that this fluid is contained in a single sac demonstrates monochorionicity. Answers A and B are not correct, as the "T" sign and the "lambda" sign indicate mono- and dichorionicity, respectively, after the fusion of the amnion and chorion. Answer C is not as good an answer. A single placenta is required for a diagnosis of monochorionic twins, but dichorionic twins may have placentas that are so close together that they appear to be a single placenta on ultrasound. Therefore, single placenta is not the best criterion for the diagnosis of chorionicity.

 ### NEED TO KNOW

Physiology of Twinning

Twin gestations can occur after two ova are fertilized separately (dizygotic twins) or after the division of a single fertilized ovum (monozygotic twins). Dizygotic twins are always dichorionic/diamniotic, which means that each embryo has an individual placenta and amniotic sac. However, monozygotic twins can be dichorionic/diamniotic (two placentas, two amniotic sacs), monochorionic/diamniotic (one placenta, two amniotic sacs), monochorionic/monoamniotic (both embryos share the same placenta and amniotic sac), or conjoined twins depending on the time of division of the single gestation into two (Fig. 19.2).

Since you are able to visualize that the twins are monochorionic and diamniotic on the ultrasound, you can estimate the time of division to be between 4 and 8 days after fertilization.

 ## CASE CONTINUES

Your ultrasound establishes that the pregnancy is presently at 8 weeks of gestational age. Ms. Jason is very anxious regarding twin pregnancy and she wants to know what to expect.

 ### NEED TO KNOW

Maternal and Fetal Risks of Twin Gestation

Twin gestation exaggerates the normal maternal physiologic adaptation to pregnancy. Maternal blood volume expansion is greater, and the cardiac output at term is increased by about 20% over singleton pregnancy.

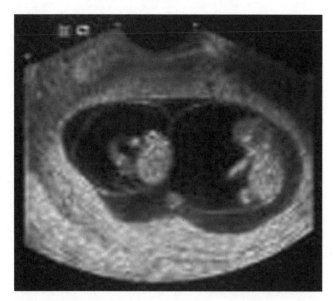

Figure 19.1 First trimester twin pregnancy. (Reproduced with permission from www.peninsulaultrasound.com/prenatal/389.jpg.)

Oxygen consumption is increased. Weight gain is also increased; normal-weight women are advised to gain 25 to 35 lb during a singleton pregnancy, whereas during a twin pregnancy the recommended weight gain is 37 to 54 lbs. These changes make pregnancy riskier for the mother when she is carrying twins, especially for the mother with heart or lung disease. Twin pregnancy is also associated with an increase in the number of maternal pregnancy complications in all patients, including anemia and preeclampsia (Table 19.1).

Given the increased demands of twin gestation, women pregnant with twins may benefit from nutritional consultation in pregnancy. The recommended daily calorie intake for a normal-weight mother pregnant with

Figure 19.2 Timing of division of the gestation in monozygous twinning and the degree of separation of the twins. Earlier division of the zygote leads to the most complete separation of the twins, with two placentas and gestational sacs. Incomplete separation of the bodies of the fetuses (conjoined twins) is due to late division, at the embryonic disc stage. Image by Kevin Dufendach, MD (2008). Used by permission. Dufendach, K. (Artist). (2008). Placentation. [Web]. Retrieved from http://commons.wikimedia.org/wiki/File:Placentation.svg

TABLE 19.1

MATERNAL COMPLICATIONS INCREASED IN TWIN PREGNANCY

Complication	Relative Risk, Twin Versus Singleton Pregnancy
Anemia	1.8
Urinary tract infection	1.3
Gestational diabetes	1.3
Preeclampsia	2.2
Eclampsia	3.0
Acute fatty liver of pregnancy	About 7
Cesarean delivery	2.5
Postpartum hemorrhage	2.0
Maternal death	1.7

Adapted from Conde-Agudelo A, Belizán JM, Lindmark G. Maternal morbidity and mortality associated with multiple gestations. Obstet Gynecol. 2000;95(6 Pt 1):899–904.

twins is 3,500 kcal at term, and these patients should be supplemented with both iron and folate. Bedrest is discouraged, except for specific obstetrical complications.

All twin pregnancies involve some increased risk to the fetuses as well. Twins are associated with an increased risk of major congenital malformations (2.12% compared with 1.05% in singletons). Monozygotic twins in particular have a higher rate of congenital malformations (4.13%) compared with dizygotic twins (1.9%). There is also a significant risk of fetal loss, as multifetal pregnancies comprise 12% of all natural conceptions but only 2% of eventual births. The fetal loss rate in the first and early second trimesters (<24 weeks) is 12.2% in monochorionic pregnancies and only 1.8% in dichorionic gestations. Twins are more likely to be growth restricted. After about 32 weeks of gestation, the average growth of twin fetuses diverges from normal singletons, and evidence suggests that the effect of this diminished growth in twins is the same as it would be in a singleton gestation. In addition, one twin of a pair may demonstrate further reduced growth due to poor placentation, genetic differences between dizygotic siblings, or intertwin transfusion (see below). All twins incur an increased risk of preterm delivery. Some of the risk of prematurity results from elective preterm delivery due to maternal or fetal complications. However, much of the prematurity risk results from spontaneous preterm labor. Overall, the average age at delivery of a twin gestation is 36 weeks. Unfortunately, progesterone supplementation and cervical cerclage, interventions that help to prevent preterm delivery in high-risk singleton gestations, are ineffective in twin gestations, although interventions to improve maternal nutrition and reduce maternal stress appear to be of benefit. Once preterm labor ensues, it is treated in the same manner as preterm labor in singletons. Finally, the risk of fetal malpresentation is increased in twins, contributing to the overall increased risk of cesarean delivery in twin gestations.

In addition to the risks common to all twins, monochorionic/diamniotic and monochorionic/monoamniotic twin gestations carry significant risks specific to their unique anatomy. Monochorionic/diamniotic twins are at increased risk of twin–twin transfusion syndrome (TTTS). TTTS occurs in about 25% of monochorionic twin gestations secondary to unbalanced vascular communications between placental vessels. Essentially all monochorionic twins have vascular connections between twins within the placenta; most vascular communications are balanced and therefore are not a risk to the fetuses. However, occasionally monochorionic twin placentas will contain deep arteriovenous anastomoses through which blood preferentially passes from one twin (the donor) to the co-twin (the recipient) (Fig. 19.3). Eventually, the donor twin becomes anemic and growth restricted with oligohydramnios due to decreased fetal urine output. At the same time, the recipient twin receives an excess share of blood, which results in polycythemia and strain on the fetal heart leading to hydrops fetalis.

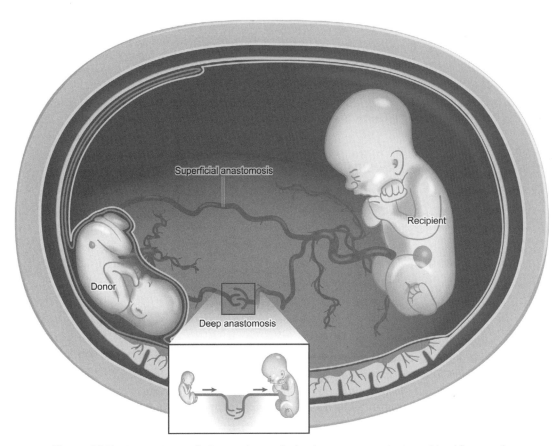

Figure 19.3   Twin–twin transfusion syndrome. At the deep anastomosis, donor blood flows to the recipient. The donor is "stuck" with no amniotic fluid and a small or absent bladder. The recipient is larger and has polyhydramnios and a large bladder. (Reproduced with permission from http://www. texaschildrens.org/carecenters/fetalsurgery/twin_twin_transfusion_syndrome.aspx.)

Monochorionic/monoamniotic twins comprise only about 1% of monozygotic twin pregnancies but contribute significantly to the rates of fetal mortality. Since monochorionic/monoamniotic twins develop in the same amniotic sac there is always the chance of cord entanglement. The risk of cord accident is so great that approximately 50% of all monochorionic/monoamniotic twin pregnancies result in fetal mortality.

 CASE CONTINUES

Ms. Jason has a normal ultrasound survey of the fetal anatomy at 18 weeks that shows no evidence of fetal anomalies and concordant growth. Her serum screen gives a low risk for fetal Down syndrome. She is concerned about the amount of time she has taken off work, and she wants to know how many doctor's appointments she will have.

 Decision 2: Follow-up

In an otherwise uncomplicated monochorionic twin pregnancy, how do you monitor the pregnancy and when do you deliver?

 A. Ultrasound for growth every 2 weeks, modified biophysical profile weekly beginning at 22 weeks, deliver at 36 weeks
 B. Ultrasound for growth every 4 to 6 weeks, biophysical profile weekly beginning at 28 weeks, deliver at 38 weeks
 C. Ultrasound for growth every 4 to 6 weeks, modified biophysical profile weekly beginning at 34 weeks, deliver at 40 weeks
 D. Ultrasound for growth at 34 weeks, modified biophysical profile weekly beginning at 40 weeks, deliver at 41 weeks

The correct answer is C: Ultrasound for growth every 4 to 6 weeks, modified biophysical profile weekly beginning at 34 weeks, deliver at 40 weeks. Although there is a lack of scientific evidence in this field, most authorities recommend serial ultrasound for fetal growth, though the time of initiation of the serial growth scans is controversial. Answer A: Ultrasound every 2 weeks is excessive in an uncomplicated twin gestation, and answer D: Ultrasound once during the pregnancy is probably not sufficient. There is no good evidence that serial antenatal testing in uncomplicated twin gestation improves outcomes, although this has become a common practice. Given this, answer B: Testing beginning at 28 weeks is not as good an answer as beginning at 34 weeks. Finally, the nadir of perinatal mortality for twin gestations is at 38 weeks. Although there is no recommendation to

deliver twins at 38 weeks, it may be prudent not to allow an uncomplicated twin gestation to progress beyond 40 weeks.

 CASE CONTINUES

Ms. Jason continues under your care, with serial ultrasounds for fetal growth every 4 to 6 weeks beginning at 24 weeks. On a repeat ultrasound performed at 28 weeks of gestation, twin A's measurements are consistent with 28 weeks and the largest vertical pocket of amniotic fluid is increased (10 cm). However, the measurements for twin B are consistent with 25 weeks of gestation and the largest vertical pocket of amniotic fluid is reduced (1.5 cm). The bladder of the smaller twin is visible and Doppler studies are normal. You are concerned about developing TTTS.

 Decision 3: Management

What are the options for treatment of TTTS at 28 weeks of gestation?

 A. Serial amnioreduction and ultrasound monitoring of fetal growth
 B. Laser ablation of placental anastomoses
 C. Immediate cesarean delivery
 D. Repeat ultrasound in 4 to 6 weeks

The correct answer is A: Serial amnioreduction and ultrasound monitoring of fetal growth. A full discussion of the treatment options for TTTS follows; however, answer B: Laser ablation of placental anastomoses is generally not recommended above 26 weeks of gestation. Answer C: Immediate cesarean delivery is not advisable in the absence of other indications that one or the other twin is gravely ill. Answer D: Expectant management, with a repeat ultrasound in 4 to 6 weeks is not acceptable, as the disorder may progress to fetal demise in that period of time.

When a pregnancy is complicated by TTTS, there is a significant risk of central nervous system (CNS) injury (multicystic encephalomalacia and cerebral palsy), preterm delivery, and fetal death. Severe TTTS is associated with a 60 to 100% fetal mortality rate and the neurological outcome of a surviving twin is typically poor. CNS injury can occur in both the donor and recipient twins and is thought to be due to blood pressure instability and severe hypotension resulting in ischemic lesions. The more premature the twins are at birth, the worse the neurodevelopmental outcome. The most important factors that contribute to perinatal outcome are the gestational age at diagnosis, the gestational age at delivery, and severity of the disease at delivery. The severity of TTTS is graded on the basis of the Quintero system (Table 19.2).

TABLE 19.2
QUINTERO SYSTEM FOR STAGING TWIN–TWIN TRANSFUSION SYSTEM

Stage	Twin	Description	Survival of Both Fetuses (with Treatment)
Stage 1	Donor	Oligohydramnios, fetal bladder visible	75%
	Recipient	Polyhydramnios	
Stage 2	Donor	"Stuck" twin, bladder not visible	60%
	Recipient	Same as stage 1	
Stage 3	Either	Abnormal Doppler's: Absent or reversed end-diastolic flow in umbilical artery. Abnormal ductus venosus, or umbilical vein flow	54%
Stage 4	Either	Ascites or hydrops	50%
Stage 5	Either	Death of either twin	

Data from Huber A, Diehl W, Bregenzer T, Hackelöer BJ, Hecher K. Stage-related outcome in twin-twin transfusion syndrome treated by fetoscopic laser coagulation. Obstet Gynecol. 2006;108(2):333–7.

Options for the management of TTTS include expectant management, amnioreduction, septostomy, selective feticide, and fetoscopic laser ablation. Expectant management is associated with an unacceptably high fetal mortality rate (67%–73%). One of the mainstays of treatment has been serial amnioreduction, which involves removing amniotic fluid from the polyhydramniotic sac containing the recipient twin. This is believed to relieve the intraamniotic pressure associated with polyhydramnios, therefore allowing increased blood flow to the donor twin. This has been associated with survival rates of 21% to 83%; in patients who deliver after 28 weeks, the survival rates are as high as 69% to 83%. However, serial amnioreduction can be associated with complications including placental abruption (1.3%), preterm rupture of membranes (6%), chorioamnionitis (1%), spontaneous delivery (3%), and fetal death (2%). Therefore, amnioreduction is typically recommended for mild TTS in gestations already past 26 weeks of gestation.

Septostomy is the intentional perforation of the intertwin membrane in an attempt to equilibrate the amniotic fluid volumes and pressure. Septostomy has similar reported neonatal outcomes compared with serial amnioreduction but is performed less often since it requires technical expertise. It is also associated with the above complications. Importantly, septostomy creates an effective "monoamniotic" pregnancy and thus increases the risk of cord entanglement.

A newer highly specialized treatment is fetoscopic laser coagulation of the placental vascular communications. First described in 1990, it is now considered the treatment of choice for severe (Quintero stage II–IV) TTTS in gestations between 16 and 26 weeks. The procedure is performed by the insertion of a 2- to 3-mm fetoscope with mapping and laser coagulation of the anastomotic vessels. In severe cases, laser ablation results in less perinatal death (26% vs. 44%)

and fewer neonatal deaths (8% vs. 26%) compared with amnioreduction. Infants with a history of TTTS treated with laser ablation have improved long-term neurologic outcomes compared with amnioreduction. Currently, the Food and Drug Administration restricts this procedure to gestations under 26 weeks, and there are technical limitations that limit the success of the procedure in the third trimester (greater distance for the fetoscope to traverse, larger placental vessels, and decreased visibility due to vernix).

Selective feticide can occasionally be the best options in cases of a serious anomaly in one of the twins or in cases of failed laser ablation or recurrent severe TTTS after laser ablation. Outcomes are not different if the procedure is performed on the donor or recipient twin, though it is often technically easier to perform on the recipient twin. The cord must be occluded completely to prevent severe hypotension in the surviving twin. Cord occlusion is typically performed with bipolar cautery forceps under ultrasound guidance. Overall survival rates for the remaining twin range from 77% to 91%.

 ## CASE CONCLUSION

Ms. Jason undergoes amnioreduction at 28 weeks, with removal of 1 L of amniotic fluid. Amnioreduction is then repeated weekly, with ultrasound evidence of improvement in growth and amniotic fluid volume in the donor twin. She receives close monitoring, and at 35 weeks the donor twin is noted to have reversed end-diastolic flow in the umbilical artery, suggesting deterioration. She is delivered by cesarean section and after a stay in the special care nursery both babies are discharged home in good condition.

SUGGESTED READINGS

American Academy of Pediatrics, American College of Obstetricians and Gynecologists. Guidelines for Perinatal Care. 6th ed. Washington, DC: ACOG; 2008.

American College of Obstetricians and Gynecologists Committee on Practice Bulletins-Obstetrics; Society for Maternal-Fetal Medicine; ACOG Joint Editorial Committee. ACOG Practice Bulletin #56: Multiple gestation: complicated twin, triplet, and high-order multifetal pregnancy. Obstet Gynecol. 2004;104(4):869–83.

Ayres A, Johnson TR. Management of multiple pregnancy: prenatal care – part I. Obstet Gynecol Surv. 2005;60(8):527–37.

Ayres A, Johnson TR. Management of multiple pregnancy: prenatal care – part II. Obstet Gynecol Surv. 2005;60(8):538–49.

Conde-Agudelo A, Belizán JM, Lindmark G. Maternal morbidity and mortality associated with multiple gestations. Obstet Gynecol. 2000;95(6 Pt 1):899–904.

Gyamfi C, Stone J, Eddleman KA. Maternal complications of multifetal pregnancy. Clin Perinatol. 2005;32(2):431–42, vii.

Huber A, Diehl W, Bregenzer T, Hackelöer BJ, Hecher K. Stage-related outcome in twin-twin transfusion syndrome treated by fetoscopic laser coagulation. Obstet Gynecol. 2006;108(2):333–7.

Modena AB, Berghella V. Antepartum management of multifetal pregnancies. Clin Perinatol. 2005;32(2):443–54, vii.

Intrauterine Growth Restriction

20

Michael G. Ross

CASE PRESENTATION

Your next patient is Ms. Gordo, a 34-year-old G2 P1, who is currently at 15 weeks of gestation. The midwife has referred her to you because of her obstetrical history.

Ms. Gordo reports no problems in the current pregnancy. In her last pregnancy she had labor induced at 35 weeks because her fetus was small for dates. At delivery, the baby weighed 1,700 g. This child is now 2 years old and at the 35th percentile for weight; she is otherwise apparently normal. Ms. Gordo reports that she has had hypertension for several years and that she is currently being treated with labetalol 400 mg BID. She denies other significant past medical history or other medication use. She reports that she used to smoke cigarettes, but stopped recently; on further questioning she admits that her last cigarette was yesterday. She reports that her mother and aunt have hypertension and her aunt has diabetes.

On physical examination, Ms. Gordo is an obese Caucasian female who is in no distress. Her blood pressure is 145/80 mm Hg, her pulse is 95 bpm, and she is afebrile. Her height is 64 inches and her weight is 243 lb. The remainder of her physical examination is unremarkable. Her uterine size accorded with her dates. Laboratory examination previously obtained is unremarkable and a first trimester screen revealed a fetal size consistent with dates at 12 weeks, and a low risk for fetal Down syndrome or trisomy 18.

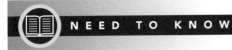
NEED TO KNOW

Risk Factors for Fetal Growth Restriction

A fetus may be small compared with others either because its capacity for growth is reduced (constitutionally small), or because its growth has been stunted (intrauterine growth restriction or IUGR). This distinction is important, as the constitutionally small fetus is not endangered by the intrauterine environment, and generally does not benefit from early delivery, whereas the IUGR fetus may be compromised and die in utero due to the same process that is causing the poor fetal growth. Tables 20.1 and 20.2 list causes of constitutionally small fetus and IUGR. Of note, we have placed viral illness and single-time teratogen exposure in the category of constitutionally small fetus, as there is no ongoing intrauterine insult that further endangers the pregnancy, and these pregnancies can be managed as constitutionally small.

An IUGR fetus will initially redirect the flow of oxygenated blood so as to protect the growth of critical organs (e.g., brain, heart) at the expense of the body corpus. Specifically, the resistance of the cerebral vasculature decreases, increasing blood flow and oxygen extraction. The brain continues to grow at normal, or near-normal rates, while the remainder of the body grows more slowly, leading to "asymmetrical" IUGR. This condition is also called head-sparing. Fetuses that are constitutionally small are not typically asymmetrical, and this finding is an important clue to the diagnosis of IUGR. Unfortunately, with continuing growth restriction, brain growth may ultimately slow, and thus the severely IUGR fetus may also be symmetrically small.

Decision 1: Management

How should this patient be followed?

A. Anatomy survey at 18 to 20 weeks, growth ultrasound every 4 to 8 weeks
B. Anatomy survey at 18 to 20 weeks, growth ultrasound every 2 weeks
C. Ultrasound for growth beginning at 34 weeks
D. Doppler of middle cerebral artery (MCA) weekly

The correct answer is A: Anatomy survey at 18 to 20 weeks and a growth ultrasound every 4 to 8 weeks. Growth scans are generally not performed more often than every 4 weeks as a screen, as the expected incremental growth is less than the expected variation in the measurements, meaning that growth scans every 2 weeks (Answer B) would not be expected to yield additional information. The prior fetus

TABLE 20.1

ETIOLOGIES OF CONSTITUTIONALLY SMALL FETUS

- Fetal ethnicity
- Fetal chromosomal anomaly
  - Fetuses with trisomy 18 average <2,000 g at term
  - Trisomy 13
  - Trisomy 21
- Fetal genetic disease
- Fetal teratogen exposure (single episode)
  - X irradiation
  - Viral illness

TABLE 20.2

ETIOLOGIES OF INTRAUTERINE GROWTH RESTRICTION (IUGR)

- Maternal vascular disease
  - Hypertension
  - Severe diabetes
- Maternal illness
  - Thrombophilia
  - Severe anemia
  - Renal disease
- Maternal undernutrition
- Maternal hypoxemia
  - Asthma
  - Cyanotic heart disease
- Maternal habits
  - Smoking
  - Alcohol abuse

was growth restricted at 35 weeks, meaning that delaying ultrasound evaluation of growth to 34 weeks (Answer C) may potentially miss the early stages of the condition. Doppler of the MCA (Answer D) has been used investigationally, but it is not a first-line study in the diagnosis of IUGR in clinical practice.

CASE CONTINUES

Ms. Gordo has a normal second trimester screen, and an anatomy survey at 20 weeks is unremarkable. Her blood pressure continues to average 145/80 mm Hg. At 24 weeks, she returns for an ultrasound for fetal growth; the fetal weight is in the 35th percentile, and all measurements are symmetric. She asks if she should be concerned that the weight is less than average.

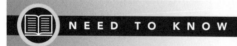

Fetal Weight Estimation by Ultrasound

Fetal weight is estimated at ultrasound by inserting fetal measurements into a formula. Most formulas use some or all of the following measures to estimate the fetal weight:

fetal biparietal diameter, head circumference, abdominal circumference, and femur length. There are a variety of published algorithms for calculating fetal weight (Table 20.3), and these may yield somewhat different weight estimates from the same basic measurements. Once the weight estimate is calculated, it is expressed as a percentile of the expected weight for gestational age. The percentile given depends on two additional issues:

1. The gestational age. In the present case, the patient is well dated based on a 12-week ultrasound. In other cases, this may not be true, and there is the concern that the original ultrasound may already reflect a fetus that is undergrown. In such a case, fetal asymmetry may provide a clue to IUGR. In other cases, it will be necessary to perform serial ultrasound and follow fetal growth. The expectation is that an IUGR fetus will continue to lag in growth and will become progressively smaller as compared with the mean.
2. The expected weights of fetuses or infants at different gestational ages in the population. The table chosen can greatly change the percentile assigned; for example, a common table uses data from Denver, where infants are significantly smaller than those born at sea level.

TABLE 20.3

FETAL WEIGHT CALCULATION ALGORITHMS. MANY OTHER PUBLICATIONS HAVE ALSO ADDRESSED THIS ISSUE, BUT THESE ARE AMONG THE MOST COMMONLY USED CALCULATIONS

1. Hadlock et al.　$Log_{10}BW = 1.5622 - 0.01080HC + 0.04680AC + 0.171FL + 0.00034HC^2 - 0.003685AC \times FL$
2. Ott et al.　$Log_{10}BW = 2.0660 + 0.04355HC + 0.05394AC - 0.0008582HC \times AC + 1.2594FL/AC$
3. Shepard et al.　$Log_{10}BW = -1.7492 + 0.166BPD + 0.046AC - 0.00246BPD \times AC$

All measurements are in centimeters.
AC, abdominal circumference; BPD, biparietal diameter; BW, birth weight (g); FL, femur length; HC, head circumference.
Adapted from Ott WJ. Sonographic diagnosis of fetal growth restriction. Clin Obstet Gynecol. 2006;49(2):295–307.

Optimally, fetal weight and weight percentile will be calculated using the same technique at every examination, so that valid comparisons can be made.

 CASE CONTINUES

You reassure Ms. Gordo that a 35th percentile fetus is within the normal range. You note that the fetal measurements are symmetrical, and that the amniotic fluid volume and placenta are normal. You continue to follow her for prenatal care, but note that the fundal height is difficult to assess due to her obesity. At 26 weeks, Ms. Gordo has a normal 50-g glucose screen for diabetes. At 28 weeks, Ms. Gordo returns for another ultrasound fetal weight estimate. At this time, the head measurements are consistent with 28 weeks, the femur is consistent with 27 weeks, and the abdomen with 26.5 weeks. The fetal weight is at the 20th percentile. You are suspicious that the fetal growth may be lagging, and schedule her for a repeat ultrasound in 3 weeks. At 31 weeks, the fetal weight is at the eighth percentile, and the fetus is asymmetric, with the head having a size of 30 weeks and the abdomen at 27 weeks. A biophysical profile (BPP) performed at the time of ultrasound is 8/8 (no nonstress test [NST] performed).

 Decision 2: Management

What are the appropriate components of monitoring in this patient?

A. NST once or twice a week
B. BPP three times weekly
C. Uterine artery Doppler weekly
D. Umbilical artery (UA) Doppler daily

The best answer is A: NST once or twice a week. With the diagnosis of IUGR, the fetus is at risk from the intrauterine environment, and fetal testing is indicated to evaluate whether the fetus is in imminent danger of intrauterine death. The most common testing modality is the NST, which can be performed once or twice a week. One may include a BPP or, more commonly, an amniotic fluid volume assessment on a weekly basis. With a normal NST and/or BPP, the risk of fetal death is low in the next several days. A daily NST (Answer A) or thrice weekly BPP (Answer B) would not be indicated. Uterine artery Doppler values (Answer C) may be abnormal in IUGR, but there is presently no protocol incorporating uterine artery Doppler for the management of the IUGR pregnancy. UA Doppler may be of additional value, although it would not be performed daily.

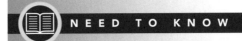

Fetal Testing

In general, the object of antenatal fetal testing is to reassure the practitioner that the fetus is unlikely to die in utero from chronic causes in the ensuing 5 to 7 days. Commonly used methods of antenatal testing include the NST, BPP, modified BPP, and contraction stress test (Table 20.4).

In a fetus with IUGR, Doppler interrogation of fetal vessels can also help to predict the fetal course and the onset of fetal hypoxic compromise (Table 20.5). Research has indicated that alterations in the diastolic flow in the UA are among the first Doppler findings; a decrease in umbilical arterial diastolic flow would indicate an increase in resistance in the placenta. The most concerning finding is the presence of absence or reversal of flow in the UA in diastole. Head-sparing can be demonstrated by an increase in diastolic flow in the MCA, indicating reduced resistance in the cerebral circulation. Venous findings occur later in the course of IUGR; the most commonly used venous study is Doppler of the ductus venosus (DV). The DV is where the umbilical vein connects to the inferior vena cava, and DV pressures reflect pressures in the right atrium. A concerning finding is absence or reversal of flow in the DV at the end of diastole, indicating poor cardiac compliance. The combination of Doppler findings and traditional fetal testing has been used to determine the time of delivery in the IUGR fetus, so as to avoid fetal death in utero. Unfortunately, there remains uncertainty as to the optimal timing of delivery so as to achieve the best long-term outcome in the IUGR fetus. Recent work makes it clear that the IUGR fetus remains at life-long risk for postnatal diseases such as obesity, diabetes, and hypertension, as a result of gestational programming. Other work suggests that there may be neurologic consequences associated with Doppler abnormalities that are not preterminal. As the fetal testing modalities currently available do not address long-term morbidity, the timing of delivery remains a problem even in fetuses with reassuring testing.

 CASE CONTINUES

You elect to follow Ms. Gordo using a regimen of twice weekly modified BPP and once weekly UA and DV Doppler values. At 33 weeks of gestation, you are called by the antenatal testing unit, because the UA Doppler has revealed absent end-diastolic flow for the first time. Her NST is nonreactive and her BPP is 6 of 10, with reduced amniotic fluid volume.

TABLE 20.4
FETAL TESTING MODALITIES

Test	Method	Interpretation	False-Negative Rate[a]
Nonstress test (NST)	Fetal heart rate monitored	Reactive (normal) if there are two fetal heart rate accelerations of 15 bpm lasting 15 seconds in 20 minutes	1.9/1,000
Biophysical profile (BPP)	NST performed and fetal ultrasound. Two points assigned for achieving five criteria in 30 minutes (10 possible points): 1. Reactive NST 2. Normal amniotic fluid index (AFI) >5 cm or single pocket >2 cm 3. Fetal breathing: an episode of 30 seconds. 4. Fetal movements: three or more 5. Fetal tone: flexion/extension of an extremity or opening/closing of hand	Normal: 8–10 with normal fluid Equivocal: 6–8 Abnormal: <6	0.8/1,000
Modified BPP	NST plus amniotic fluid assessment		0.8/1,000
Contraction stress test (CST)	Fetal heart rate monitored during natural or induced contractions (three in 10 minutes)	Positive (abnormal) if there are late decelerations after >50% of contractions	0.3/1,000

[a]False-negative rate is the risk of stillbirth within 1 week of a normal test, excluding lethal congenital anomalies and nonpredictable causes of stillbirth.

TABLE 20.5

MANAGEMENT OF IUGR USING FETAL TESTING AND DOPPLER INDICES. THIS MANAGEMENT SCHEME IS BASED ON THE FULL BPP AND THE PERFORMANCE OF FETAL ARTERIAL AND VENOUS DOPPLER'S. THIS REPRESENTS THE MOST AGGRESSIVE USE OF DOPPLER TECHNOLOGY IN THE MANAGEMENT OF IUGR

Finding	Interpretation	Action
Blood Flow Redistribution Abnormal UA indices Low MCA, normal veins BPP ≥8/10, AFV normal	Hypoxemia possible, asphyxia rare Increased risk for interapartum distress	Deliver for obstetric or maternal factors only, weekly Doppler BPP 2 times/week
Significant Blood Flow Redistribution UA A/REDV, normal veins BPS ≥6/10, oligohydramnios	Hypoxemia common, acidemia or asphyxia possible Onset of fetal compromise	>34 wk: deliver <32 wk: consider antenatal steroids frequent
Fetal Compromise Increased DV pulsatility BPP ≥6/10, oligohydramnios	Hypoxemia common, acidemia or asphyxia likely	>32 wk: deliver <32 wk: admit, steroids, individualize testing
Fetal Decompensation Compromise by above criteria Absent or reversed DV a-wave, pulsatile UV BPP <6/10, oligohydramnios	Cardiovascular instability, metabolic compromise, stillbirth imminent, high perinatal mortality irrespective of intervention	Deliver at tertiary care center with the highest level of NICU care

A/REDV, absent/ reversed end-diastolic velocity; BPP, biophysical profile DV, ductus venosus; MCA, middle cerebral artery; NICU, neonatal intensive care unit; UA, umbilical artery; UV, umbilical vein.
Adapted from Baschat AA. Fetal growth restriction – from observation to intervention. J Perinat Med. 2010;38(3):239–46.

Decision 3: Management

What is the appropriate management of absent end-diastolic flow in the UA?

- **A.** Emergent cesarean delivery
- **B.** Immediate induction of labor
- **C.** Amniocentesis, delivery if mature
- **D.** Immediate maternal glucocorticoid therapy, delivery after 48 hours

The correct answer is D: Immediate maternal glucocorticoid therapy, delivery after 48 hours. There is little scientific evidence to guide management in this case, but the preponderance of expert opinion favors option D. Others would opt for immediate delivery (Answer B), arguing that there is little evidence for a benefit of steroids in IUGR. The scenario as presented does not justify immediate cesarean delivery (Answer A), and delaying delivery to pulmonary maturity (Answer C) is outside of the usual recommendations, given the equivocal fetal testing and may involve an increased risk of intrauterine fetal demise.

CASE CONCLUSION

You administer betamethasone and maintain Ms. Gordo on fetal heart rate monitoring for the next 48 hours. You then attempt to induce labor; however, the fetus does not tolerate uterine contractions, and you perform a cesarean delivery of a 1,780-g male infant with Apgar score of 6/8 at 1 and 5 minutes. Ms. Gordo does well and is discharged on the fourth postpartum day. Her son remains in the special care nursery for 2 weeks due to poor feeding efforts but is eventually discharged home in good condition.

SUGGESTED READINGS

Baschat AA. Doppler application in the delivery timing of the preterm growth-restricted fetus: another step in the right direction. Ultrasound Obstet Gynecol. 2004;23(2):111–8.

Baschat AA. Fetal growth restriction – from observation to intervention. J Perinat Med. 2010;38(3):239–46.

Grivell RM, Wong L, Bhatia V. Regimens of fetal surveillance for impaired fetal growth. Cochrane Database Syst Rev. 2009;(1): CD007113.

Hoffman C, Galan HL. Assessing the 'at-risk' fetus: Doppler ultrasound. Curr Opin Obstet Gynecol. 2009;21(2):161–6.

Mozurkewich E, Chilimigras J, Koepke E, Keeton K, King VJ. Indications for induction of labour: a best-evidence review. BJOG. 2009;116(5):626–36.

Manning FA. Antepartum fetal testing: a critical appraisal. Curr Opin Obstet Gynecol. 2009;21(4):348–52.

Ott WJ. Sonographic diagnosis of fetal growth restriction. Clin Obstet Gynecol. 2006;49(2):295–307.

Torrance HL, Derks JB, Scherjon SA, Wijnberger LD, Visser GH. Is antenatal steroid treatment effective in preterm IUGR fetuses? Acta Obstet Gynecol Scand. 2009;88(10):1068–73.

Macrosomia

Marquis Jessie

CASE PRESENTATION

Ms. Hernandez, a 30-year-old Hispanic G2 P1 presents for her first prenatal visit. By her last menstrual period she is 15 weeks pregnant. She reports no problems in this pregnancy up to this point. She further reports no significant medical history and no prior surgeries. She does state that in the past 18 months she has successfully participated in a weight loss program and has lost 75 lbs. In her last pregnancy she was diagnosed with gestational diabetes. In that pregnancy, she had a vaginal delivery of a 4,600-g infant, which was a difficult delivery that included a tear into her rectum.

On physical examination, she is an obese woman in no distress. Her blood pressure is 130/60 mm Hg, and her pulse is 95 bpm. Her height is 62 inches and her weight is 240 lb; her current body mass index (BMI) is 44. Her physical examination is unremarkable. Her fundal height is difficult to assess, but an ultrasound is consistent with her last period. She asks if this baby will also be large.

 NEED TO KNOW

Fetal Macrosomia

In relation to macrosomia, there are three terms/criteria that are relevant. Macrosomia is not formally defined, although most clinicians refer to a macrosomic infant as growth of a fetus beyond 4,000 or 4,500 g, irrespective of gestational age. Large for gestational age refers to a fetus with an estimated fetal weight above the 90th percentile for gestational age. The third criterion is the estimated fetal weight at which an elective cesarean delivery should be offered to the patient. As defined by the American Congress of Obstetricians and Gynecologists (ACOG), this is 4,500 g for a gestational diabetics and 5,000 g for nondiabetics.

Fetal macrosomia is associated with an increase in fetal and maternal morbidities related to difficult delivery. For the mother, delivery of a macrosomic fetus increases the risk of cesarean delivery, perineal tears, sphincter injuries,

and postpartum hemorrhage. The fetus is at increased risk of a brachial plexus injury and clavicular fracture, as well as low Apgar scores and neonatal intensive care unit admission. Although a 4,000-g fetus is at increased risk of delivery complications, the risk increases significantly above 4,500 g (Table 21.1). Despite the increased risk of complications above 4,500 g, the number of cesarean deliveries that would need to be performed to prevent one fetal brachial plexus injury does not justify operative delivery until 5,000 g. In addition to immediate complications due to birth trauma, macrosomic infants are at risk for long-term health problems. Macrosomic infants are more likely to develop diabetes, obesity, and metabolic syndrome, especially if macrosomia is associated with maternal diabetes.

Macrosomia can be attributed to three causes: (1) an increased intrinsic growth potential of the fetus, accounting for 50% to 60% of cases, (2) increased fetal growth due to maternal metabolic derangements (most commonly diabetes), accounting for 35% to 40% of cases, and (3) certain genetic diseases that are rare.

Intrinsic growth potential, the most common reason cited for macrosomia, is partially genetically defined, as the rate of macrosomia varies depending on the population studied. The rate (defined as birth weight >4,000 g) is 4% in Japanese, 11% in Latinas, and 20% in Scandinavians and Samoans.

The most common genetic cause of macrosomia is Beckwith-Weidemann syndrome (BWS), occurring in 1:12,000 births. In addition to large fetal size, BWS is associated with omphalocele, macroglossia, and an increased risk for neoplasms.

Fetal macrosomia due to maternal metabolic derangement is of special interest both because it is a potentially avoidable cause of macrosomia and because the increased fetal growth may be nonsymmetrical. Specifically, infants of diabetic mothers with poor glycemic control may experience disproportionate trunk growth with chest/head and shoulder/head ratios larger than that in infants of normoglycemic mothers. This disproportionate growth of the abdomen and thorax of the poorly controlled diabetic fetus forms the basis for the increased incidence of shoulder dystocia in infants born to diabetic mothers. Insulin levels are predictive of fetal size: amniotic fluid and cord

TABLE 21.1

RATE OF BIRTH INJURY WITH INCREASING FETAL MACROSOMIA

Risk Factor	Odds Ratio	Confidence Limits[a]	
		Lower	Upper
Diabetes	3.19	1.62	6.27
Cesarean delivery	0.05	0.01	0.20
Birth weight (g)[b]			
≥4,000 vs. <4,000	9.56	6.15	14.86
≥4,500 vs. <4,500	17.94	10.29	31.28
≥5,000 vs. <5,000	45.15	15.81	128.75

[a]95% confidence intervals.
[b]Multivariate analyses examining separately three birth-weight thresholds as risk factors for brachial plexus injury.
Adapted from Wikström I, Axelsson O, Bergström R, Meirik O. Traumatic injury in large-for-date infants. Acta Obstet Gynecol Scand. 1988;67(3):259–64.

blood insulin and C-peptide levels in diabetic mothers at term correlate directly with neonatal fat mass, and umbilical cord insulin levels at delivery correlate directly with fetal weight. Even in the absence of overt hyperglycemia, increased maternal plasma insulin (caused by maternal insulin resistance) is associated with an increased risk of fetal macrosomia. In addition to insulin, insulin-like growth factor (IGF) has been shown to be associated with fetal overgrowth. Cord serum IGF I and II levels in macrosomic neonates of diabetic mothers have been reported to be seven times that of nonmacrosomic infants of nondiabetic mothers.

In addition to glucose and insulin, maternal serum lipids have been linked to fetal macrosomia. In fact, midtrimester triglyceride levels have been shown to be more predictive of macrosomia than measures of glucose tolerance. Triglyceride levels have also been shown to correlate with birth weight.

Finally, apparent macrosomia may be due to an erroneous estimate of the fetal weight. This is not a trivial matter, as an erroneous diagnosis of macrosomia in itself is associated with an increased rate of cesarean delivery. The accuracy of fetal weight estimation is discussed below.

 Decision 1: Counseling

Given this history, what factor confers the highest risk for macrosomia in the current pregnancy?

A. Obesity
B. Prior gestational diabetes
C. Prior macrosomic fetus
D. Maternal age

TABLE 21.2

INSTITUTE OF MEDICINE GUIDELINES FOR WEIGHT GAIN IN PREGNANCY

Initial Body Mass Index	IOM Recommended Weight Gain, lb
<19.8 (underweight)	28–40
19.8–26.0 (normal)	25–35
26.1–29.0 (overweight)	15–25
>29.0 (obese)	At least 15

The correct answer is C: A prior macrosomic fetus. The recurrence rate for fetal macrosomia is up to 32%, or about 10 times the background rate. Maternal weight (Answer A): both prepregnancy obesity and excessive weight gain during pregnancy are risk factors for macrosomia. The incidence of macrosomia is triple that of normal-weight mothers when the maternal prepregnancy BMI is more than 40. In addition, the risk of macrosomia is increased by onefold to twofold if the mother gained excessive weight during pregnancy, regardless of her prepregnancy BMI. Table 21.2 shows the Institute of Medicine's recommendations for optimal weight gains based on prepregnancy BMI. Gestational diabetes (Answer B) may recur in this patient and may be associated with increased fetal growth and macrosomia, but optimal treatment of the diabetes can reduce this risk (from about 14%–6% in one study). Although several studies have linked maternal age (Answer D) to an increased risk of macrosomia, much of the data is confounded by variables such as obesity and a higher incidence of diabetes (both pregestational and gestational diabetes). One of the largest studies of fetal macrosomia and associated shoulder dystocia did not find a correlation between maternal age and fetal birth weight when corrected for other variables such as diabetes and maternal obesity.

As noted above, an increased risk of macrosomia (whether defined as 4,000 or 4,500 g) does not justify an elective cesarean delivery, unless the ACOG fetal weight criteria are met.

 CASE CONTINUES

At Ms. Hernandez' initial intake visit, prenatal labs are performed, including a 1-hour glucose challenge test because of her previous prenatal history and current risk factors for gestational diabetes. The blood glucose level is 128 mg/dL after a 50-g glucose load, which is interpreted as normal. Her second trimester serum screen predicts a low risk for fetal Down syndrome, and a 20-week fetal anatomy survey is unremarkable.

Decision 2: Follow-up

Given this patient's history and prenatal course, how would you go about monitoring her fetal growth?

A. Fundal height assessment at each visit
B. Ultrasound for fetal growth at 2-week intervals
C. Maternal glucose monitoring fasting and postprandial
D. Maternal weight gain monitoring

The correct answer is A: Fundal height assessment at each visit. Fundal height assessment, in conjunction with palpation of the fetus is an inexpensive and reasonably accurate method of assessing fetal growth. Serial ultrasound (Answer B) is also a reasonable choice for following fetal growth, but it would not be performed every 2 weeks. In the absence of maternal diabetes, frequent maternal blood glucose monitoring (Answer C) is not useful. Although excessive maternal weight gain (Answer D) may increase the risk of macrosomia, monitoring maternal weight is not an effective method of assessing fetal weight gain.

CASE CONTINUES

Ms. Hernandez' repeat glucose challenge test at 25 weeks remains negative. Her follow-up growth scans at 28 and 32 weeks reveal an infant that is in the 85th and 91st percentile for estimated fetal weight, respectively. She has gained 28 lb throughout the pregnancy, and by 37 weeks, clinical estimation of her baby's weight is 4,200 g.

Decision 3: Delivery planning

Given this patient's history and prenatal course, what is the best management?

A. Immediate cesarean delivery
B. Immediate induction of labor
C. Cesarean delivery at 39 weeks
D. Allow the patient to go into spontaneous labor

The correct answer here is D: Allow the patient to go into labor. At this point (37 weeks), there is no intervention that can be shown to improve outcome when compared with allowing the natural processes of labor and delivery to occur. Immediate cesarean delivery (Answer A) at 37 weeks would not be appropriate in any pregnancy without an indication for shortening the pregnancy, which does not exist in this case. Induction of labor (Answer B)

for a large fetus with "impending" macrosomia has been studied previously, with several studies concluding that labor induction to avoid macrosomia does not appear to reduce the cesarean delivery rate. In some studies, the cesarean delivery rate was actually increased. Cesarean delivery at 39 weeks (Answer C) is not currently indicated. With an estimated fetal weight of 4,200 g at 37 weeks, one would expect a fetal weight of 4,600 to 4,700 g at 39 weeks, a value that would not indicate operative delivery. Issues that would indicate a planned cesarean delivery would include the following:

■ An estimated fetal weight above 5,000 g. As discussed above, ACOG recommends that women be offered an elective cesarean delivery when the fetal size exceeds 5,000 g. This recommendation reflects the increase in fetal injuries with this fetal size, as well as the risk of indicated cesarean delivery should labor be attempted. Given the increase in maternal and fetal morbidity when cesarean follows labor, planned cesarean may be the safest delivery option for many of these patients. When the mother has diabetes, a threshold of 4,500 g is utilized because of the increase in shoulder dystocia associated with the diabetic fetal body habitus.

■ A past history of rectal tear or maternal procedures for urinary or fecal incontinence. A patient with a rectal tear at a previous delivery is at increased risk of a recurrence of a rectal tear at a subsequent vaginal delivery. In addition, pregnancy and vaginal delivery may be associated with failure of a previous incontinence procedure. In a patient with a prior procedure who is currently continent, a planned cesarean delivery might be considered to reduce the risk of incontinence after pregnancy.

■ A history of severe shoulder dystocia in the prior pregnancy. The risk of shoulder dystocia is increased markedly when the mother has a history of a prior shoulder dystocia. Considerations for vaginal versus cesarean delivery are dependent upon the estimated fetal weight in the current pregnancy.

■ Maternal request

CASE CONTINUES

You discuss the various delivery options with Ms. Hernandez after reviewing the records of her previous delivery. Her previous delivery was remarkable for delivery of a 4,650-g male infant vaginally. There was a mild shoulder dystocia documented, but the Apgar score was 7 and 9 at 1 and 5 minutes. A partial third-degree tear was repaired in layers. Ms. Hernandez states that her son is now 3 years old and developing normally; he remains large for his age. She feels that the current fetus is smaller than her son, and she denies any symptoms of fecal or urinary incontinence. After discussion, you and Ms. Hernandez elect to await spontaneous labor, with the plan that you will consider labor induction if she has not delivered by 41 weeks.

At 39 weeks and 4 days, Ms. Hernandez arrives in labor and delivery complaining of regular uterine contractions. She is checked by the nurse, who finds that she is 4 cm dilated and 80% effaced, with the vertex at −1 station. Upon your arrival, your estimated fetal weight is 4,800 g.

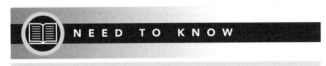

NEED TO KNOW

Fetal Weight Estimation in the Large Fetus

In the case of a macrosomic fetus, decisions about the management of labor and route of delivery are strongly affected by the estimated fetal weight. This is the reason that an erroneous diagnosis of fetal macrosomia can lead to an increase in the cesarean delivery rate. Fetal weight can be estimated by palpation of the fetus (Fig. 21.1) or by ultrasound. Manual palpation can also be used to assess fetal presentation and station. Ultrasound measurements can be used to assess the fetal weight using a variety of published algorithms (see Chapter 23, IUGR). Finally, the mother can be asked her opinion about the weight of her fetus. Somewhat surprisingly, maternal perception may have similar accuracy, although all of these methods have substantial error (Table 21.3).

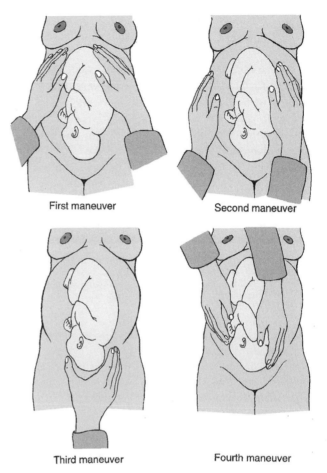

Figure 21.1 Leopold's maneuvers. First maneuver: assess the part in the fundus (vertex or breech). Second maneuver: assess the location of the fetal spine. Third maneuver: assess engagement of the presenting part. Fourth maneuver: assess attitude of the fetal head. (LifeART (and/or) MediClip image copyright 2008 Wolters Kluwer Health, Inc., Lippincott Williams Wilkins. All rights reserved.)

TABLE 21.3

THE PERFORMANCE OF VARIOUS METHODS OF FETAL WEIGHT ESTIMATION IS SIMILAR IN PREDICTING BIRTH WEIGHT >4,000 G. NOT SHOWN HERE: ALL METHODS SYSTEMATICALLY UNDERESTIMATED FETAL WEIGHTS BY 200 TO 470 G

Method	Sensitivity (%)	Specificity (%)	Positive Predictive Value (%)	Negative Predictive Value (%)
MD palpation	16	99	80	95
Mother	29	96	64	96
US: Shepherd	48	92	56	99
US: Hadlock	40	94	59	100

MD palpation, EFW by palpation by the attending physician; Mother, EFW by the pregnant woman; US, ultrasound EFW; Shepherd, Shepherd's algorithm using AC and BPD; Hadlock, Hadlock's algorithm using AC and FL.
Adapted from Peregrine E, O'brien P, Jauniaux E. Clinical and ultrasound estimation of birth weight prior to induction of labor at term. Ultrasound Obstet Gynecol. 2007;29(3):304–9.

CASE CONCLUSION

Ms. Hernandez tells you that this baby feels about the same size as her last one. Her vaginal examination is 7 cm dilated, with the fetal vertex at +1 station. She progresses in labor and delivers vaginally after a 40-minute second stage, with no perineal laceration. Her baby is a girl weighing 4,950 g, with Apgar score of 8 and 9 at 1 and 5 minutes. Mother and baby do well and are discharged home on the second day after the delivery.

SUGGESTED READINGS

ACOG Committee on Practice Bulletins–Obstetrics. ACOG practice bulletin #22, Fetal Macrosomia Nov 2000.

De Boo HA, Harding JE. The developmental origins of adult disease (Barker) hypothesis. Aust N Z J Obstet Gynaecol. 2006;46(1):4–14.

Henriksen T. The macrosomic fetus: a challenge in current obstetrics. Acta Obstet Gynecol Scand. 2008;87(2):134–45.

Landon MB, Spong CY, Thom E, et al. A multicenter, randomized trial of treatment for mild gestational diabetes. N Engl J Med. 2009; 361(14):1339–48.

Lipscomb KR, Gregory K, Shaw K. The outcome of macrosomic infants weighing at least 4500 grams: Los Angeles county + University of Southern California experience. Obstet Gynecol. 1995;85: 558–64.

Lowder JL, Burrows LJ, Krohn MA, Weber AM. Risk factors for primary and subsequent anal sphincter lacerations: a comparison of cohorts by parity and prior mode of delivery. Am J Obstet Gynecol. 2007;196(4):344.e1–5.

Peregrine E, O'Brien P, Jauniaux E. Clinical and ultrasound estimation of birth weight prior to induction of labor at term. Ultrasound Obstet Gynecol. 2007;29(3):304–9.

Sacks DA. Etiology, detection, and management of fetal macrosomia in pregnancies complicated by diabetes mellitus. Clin Obstet Gynecol. 2007;50(4):980–9.

Wikström I, Axelsson O, Bergström R, Meirik O. Traumatic injury in large-for-date infants. Acta Obstet Gynecol Scand. 1988;67(3): 259–64.

Oligohydramnios

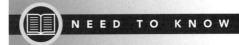

Michael G. Ross   Marie H. Beall

CASE PRESENTATION

The nurse on labor and delivery calls you to evaluate Mrs. Newton, a 42-year-old G2 P1 patient of your group who is at 26 weeks of gestation by a first trimester ultrasound. She has come in to labor and delivery with a complaint of increased vaginal discharge and is worried that she may have ruptured her membranes.

The patient's prenatal records are available. You learn that in her previous pregnancy she delivered at 32 weeks. The infant was moderately growth restricted, with a fetal weight in the ninth percentile. She reports that she ruptured her membranes in that pregnancy and went to hospital, where the baby died soon after delivery. She does not know the baby's diagnosis. Mrs. Newton denies other significant past medical history, and specifically denies any history of hypertension or lupus. This pregnancy has been uneventful. Her prenatal labs and Down syndrome screening results have been normal. She had a first trimester dating ultrasound that agreed with her last menstrual period, and at 20 weeks she was seen by the maternal–fetal medicine (MFM) specialist. The MFM's ultrasound revealed a normally grown fetus with no observed anomalies. The MFM recommended that Mrs. Newton be tested for antiphospholipid syndrome and that she be followed with ultrasounds for fetal growth every 6 weeks and with weekly biophysical profiles (BPPs) beginning at 26 weeks. Testing for antiphospholipid syndrome has not yet been done, and the first BPP is scheduled for 2 days from now.

On physical examination, the patient is a thin, anxious white female. Her fundal height is 22 cm; her fundus is not tender, and there is no evidence of contractions. Fetal heart tones are heard at 145 bpm; they are nonreactive with normal variability and no decelerations are seen. Clinically, you suspect that the amniotic fluid volume may be decreased. You ask for an ultrasound to evaluate the amniotic fluid volume.

Definition of Oligohydramnios

Oligohydramnios is an amniotic fluid volume that is less than normal. The expected amount of amniotic fluid varies during and between pregnancies, making the absolute definition of this problematic; however, an amniotic fluid volume of <250 to 300 cc appears to be abnormal at any time during the second half of human pregnancy (Fig. 22.1). Detecting low amniotic fluid volumes is also problematic. In clinical practice, ultrasound measurement of amniotic fluid pockets is commonly used as an estimate of amniotic fluid volume. A pregnancy lacking a single deepest pocket of 2 cm (Fig. 22.2), or one with an amniotic fluid index (AFI) <5 cm (Fig. 22.3), is deemed to demonstrate oligohydramnios. Unfortunately, two-dimensional estimates of amniotic fluid volume correlate poorly with actual volume, and in particular the measurements above demonstrate poor specificity for the diagnosis of oligohydramnios. When the two measures were compared, a meta-analysis suggested that the single deepest pocket method yields a similar perinatal outcome with increased specificity for the diagnosis of oligohydramnios when compared with AFI. Some authors have also suggested that the subjective finding of diminished amniotic fluid is at least as accurate as the various measurement scenarios.

Decision 1: Diagnosis

What is the most likely etiology for Mrs. Newton's oligohydramnios?

A. Fetal anomaly
B. Preterm premature rupture of the membranes (PPROM)
C. Placental abruption
D. Reduced fetal growth

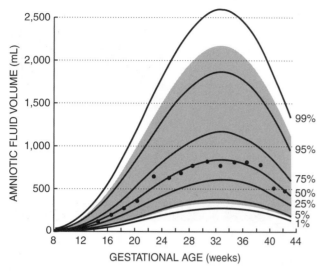

Figure 22.1 Normal amniotic fluid volume in human pregnancy. (Used with permission from: Brace RA, Wolf EJ. Normal amniotic fluid volume changes throughout pregnancy. Am J Obstet Gynecol. 1989 Aug;161(2):382–8.)

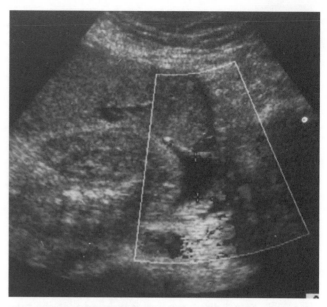

Figure 22.2 Single deepest pocket of amniotic fluid of 1.8 cm, demonstrating oligohydramnios. (Reproduced with permission from http://www.iame.com/learning/olig/oligi_images/cmeoli_fig4.jpg.)

The correct answer is B: PPROM. Although a fetal anomaly may be an etiology for oligohydramnios, it is important to remember that Mrs. Newton had a normal ultrasound, including a normal amniotic fluid assessment, at 20 weeks, reducing the likelihood of a fetal anomaly. In general, fetal anomalies are a common cause of oligohydramnios in the second trimester, while preterm rupture of the membranes is a much more likely diagnosis when oligohydramnios is found in the third trimester. Although, in theory, placental abruption may disrupt placental function sufficiently to cause oligohydramnios, this is very unlikely, and the abruption per se is not a cause. Similarly, reduced fetal growth may be a marker of the same condition that also leads to oligohydramnios, but fetal growth disturbances by themselves, are not a cause of oligohydramnios.

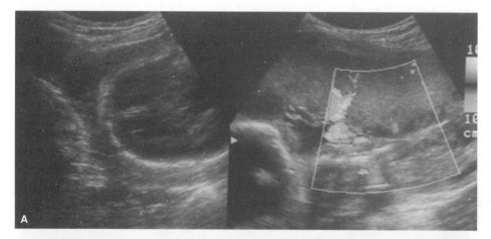

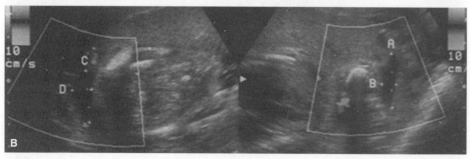

Figure 22.3 Four-quadrant AFI of 4.2 cm, demonstrating oligohydramnios. (Reproduced with permission from http://www.iame.com/learning/olig/oligi_images/cmeoli_fig6at.jpg.)

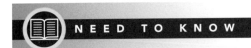

NEED TO KNOW

Pathophysiology of Oligohydramnios

By far the most common cause of decreased amniotic fluid volume in the third trimester is leakage of fluid from the vagina. PPROM occurs in about 3% of pregnancies, and is implicated in one-third of preterm births. Premature rupture of the membranes is covered in Chapter 28. In the absence of membrane rupture, oligohydramnios is due to a defect in the normal production and resorption of amniotic fluid. Amniotic fluid dynamics are described in Chapter 23 (polyhydramnios). Briefly, amniotic fluid in the second half of pregnancy is formed by the fetal kidneys and lungs and is returned to the fetal circulation by fetal swallowing and by direct absorption across the amnion. Therefore, oligohydramnios that is not due to fluid loss is most often due to a defect in fetal urine production. There are no proven cases in which oligohydramnios results from increased fetal absorption of fluid, and absence of fetal lung fluid leads to a minor amniotic fluid deficit.

Fetal urine may be reduced because of abnormal production or abnormal excretion. One cause of fetal oliguria is reduced blood flow to the kidney. This is thought to be the mechanism of oligohydramnios associated with growth restriction and poor placental function. A number of authors have described alterations in fetal renal artery flow associated with oligohydramnios, both preterm and postterm, suggesting that with marginal placental function, fetal blood flow is redirected to vital organs, including the brain. The fetal kidneys are less well perfused, reducing fetal urine volume. The donor twin in the setting of twin–twin transfusion will also demonstrate oligohydramnios due to poor renal perfusion. Finally, maternal dehydration may be associated with oligohydramnios probably due to reduced flow of water from the maternal to the fetal compartment leading to fetal dehydration and reduced renal blood flow.

Fetal renal function may also be impaired as a consequence of renal disease. Maternal use of angiotensin-converting enzyme inhibitors has been associated with fetal renal damage, including renal failure. Infantile polycystic kidney disease is an autosomally inherited disease (usually recessive) characterized by impaired function of the fetal kidneys and oligohydramnios. The pregnancy may also be complicated by fetal renal agenesis, which is associated with profound oligohydramnios. Renal agenesis is occasionally found with many chromosomal abnormalities, and with a variety of other syndromes, as well as an isolated finding. There are a very large number of heritable conditions that may be a cause of absent kidneys or impaired renal function; some of these are listed in Tables 22.1 and 22.2.

TABLE 22.1

SOME COMMON GENETIC SYNDROMES ASSOCIATED WITH UNILATERAL OR BILATERAL RENAL AGENESIS

Syndrome	Other Anomalies	Gene
Autosomal Dominant		
EEC syndrome	Ectrodactyly, ectodermal dysplasia, cleft palate	P63
Pallister–Hall syndrome	Imperforate anus, mesaxial polydactyly, hypothalamic hamartoma	GLI3
Renal coloboma syndrome	Myopia, nystagmus, optic nerve coloboma	PAX2
Autosomal Recessive		
Antley–Bixler syndrome	Craniosynostosis, bowing of ulna and femur, vertebral anomalies, thin ribs, ambiguous genitalia	FGFR2
Fryns syndrome	Diaphragmatic hernia, lung hypoplasia, cleft lip and palate, distal limb hypoplasia	Unknown
Rokitansky sequence	Vaginal atresia, rudimentary uterus	Unknown
Smith–Lemli–Opitz syndrome	Toe syndactyly, growth retardation, cardiac and cerebral malformations, genital anomalies	DHCR7
X-linked		
Kallmann syndrome	Hypogonadotropic hypogonadism, anosmia	KAL1
Sporadic/Unknown		
Caudal regression syndrome	Imperforate anus, sacral agenesis, CNS anomalies	Maternal diabetes
Goldenhar (oculoauriculovertebral) syndrome	Facial asymmetry, microphthalmia, ear anomalies, heart defect, cervical vertebral defect	Unknown
MURCS association	Uterus hypoplasia, cervical vertebral anomalies, upper limb anomalies	Unknown
VATER association	Vertebral defects, radial ray defects, heart defects, esophageal/anal atresia	Unknown

Modified from: Deshpande C, Hennekam RC. Genetic syndromes and prenatally detected renal anomalies. Semin Fetal Neonatal Med. 2008;13(3):171–80.

TABLE 22.2

GENETIC SYNDROMES PRESENTING AS CYSTIC KIDNEYS

Diagnosis	Associated Features on Scan	Gene(s)
Ellis—Van Creveld syndrome	Nuchal edema, short ribs, polydactyly, cardiac defects	EVC, EVC2
Jeune syndrome	Short ribs, short limbs, characteristic iliac spur	IFT80
Joubert syndrome	Cerebellar vermis aplasia	CEP290, RPGRIP1 L, NPH1, NPH2, MKS3
Meckel–Gruber syndrome	Posterior encephalocele, postaxial polydactyly	CEP290, MKS1, MKS3
Orofaciodigital syndromes	Cleft lip, postaxial polydactyly, cerebellar vermis aplasia	OFD1 (X-linked), others unknown
Smith–Lemli–Opitz syndrome	Microcephaly, cleft palate, cardiac, CNS, and genital anomalies	DHCR7
Zellweger syndrome	Nuchal edema, fetal hypokinesia	PEX

Modified from: Deshpande C, Hennekam RC. Genetic syndromes and prenatally detected renal anomalies. Semin Fetal Neonatal Med. 2008;13(3):171–80.

Finally, reduced amniotic fluid volume may be a consequence of a defect in urine excretion due to a blockage in the fetal urinary tract preventing fetal urine from entering the amniotic sac. Fetal urinary obstructions may occur at various points in the urinary tract with the most common sites described in Table 22.3.

Absence of the kidneys can be diagnosed on ultrasound in which absence of both the kidneys and the renal arteries are noted (Fig. 22.4). Other lesions, including multicystic dysplastic kidneys and obstructions in the urinary tract downstream from the kidney, are also amenable to ultrasound diagnosis. Amniocentesis for fetal karyotype may be helpful in diagnosis, especially in the fetus with other anomalies. When there is no amniotic fluid, fetal karyotype may be obtained from a placental biopsy. In some cases, transabdominal amnioinfusion, or injecting sterile fluid, usually lactated Ringer's solution, into the amniotic cavity may assist in visualizing the fetus.

There are few treatments available for oligohydramnios. Maternal hydration with hypotonic solution has been shown to increase amniotic fluid volume in randomized controlled trials. This intervention is unlikely to have an effect when there is fetal renal agenesis or a total urinary obstruction. All other treatments of oligohydramnios in utero are unproven. There have been a number of reports of the use of vesicoamniotic shunts in fetuses with bladder outlet obstructions, with limited success.

In addition, some authors have described repeated amnioinfusion in pregnancies with severe second trimester oligohydramnios due to premature rupture of the membranes or urinary malformations, with fetal survival. Both of these in utero treatments may be effective in reducing the risk of fetal pulmonary hypoplasia. However, both have significant risks of fetal harm, preterm labor, and infection. These interventions should be used only after a thorough discussion of the risks and benefits.

 CASE CONTINUES

An ultrasound is performed and reveals a single intrauterine gestation in the vertex presentation. Fetal growth appears to be normal. A small fetal bladder and two fetal kidneys are seen. The placenta is posterior and grade 1 to 2. The AFI is 4 cm, and the BPP is 6/8 (two points lost for the low AFI).

You return to reevaluate Mrs. Newton. She is now lying in bed and appears comfortable. She is afebrile, her blood pressure is 90/60 mm Hg, and pulse is 100 bpm. She remains anxious about the condition of her baby and expresses a fear that she has ruptured her membranes and that this pregnancy will "end up like the last one." She reports no current vaginal leakage, and no abdominal pain. She does report pain in her knees, which she has had off and on for years.

TABLE 22.3

FETAL URINARY OBSTRUCTIONS

Site	Incidence	Inheritance
Uteropelvic junction	1–5/1,000 (male:female 4:1)	Sporadic
Uterovesicle junction	1:5,000 (10%–20% bilateral)	Sporadic (rare autosomal dominant)
Posterior urethral valves	Rare	Sporadic (may be associated with chromosomal trisomies)

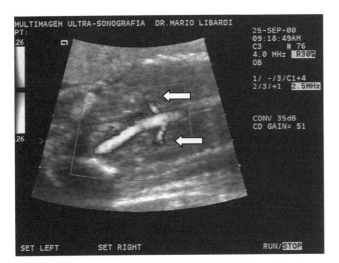

Figure 22.4 Fetal renal arteries (arrows) as demonstrated by color Doppler. (Reproduced with permission from http://www. obgyn.net/us/ gallery/OB_2_Normal_Abdominal_Vessels.jpg.)

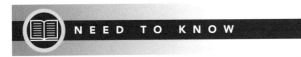

Decision 2: Evaluation

What is the best initial evaluation option?

A. Sterile speculum examination
B. Indigo carmine dye injection
C. Targeted ultrasound
D. Amniocentesis for lung maturity

The correct answer is A: sterile speculum examination. Given this patient's history and presentation, premature rupture of the membranes must be considered and ruled out. The most appropriate initial approach, of the options given, is a sterile speculum examination to evaluate for gross leakage from the cervix. The pH of the secretions and a slide test for evaluation of ferning may also be performed. If any doubt remains about the membrane status, indigo carmine dye injection into the amniotic cavity by amniocentesis is a good second-line option to confirm the diagnosis. In this case, the leakage of blue dye per vagina is diagnostic. Targeted ultrasound may be of value if there is unexplained oligohydramnios with intact membranes. Amniocentesis for lung maturity is unlikely to be helpful at 26 weeks.

NEED TO KNOW

Prognosis of Oligohydramnios

Severe oligohydramnios occurring in the second trimester of pregnancy has been associated with a high likelihood of fetal demise. In particular, severe oligohydramnios due to PPROM in the second trimester has been reported to

have a 55% to 90% mortality rate when the duration of the latency period was more than 14 days. Surviving fetuses may experience complications of pulmonary hypoplasia and orthopedic abnormalities due to fetal constraint, as well as residual impaired renal function. Pulmonary hypoplasia, in particular, presents a threat to the survival of the fetus with severe second trimester oligohydramnios, although interventions such as inhaled nitric oxide and high-frequency ventilation have improved survival in this condition. When oligohydramnios is caused by fetal renal abnormalities, it signals a grave prognosis, with a high likelihood of newborn renal failure, as well as the possibility of the Potter syndrome (pulmonary hypoplasia and evidence of in utero constraint).

The prognosis of third trimester oligohydramnios is better than that occurring in the second trimester. In one series, perinatal survival with third trimester oligohydramnios was 85% compared with 10% survival when oligohydramnios occurred in the second trimester. Most cases of severe oligohydramnios in the third trimester occurred at or near term; they were not associated with Potter-like effects, although they were often associated with fetal growth restriction. Many studies have shown an inverse relationship between amniotic fluid volume in the third trimester and the incidence of adverse pregnancy outcome (Table 22.4). In addition, oligohydramnios increases the risk of umbilical cord compression, uteroplacental insufficiency, meconium aspiration, and cesarean delivery.

CASE CONTINUES

A sterile speculum examination reveals no evidence of fluid leakage. As Mrs. Newton continues to insist that she feels leakage, you perform an indigo carmine injection,

TABLE 22.4

PERINATAL MORTALITY RELATED TO AMNIOTIC FLUID VOLUME. CORRECTED MORTALITY INCLUDES ONLY FETUSES WITHOUT ANOMALIES

Group	Amniotic Fluid Definition[a]	Perinatal Mortality Gross	Corrected
Normal	2–8 cm	4.65	1.97
Marginal	1–2 cm	56.6	37.74
Decreased	<1 cm	187.5	109.4

[a]Single vertical pocket.
Modified with permission from Chamberlain PF, Manning FA, Morrison I, et al. Untrasound evaluation of amniotic fluid volume. I. the relationship of marginal and decreased amniotic fluid volume to perinatal outcome. Am J obstet Gynecol. 1984;150:245.

with no evidence of leakage per vagina. At the time of injection, a targeted ultrasound examination is performed, and the fetus is noted to be of average size. The placenta is grade I and the AFI is 4.6 cm. Apparently normal kidneys and renal arteries are seen. Fetal bladder and stomach are seen.

Decision 3: Management

What management could be helpful?

A. Amnioinfusion
B. Maternal hydration
C. Desmopressin
D. Fetal membrane sealant

The correct answer is B: Maternal hydration. The workup to this point suggests that there are not ruptured membranes in this case, and there is no fetal anomaly responsible for the oligohydramnios. Membrane sealant would be inappropriate without ruptured membranes and would be experimental in any case. Desmopressin (synthetic antidiuretic hormone, DDAVP) has been used experimentally to lower maternal osmolality and promote water flow to the fetal compartment, but it has not been used clinically for this indication. Maternal hypotonic hydration may also improve fetal-to-maternal water flow and has been successful in raising the AFI in patients with both normal fluid volumes and with oligohydramnios. Transabdominal amnioinfusion has been used in the management of patients with severe oligohydramnios, and a number of case reports suggest that use of amnioinfusion may avoid the pulmonary hypoplasia commonly seen with early anhydramnios. Amnioinfusion carries a greater risk than maternal hydration and will therefore typically be reserved as a second-line treatment.

CASE CONCLUSION

The patient is admitted to the hospital for intravenous hydration, and the nurse consults the pharmacy database to check for other medications the patient may have been taking. She notes that the patient has filled a number of prescriptions for celecoxib (Celebrex). Upon questioning, the patient admits that she has been regularly taking celecoxib for her knee pain. She had previously denied taking medications, as she has been told that she should not be taking a nonsteroidal anti-inflammatory drug in pregnancy. On review, you find that there are no reports of oligohydramnios with celecoxib use, but that other COX-II inhibitors have been associated with oligohydramnios when used regularly in the second half of pregnancy. You advise the patient that she should discontinue use of the medication.

The AFI rises to 7.2 cm over the next 6 hours with hydration, and you elect to send the patient home with close follow-up. She is seen in the fetal testing unit 3 days later with a nonstress test appropriate for gestational age and an AFI of 12 cm. Her pregnancy continues to term, with normal fetal growth. By 39 weeks she has gained 35 lb and her activity is severely limited by pain in her knees. You agree to induce labor for this reason, and she delivers a 2,732-g female infant without incident. The pediatrician advises that the dose of celecoxib transferred to the infant in breast milk is expected to be small, and the patient returns home on celecoxib with her newborn.

SUGGESTED READINGS

Damen-Elias HA, De Jong TP, Stigter RH, Visser GH, Stoutenbeek PH. Congenital renal tract anomalies: outcome and follow-up of 402 cases detected antenatally between 1986 and 2001. Ultrasound Obstet Gynecol. 2005;25(2):134–43.

Deshpande C, Hennekam RC. Genetic syndromes and prenatally detected renal anomalies. Semin Fetal Neonatal Med. 2008;13(3): 171–80.

Harman CR. Amniotic fluid abnormalities. Semin Perinatol. 2008;32(4): 288–94.

Magann EF, Chauhan SP, Doherty DA, Magann MI, Morrison JC. The evidence for abandoning the amniotic fluid index in favor of the single deepest pocket. Am J Perinatol. 2007;24(9):549–55.

Nabhan AF, Abdelmoula YA. Amniotic fluid index versus single deepest vertical pocket: a meta-analysis of randomized controlled trials. Int J Gynaecol Obstet. 2009 Mar;104(3):184–8.

Stigter RH, Mulder EJ, Bruinse HW, Visser GH. Doppler studies on the fetal renal artery in the severely growth-restricted fetus. Ultrasound Obstet Gynecol. 2001;18(2):141–5.

Williams O, Hutchings G, Debieve F, Debauche C. Contemporary neonatal outcome following rupture of membranes prior to 25 weeks with prolonged oligohydramnios. Early Hum Dev. 2008; 85(5):273–7.

Polyhydramnios

Marie H. Beall   Michael G. Ross

CASE PRESENTATION

Your next patient is Mrs. Matthews, a 26-year-old G2 P1 at 29 weeks by her last menstrual period, confirmed by a first trimester ultrasound. Her first pregnancy was uncomplicated and ended in a vaginal delivery at term. This pregnancy has been uncomplicated except that last week she had a 1-hour glucose screen of 160. A 3-hour glucose tolerance test (GTT) has been ordered, but the results are not available. Today Mrs. Matthews complains of a feeling of heaviness, shortness of breath, and some uterine contractions; she also feels that "the baby" has grown a lot in the last few weeks. Her blood pressure is 105/66 mm Hg, her weight is 160 lb, which is a gain of 10 lb in 6 weeks. Her respiratory rate is 18, and she appears in mild respiratory distress.

On physical examination, the uterine fundal height is 40 cm. Fetal heart tones are normal at 140 bpm, and the fetus appears active, but fetal parts are difficult to appreciate by palpation. Clinically, you suspect that the amniotic fluid volume is increased.

NEED TO KNOW

Polyhydramnios

Polyhydramnios is an increased amount of amniotic fluid. The absolute definition of polyhydramnios is problematic, as there is a very wide range of amniotic fluid volumes in normal pregnancies (Fig. 23.1). In addition, although the normal amount of amniotic fluid over gestation has been described, direct measurement of the amniotic fluid volume is not available in human pregnancies, making it necessary to use indirect or semiquantitative measures.

The amount of amniotic fluid is most commonly evaluated using the amniotic fluid index (AFI) or the single deepest pocket (SDP) of amniotic fluid, both semiquantitative measures of fluid volume. In assessing AFI, the sonographer measures the deepest amniotic fluid pocket in each of the four quadrants of the abdomen (as defined by the umbilicus and the linea nigra). Pockets are measured perpendicular to the floor with the patient in supine position, and the calipers should not crossover small parts or umbilical cord. The AFI is the sum of the four measurements; the SDP is the one largest measurement. The most commonly used indication of increased amniotic fluid volume is an AFI of ≥25 cm, or an SDP of >8 cm. The 95th percentile AFI at maximum fluid volumes for normal gestations is between 18 and 20 cm (Fig. 23.2), leading some centers to use lower cutoff figures. However, there is evidence to suggest that the higher AFI cutoff selects the majority of fetuses with an abnormal outcome, with a lower false-positive rate. Polyhydramnios is often categorized as mild, moderate, or severe; although these terms are not strictly defined, they correspond roughly to AFIs of 25 to 30, 30 to 35, and >35 cm or SDPs of 8 to 12, 12 to 16, and >16 cm.

Decision 1: Differential diagnosis

Which of the following is a common cause of polyhydramnios?

- A. Fetal renal agenesis
- B. Congenital influenza
- C. Maternal diabetes
- D. Fetal skeletal anomaly

The correct answer is C: Maternal diabetes. Polyhydramnios is associated with a number of genetic, metabolic, anatomic, and infectious causes (Table 23.1). In up to 60% of cases, the polyhydramnios is idiopathic, meaning that no diagnosis can be found. The most commonly associated conditions were fetal anomalies (primarily gastrointestinal, central nervous system, and cardiac), twin gestation, and maternal diabetes. Fetal anomalies are increasingly prevalent with more severe polyhydramnios, with an incidence of 30% to 60% when the AFI is >35 cm (Table 23.2).

Fetal renal agenesis is a cause of oligohydramnios. Fetal skeletal anomalies or influenza are not common causes of polyhydramnios.

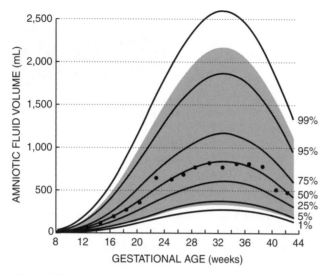

Figure 23.1 Normal amniotic fluid volume in human pregnancy. (Adapted from Brace RA, Wolf EJ. Normal amniotic fluid volume changes throughout pregnancy. Am J Obstet Gynecol. 1989;161(2): 382–8.)

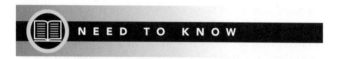

NEED TO KNOW

Amniotic Fluid Dynamics

In early pregnancy, amniotic fluid is most likely a transudate across the membranes and nonkeratinized fetal skin, although the actual source of early amniotic fluid

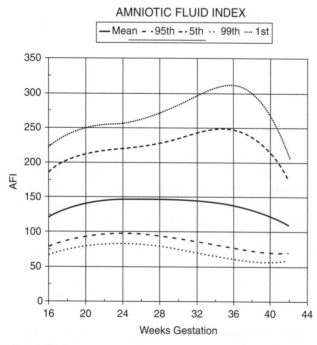

Figure 23.2 AFI over gestation in normal pregnancies. (Adapted from Moore TR. Clinical assessment of amniotic fluid. Clin Obstet Gynecol. 1997;40(2):303–13.)

TABLE 23.1

ABNORMALITIES ASSOCIATED WITH POLYHYDRAMNIOS

Chromosomal Abnormalities
   Trisomy 13
   Trisomy 18
   Trisomy 21

Structural Abnormalities
   Anencephaly
   Tracheoesophageal fistula
   Duodenal atresia
   Other bowel abnormalities
   Skeletal dysplasia
   Other genetic disease
   Cystic adenomatoid malformation of the lung
   Other thoracic tumors
   Pharyngeal teratoma

Inherited Diseases
   Bartter syndrome (fetal polyuria due to sodium resorption defect)
   Fetal overgrowth syndromes (Beckwith–Wiedemann syndrome, Perlman syndrome)
   Myotonic dystrophy

Hydrops
   Isoimmunization
   Fetal infection
   Cardiac arrhythmia
   Placental tumors

Maternal
   Diabetes
   Twin–twin transfusion syndrome

Idiopathic
Adapted from Carlson DE, Platt LD, Medearis AL, Horenstein J. Quantifiable polyhydramnios: diagnosis and management. Obstet Gynecol. 1990; 75(6):989–93.

has not been demonstrated. In later pregnancy, evidence from animal models suggests that the amniotic fluid is actively produced and resorbed by the fetus, and the fetus may be able to regulate the fluid volume. During the second half of pregnancy, fluid circulates between the fetus and the amniotic cavity. Fluid is produced by the fetal lungs and kidneys, and resorbed by fetal swallowing. Fluid may also be resorbed directly across the amnion into the fetal vessels. There are a number of minor contributors to fluid production, including transudation across the umbilical cord and skin, fetal saliva, and water produced as a result of fetal metabolism. Derangements in amniotic fluid volume may result from alterations in either fluid production or resorption. The pathophysiology of polyhydramnios is discussed here. Oligohydramnios is the subject of Chapter 22.

Increased urine production may be a source of polyhydramnios. Based on ultrasound measurements of the fetal bladder, the human fetus is estimated to produce approximately 1,000 mL/d of urine at term, representing

TABLE 23.2

SEVERITY OF POLYHYDRAMNIOS AND RISK OF FETAL ABNORMALITIES. POLYHYDRAMNIOS IS ASSOCIATED WITH AN INCREASED RISK OF PERINATAL MORTALITY AND FETAL ANOMALIES, AND THE RISK INCREASES WITH INCREASING AMOUNTS OF AMNIOTIC FLUID

Degree	SDP	Frequency (%)	Perinatal Mortality (per 1,000)	Anomalies
Mild	>8	68	50	6% or less
Moderate	>11	19	190	Up to 45%
Severe	>15	13	540	Up to 65%

SDP, single deepest pocket.

the majority (about 80%) of amniotic fluid. Fetal urine flow can be increased in infants of diabetic mothers, presumably due to an osmotic dieresis resulting from increased fetal plasma glucose. Human fetal urine flow can also be increased in conditions of circulatory overload, as may occur with a twin transfusion syndrome or in severe fetal anemia, possibly an effect of increased fetal plasma atrial natriuretic factor. In theory, conditions leading to maternal hypoosmolality or low serum oncotic pressure might increase water transfer to the fetus across the placenta, with a resultant fetal volume overload, although this has not been described in clinical practice.

Fluid produced in the fetal lungs accounts for about 20% of amniotic fluid volume. Although there are no human data, studies on sheep suggest that lung fluid production is normally at the maximum rate, and increased lung fluid production is rarely a cause of polyhydramnios in clinical practice. Similarly, the minor sources of fluid mentioned are not significant sources of amniotic fluid and are not sources of polyhydramnios.

Absent or reduced fetal swallowing is a common cause of polyhydramnios. Although data are scanty, evidence suggests that the term human fetus swallows up to 750 mL/d, making this the major route of amniotic fluid resorption. Swallowing may be compromised both by neurologic lesions that prevent or impair swallowing activity, and by anatomic lesions that block passage of the fluid into the fetal intestine, where it is normally absorbed.

Amniotic fluid may also be absorbed directly through the amnion into the fetal vessels, a phenomenon called intramembranous flow. In the sheep, intramembranous flow can be inferred from experimental results; however, intramembranous flow has not been directly demonstrated in the human. In the mouse, a defect in membrane water channels has been reported to result in increased amniotic fluid volumes. However, there is no clinical condition where a defect in intramembranous flow can be shown to cause human polyhydramnios.

 CASE CONTINUES

You perform a brief office ultrasound, which reveals an AFI of 45 cm. The patient is not having uterine contractions; her cervix is 50% effaced and 1 cm dilated with the presenting part ballotable. You elect to send Mrs. Matthews to labor and delivery for monitoring, and you plan a workup in the hospital.

 Decision 2: Patient evaluation

What are the different evaluation options?

A. Targeted fetal ultrasound
B. Maternal serum sodium
C. Fetal bladder measurement
D. Fetal middle cerebral artery (MCA) Doppler

The best initial options for evaluation of this pregnancy are A and D. In general, the preliminary clinical evaluation of this patient will include the following:

An Evaluation by Targeted Ultrasound

- For fetal structural abnormalities, especially in the gastrointestinal tract and brain, which may impair fetal swallowing
- For intermittent fetal tachycardia that may result in high-output cardiac failure
- For evidence of fetal hydrops that may indicate anemia or cardiac failure
- For MCA peak flow velocity that may be elevated in fetal anemia
- To exclude twin pregnancy with twin–twin transfusion or twin reversed arterial perfusion

Maternal Blood Work

- Blood type and antibody screen on the mother will identify the fetus at risk from maternal isoimmunization.
- Maternal serology will exclude a fetus affected by maternal syphilis.
- GTT will exclude maternal diabetes.

Additional testing will be guided by the results of the primary tests and by the patient's history and presentation:

Fetal Anemia (Suspected Due to Elevated MCA Peak Flow)
- Consider maternal titers for parvovirus B19, especially if history of exposure.
- Consider evaluation for fetal–maternal bleeding, especially if history of trauma
- Consider evaluation for thalassemia, especially if family history or parental consanguinity.
- Might consider amniocentesis for delta OD 450 Å if evidence of maternal isoimmunization.

Nonanemic Hydrops
- Consider fetal echocardiogram.
- Consider fetal karyotype.

Fetal Anomaly
- Consider fetal karyotype.
- Other workup depends on anomaly seen.

Normal Fetus Seen
- Consider fetal karyotype if polyhydramnios severe (AFI >35 cm)
- Consider fetal biophysical profile (BPP) to evaluate for movement disorders.
- Consider evaluation for inborn error of metabolism if family history or parental consanguinity.

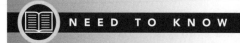

Prognosis of Polyhydramnios

The outcome of a pregnancy complicated by polyhydramnios is often a function of the underlying cause. For fetuses with treatable lesions, attention to treating the underlying pathology may improve outcome. Examples of treatment might include control of maternal diabetes, fetal transfusion for fetal anemia, treatment of infections, and control of fetal heart rate. A number of abnormal outcomes have, however, been associated with polyhydramnios per se. In the mother, idiopathic polyhydramnios is associated with an increased risk of preeclampsia, preterm delivery, ineffective contractions (due to uterine overdistention), cesarean delivery, placental abruption, and postpartum hemorrhage. For the fetus, polyhydramnios increases the risk of prematurity and malpresentation. There is a 3% to 5% risk of fetal death, which is greater when the polyhydramnios is more severe. The increase in fetal death may be due to increased intrauterine pressure that interferes with normal placental blood flow. Severe polyhydramnios is also associated with a risk of about 10% of undiagnosed fetal anomalies.

The risk of fetal death has lead to a recommendation that all pregnancies complicated by polyhydramnios be followed with antenatal testing. There is no evidence to suggest an optimal testing regimen. Because the modified BPP (NST and AFI) is compromised by the amniotic fluid abnormality many practitioners have chosen to perform testing with the full BPP on a regular basis.

 CASE CONTINUES

On labor and delivery Mrs. Matthews is put on the monitor, where she is found to have a normal fetal heart rate of 135 bpm, with accelerations. No decelerations are seen. She is having difficulty breathing when flat in bed.

 Decision 3: Management

What would your response be to the patient's symptoms?

A. Amnioreduction
B. Indomethacin
C. Furosemide
D. Magnesium sulfate

The best answers are A: *Amnioreduction* **and B:** Indomethacin. Amnioreduction is the removal of amniotic fluid via a needle inserted through the maternal abdomen. It is an effective means of reducing amniotic fluid volume, but it has not been shown to reduce the rate of preterm delivery. Amnioreduction is, therefore usually reserved for circumstances where the fluid volume itself is the problem, as when there is maternal respiratory compromise. As the amniotic fluid volume in the human fetus is replenished on a daily basis, one-time removal of the fluid is unlikely to provide lasting relief of the patient's symptoms. Many practitioners will use indomethacin to maintain the reduction in amniotic fluid volume. Although it has not been studied in randomized controlled trials, several studies have described the utility of indomethacin in patients with polyhydramnios The reduction in fluid volume is thought to be due to the effect of indomethacin on the fetal kidney. The most commonly used dose is 50 mg per rectum once, then 25 mg orally every 6 hours to complete a 48-hour course. As indomethacin and other nonsteroidal anti-inflammatory agents have been associated with constriction of the ductus arteriosus, and with closure of the ductus in fetuses above 32 to 34 weeks, it is not recommended to use indomethacin for more than 48 hours without imaging of the fetal ductus by ultrasound. Many authors also do not

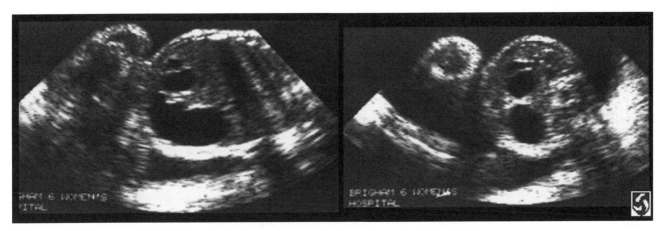

Figure 23.3 Fetal examination with "double bubble" sign of duodenal atresia. S = stomach, D = duodenum. (Reproduced with permission from Miller, Frank H and Laing, Faye C. Duodenal Atresia. Brigham and Women's Hospital, Department of Radiology Teaching Case Database. June 8, 1994.)

recommend the use of indomethacin in pregnancies of more than 32 weeks gestational age. In contrast, maternal side effects of indomethacin are few and limited to gastric upset and a slightly increased blood loss if surgical delivery is necessary.

Although maternal hyperosmolarity will theoretically reduce water flow to the fetus, maternal use of diuretics such as furosemide has not been shown to have an effect on the amniotic fluid volume.

Magnesium sulfate may be used in the treatment of premature labor, although randomized trials have not demonstrated effectiveness for this indication. It will not, however, affect the amniotic fluid volume.

 CASE CONCLUSION

Mrs. Matthews is given indomethacin 50 mg PR. A targeted ultrasound and amnioreduction are performed. Prior to amnioreduction, the AFI is 42 cm. There are normal fetal kidneys and bladder. The fetus is active, and the fetal heart rate is 142 bpm. Fetal MCA Doppler reveals a peak flow velocity that is in the normal range. The fetal stomach bubble is abnormal (Fig. 23.3). Two liters of amniotic fluid are removed over 45 minutes, with good resolution of the maternal symptoms. Other workup includes a blood type of O+ with negative antibody screen, negative VDRL and negative IgM antibodies to TORCH organisms. The mother's 3-hour GTT is normal.

You make a diagnosis of fetal duodenal atresia. You refer Mrs. Matthews for care to the University hospital, where there is a pediatric surgeon. She is admitted there with intermittent premature labor, and at 34 weeks she ruptures her membranes and subsequently delivers a 2,200-g female infant. Evaluation of the newborn reveals an isolated duodenal atresia. The infant undergoes repair of the lesion on day of life number 2 and recovers uneventfully. At 6 months of age, the baby appears to be developing normally.

SUGGESTED READINGS

Brace RA, Wolf EJ. Normal amniotic fluid volume changes throughout pregnancy. Am J Obstet Gynecol. 1989;161(2):382–8.

Carlson DE, Platt LD, Medearis AL, Horenstein J. Quantifiable polyhydramnios: diagnosis and management. Obstet Gynecol. 1990;75(6): 989–93.

Dashe JS, McIntire DD, Ramus RM, Santos-Ramos R, Twickler DM. Hydramnios: anomaly prevalence and sonographic detection. Obstet Gynecol. 2002;100(1):134–9.

Golan A, Wolman I, Sagi J, Yovel I, David MP. Persistence of polyhydramnios during pregnancy–its significance and correlation with maternal and fetal complications. Gynecol Obstet Invest. 1994; 37(1):18–20.

Harman CR. Amniotic fluid abnormalities. Semin Perinatol. 2008;32(4): 288–94.

Magann EF, Chauhan SP, Doherty DA, Lutgendorf MA, Magann MI, Morrison JC. A review of idiopathic hydramnios and pregnancy outcomes. Obstet Gynecol Surv. 2007;62(12):795–802.

Magann EF, Sanderson M, Martin JN, Chauhan S. The amniotic fluid index, single deepest pocket, and two-diameter pocket in normal human pregnancy. Am J Obstet Gynecol. 2000;182(6): 1581–8.

Maymon E, Ghezzi F, Shoham-Vardi I, et al. Isolated hydramnios at term gestation and the occurrence of peripartum complications. Eur J Obstet Gynecol Reprod Biol. 1998;77(2):157–61.

Moore TR. Clinical assessment of amniotic fluid. Clin Obstet Gynecol. 1997;40(2):303–13.

Teratogens in Pregnancy

Noelia Zork

 CASE PRESENTATION

Ms. Sorenson, a 29-year-old G1 P0 was admitted by the internist to the intensive care unit (ICU) 15 days ago for severe pneumonia that progressed to adult respiratory distress syndrome and required intubation. Yesterday, hospital day 14, the patient was extubated successfully and was completely oriented. In discussing her hospital course and her illness the patient mentions that she had not had her period in about 2 months. A serum β-hCG (the beta subunit of human chorionic gonadotropin) was drawn and was 84,000 mIU. A pelvic ultrasound was performed that day and revealed an intrauterine pregnancy at 9 weeks and 2 days with cardiac activity at 162 bpm. The pregnancy was unplanned but desired. Realizing the potential problems, the ICU team consults you, the obstetrician, to evaluate Ms. Sorenson and her risk of congenital anomalies given the treatment provided during her hospitalization.

In reviewing Ms. Sorenson's chart, you note that she had multiple imaging studies, including multiple chest x-rays and computed tomography (CT) scans and a procedure under fluoroscopy. In addition, you see that she had a near constant fever, the maximum being 101.0°F, during her first 3 days of hospitalization and during this time the patient was suboptimally oxygenated, with an arterial PO$_2$ at about 60 mm Hg. When you interview Ms. Sorenson, she asks you if any of the medications or procedures performed so far could have "hurt the baby."

 Decision 1: Identification of risks

Which of the following is a potential teratogen in this patient?

A. Ionizing radiation
B. Hyperthermia
C. Medications
D. Hypoxia

The correct answer is A: Ionizing radiation. Prolonged maternal hyperthermia may increase the risk of neural tube defects during the first 4 weeks of gestation; however, the risk is best established for higher temperatures. Temporary hypoxia has not been shown to be a teratogen, although chronic hypoxia throughout the pregnancy such as in severe asthma, chronic obstructive pulmonary disease, or cyanotic heart disease, increases the risk of severe fetal growth restriction. Lastly, most medications used for intubation, thromboembolism and gastrointestinal ulcer prophylaxis, cardiovascular support, and sedation are nonteratogenic, especially given their short-term use in this case. Some classes of antibiotics that may have been used are potential teratogens but are not as well linked to fetal anomalies as ionizing radiation.

NEED TO KNOW

Fetal Effects of Exposure to Radiation

Most of the information available on the effects of intrauterine exposure to radiation has been gathered from survivors of the atomic bombs in Nagasaki and Hiroshima, Japan. The most commonly encountered effects are in the central nervous system (CNS), specifically microcephaly and mental retardation, but effects also include intrauterine growth restriction. Although this population was exposed to extremely high doses of radiation, there is still cause for concern when exposing both mother and fetus to radiation through diagnostic tests such as radiography, CT, angiography, and imaging with radioisotopes. Cumulative exposure to these and other types of ionizing radiation increase the fetal risks of cell death, teratogenicity, germ cell mutations, genetic damage, and carcinogenesis.

In assessing the risks of intrauterine exposure to radiation, two factors must be considered; fetal absorbed dose and timing of the exposure. The fetal dose is expressed in radiation absorbed dose (rad) or gray (1 gray equals 1 joule of radiation energy absorbed by 1 kg of matter), with 100 rad equaling 1 gray. Risks of anomalies, growth restriction, or spontaneous abortions are likely not increased at doses <5 rad,

TABLE 24.1

ESTIMATES OF FETAL DOSE FOR VARIOUS RADIOLOGIC PROCEDURES

Procedure	Dose/Study (rad)
X-ray	
Skull X-ray (three views)	<0.00005
Chest X-ray (AP/Lat)	0.00002–0.00007
Mammogram	0.007–0.02
Abdomen	0.122–0.245
Lumbosacral spine	0.168–0.359
Intravenous pyelogram	0.686–1.398
Hip (two views)	0.103–0.213
Computed Tomography	
Head	<0.001
Chest	<0.001
Abdomen and pelvis	2.5–3.2
Renal stone protocol	2.2–2.5
Fluoroscopy	
Upper GI series	0.056
Barium swallow	0.006
Barium enema	1.945–3.986
Cerebral angiography	<0.01
Cardiac angiography	0.065
Single vessel PTCA (Percutaneous transluminal coronary angioplasty)	0.06
Double-vessel PTCA	0.09
Nuclear Medicine	
Ventilation–perfusion scan	0.045–0.057
Thyroid ^{123}I	0.01
Thyroid ^{131}I at 20 weeks	3 (whole body)
590 (fetal tissue)	

Data from Cunningham FG, Leveno KJ, Bloom SL, Hauth JC, Gilstrap LC III, Wenstrom KD. General considerations and maternal evaluation. In: Williams Obstetrics. 22nd ed. New York, NY: McGraw-Hill; 2005, pp. 974–84.

at any gestational age, and 5 rad represents a significant number of diagnostic studies. For example, a chest x-ray (PA/lateral) results in a fetal dose of approximately 0.00007 rad. To achieve 5 rad, more than 70,000 chest x-rays would have to be performed. Using CT scanners that use higher doses of radiation, a chest CT would result in an exposure of 0.025 rad (200 chest CT = 5 rad) whereas abdomen or pelvic CTs result in 2.4 rad (two abdomen/pelvis CT = 5 rad). Table 24.1 summarizes the fetal dosage of common imaging techniques.

If there is high-dose exposure from 2 to 4 weeks of gestation, animal studies suggest that this would more likely result in spontaneous abortion or failure of implantation than a fetal anomaly. If the embryo survives this early exposure, it will continue to develop as a normal fetus. The greatest risk to the CNS appears to be between 8 and 15 weeks of gestation, with less risk at <8 weeks or >25 weeks. Although an absolute

threshold has not been established, some suggest that risk of mental retardation begins around 20 to 40 rad. The risk increases as the fetal dose increases beyond this threshold.

The risk of developing germ cell mutations after exposure to 1 rad has been estimated to be at most 0.1%, but no inherited gene mutations resulting from radiation exposure have ever been shown in humans. In addition, the rates of intrauterine fetal death are not increased in those exposed to even very high levels of radiation.

It has been reported that radiation exposure to the fetus increases the risk of cancer later in life. However, if there is a carcinogenic effect, it is likely small. Fetal exposure of 1 to 2 rad has been suggested to increase the risk of childhood leukemia by 1.5- to 2.0-fold over baseline risk. This is estimated to represent 1 in 2,000 children exposed to ionizing radiation in utero who will develop childhood leukemia.

Nuclear medicine studies are also potential teratogens because they use radioactive materials in addition to ionizing radiation. If indicated, many studies can be performed with little fetal exposure to radiation if the lowest dose of radionuclide is used. The fetus may be exposed to a concentrated dose of the radionuclide through concentration in fetal tissues (as for radioactive iodine). For iodine, the fetal dose is greatest after 10 weeks, at which time the fetus begins to concentrate iodine in its own thyroid. Radioactive ablation of the thyroid is contraindicated during pregnancy because it may cause ablation of the fetal thyroid. Radioactive agents may also affect the fetus without passage across the placenta, as concentration in the maternal bladder as the agent is excreted may result in increased exposure at earlier gestational ages.

There is also concern for teratogenicity of nonradioactive contrast materials used in radiography studies. There are various types of contrast medium, but they can simply be placed into two groups: iodine-based materials and non–iodine-based materials. Examples of some iodine-based materials that are most commonly used include iohexol (Omniopaque), iopamidol (Isovue), ioversol (Optiray), and iopromide (Ultravist). These substances are those used orally or intravascularly in CT scan, angiography, venography, and hysterosalpingogram. The non–iodine-based materials include barium, used in gastrointestinal studies, and gadolinium, used for magnetic resonance imaging studies. Both iodinated materials and gadolinium may cross the placenta. The effects of fetal exposure to these contrast materials have not been studied in humans, but no fetal harm was seen in animal studies for iohexol, iopamidol, iothalamate, ioversol, ioxaglate, and metrizamide. Animal studies using gadolinium at several times the recommended human dose did show deleterious effects. However, with iodinated contrast material there is the theoretical risk of neonatal hypothyroidism. In additional to pregnancy risks, some of these agents pass into breast milk. Although they have not been shown to cause adverse effects in nursing infants, the recommendations are for the mother to discard her breast milk for 24 hours following the procedure. Barium is not systemically absorbed, although its effects during pregnancy have also not been studied in humans.

When considering the fetal dosage for certain procedures, it is important to note that the exposure can be affected by several variables including maternal weight, radiographic technique, and type of equipment used. If more customized estimations are desired, a radiation physicist should be consulted.

 ## CASE CONTINUES

In telling Ms. Sorenson about the potential effects of radiation on her baby, she becomes concerned and states that if there was a strong likelihood that the fetus was affected she would consider termination. To give her a more definite answer, you consult a radiation physicist who calculates the total fetal dose to be 4.5 rad since admission.

Further review of the chart for other teratogen exposures reveals that Ms. Sorenson has a known history of epilepsy and has been receiving phenytoin.

 ### NEED TO KNOW

Drug Teratogen Categorization

There is a 2% to 4% risk of significant congenital defects among all pregnancies. Even though these defects can be caused by external factors such as medications or infections, only 5% of all clinically significant anomalies can be attributed to known teratogens. Of all potential teratogens, the most commonly encountered are medications. In an effort to provide guidance to clinicians, the U.S. Food and Drug Administration (FDA) released a standardized category system in 1979 that is based on the level of risk to the fetus. Table 24.2 provides these ratings.

One of the problems with using the FDA category system to guide which medications are given to pregnant patients is that it incorrectly assumes that all drugs in a category pose equal threats to a fetus. For example, both oral contraceptive pills (OCPs) and isotretinoin are in category X. OCPs pose a minimal threat to the fetus. Many patients, not knowing that they were pregnant, continued taking the pills during the early part of pregnancy and the results have been

TABLE 24.2

FDA CLASSIFICATION OF MEDICATIONS FOR TERATOGENIC POTENTIAL

Category A	Controlled studies show no risk. Adequate, well-controlled studies in pregnant women have failed to demonstrate a risk to the fetus.
Category B	No evidence of risk in humans. Either animal study shows risk, but human findings do not, or if no adequate human studies have been done, animal findings are negative.
Category C	Risk cannot be ruled out. Human studies are lacking, and animal studies are either positive for fetal risk or lacking. However, potential benefits may justify potential risk.
Category D	Positive evidence of risk. Investigational or postmarketing data show risk to the fetus. Nevertheless, potential benefits may outweigh the potential risk.
Category X	Contraindicated in pregnancy. Studies in animals or humans or investigational or postmarketing reports have shown fetal risk, which clearly outweighs any possible benefit to the patient. Or the drug has no indication in pregnancy.

well studied. OCPs are rated X because of the lack of any indication for their use rather than for any proven risk. In contrast, isotretinoin is a well-known teratogen with malformation risk of up to 20%, including craniofacial, cardiac, and CNS defects. A second issue is that the risk assessments are assigned by the pharmaceutical companies, generally on the basis of the studies done to obtain FDA approval. As most drugs have not been specifically studied during human pregnancy, most new drugs reach market with a category C rating, and no information available regarding teratogenicity. Physicians must know the characteristics of the specific drug being prescribed, not only which category it is assigned. Table 24.3 contains a list of known human teratogenic agents.

Regarding Ms. Sorenson, she was given phenytoin (Dilantin) for her seizure disorder. Phenytoin may lead to fetal hydantoin syndrome, which consists of craniofacial anomalies (i.e., cleft palate, midfacial hypoplasia), hypoplastic fingernails and distal phalanges, developmental delay, fetal growth restriction, microcephaly, and cardiac defects. The syndrome is seen in <10% of exposed fetuses but some elements of the syndrome may be seen in up to 30%. Like most other teratogens, the risk of developing this syndrome is dependent on dose and gestational age at exposure. In addition, there appear to be genetic differences in drug metabolism that place some mothers at higher risk of fetal hydantoin syndrome in their offspring.

TABLE 24.3
KNOWN HUMAN TERATOGENS

Agent	Effects
ACE inhibitors and ARBs (e.g., enalapril, lisinopril, losartan)	Fetal renal tubular dysplasia, oligohydramnios, neonatal renal failure, lack of cranial ossification, intrauterine growth restriction
Alcohol	Growth restriction before and after birth, mental retardation, microcephaly, midfacial hypoplasia, renal and cardiac defects, various other major and minor malformations
Androgens and testosterone derivatives (e.g., danazol)	Virilization of female, advanced genital development in males
Antithyroid medications (e.g., propylthiouracil, methimazole)	If used after 10 weeks, congenital goiter, fetal thyroid dysfunction, effects may be transient
Carbamazepine	Neural tube defects, minor craniofacial defects, fingernail hypoplasia, microcephaly, developmental delay, intrauterine growth restriction
Cocaine	Bowel atresia and infarcts; malformations of the heart, limbs, face, and genitourinary tract; microcephaly, IUGR, cerebral infarcts, absence of skin in an area
Coumarin	Nasal hypoplasia and stippled bone epiphyses are most common; other effects include broad short hands with shortened phalanges, ophthalmologic abnormalities, IUGR, developmental delay, anomalies of neck and CNS
Folic acid antagonists (e.g., methotrexate, aminopterin, trimethoprim)	Increased risk for spontaneous abortions, cardiac anomalies, cleft palate, urogenital anomalies
Diethylstilbestrol	Clear-cell adenocarcinoma of the vagina or cervix, vaginal adenosis, abnormalities of cervix and uterus, abnormalities of the testes, possible infertility in males and females
Lead	Increased abortion rate, stillbirths
Lithium	Congenital heart disease (Ebstein's anomaly)
Methylene blue (injected into amniotic sac)	Hyperbilirubinemia, methemoglobinemia, hemolytic anemia, blue staining of skin
Organic mercury	Cerebral atrophy, microcephaly, mental retardation, spasticity, seizures, blindness
Penicillamine	Cutis laxa
Phenytoin	IUGR, mental retardation, microcephaly, dysmorphic craniofacial features, cardiac defects, hypoplastic nails, and distal phalanges
Streptomycin and kanamycin	Hearing loss, eighth-nerve damage
Tetracycline	Hypoplasia of tooth enamel, incorporation of tetracycline into bone and teeth, permanent yellow-brown discoloration of deciduous teeth
Thalidomide	Bilateral limb deficiencies, anotia and microtia cardiac and gastrointestinal anomalies
Trimethadione and paramethadione	Cleft lip or cleft palate; cardiac defects; growth deficiency; microcephaly; mental retardation; characteristic facial appearance; ophthalmic, limb, genitourinary tract abnormalities
Tobacco	Low birth weights, spontaneous abortion, cleft lip and palate, microcephaly (effects seen also with smokeless tobacco and second-hand smoke)
Valproic acid	Neural tube defects, especially spina bifida, minor facial defects
Vitamin A and its derivatives (e.g., isotretinoin, etretinate, retinoids)	Increased abortion rate, microtia, central nervous system defects, thymic agenesis, cardiovascular effects, craniofacial dimorphism, microphthalmia, cleft lip and palate, mental retardation

ACE, angiotensin-converting enzyme; ARBs, angiotensin II receptor blockers; CNS, central nervous system; IUGR, intrauterine growth retardation

Decision 2: Fetal Diagnosis

What is the best option for early testing in this patient?

A. Fetal nuchal translucency screen at 10 weeks
B. Maternal quadruple serum screen at 15 weeks
C. Chorionic villus sampling (CVS) at 11 weeks
D. Ultrasound at 13 weeks

The correct answer is D: Ultrasound at 13 weeks. Ms. Sorenson has been exposed to both known and unknown

teratogens, and the best way to identify any abnormalities would be a fetal anatomy scan. The remaining choices would be more appropriate if the patient was at an increased risk of a genetic or chromosomal abnormality.

Nuchal translucency screening, performed at 10 to 14 weeks, measures the thickness of the lucency at the back of the fetus' neck and is used, with the level of hCG and pregnancy-associated plasma protein A to predict fetal aneuploidy. Maternal quadruple serum screen uses the levels of four maternal serum analytes (hCG, alpha-fetoprotein, estriol, and inhibin A) between 15 and 20 weeks to predict the risk for chromosomal abnormalities and neural tube defects. If aneuploidy is suspected with either screen, the patient can be offered a definitive diagnosis through CVS or amniocentesis, both of which are more than 99% accurate. CVS is done at 10 to 12 weeks and consists of removing a piece of placental villi either transcervically or transabdominally. Amniocentesis is commonly performed between 15 and 20 weeks and is done transabdominally to obtain a sample of amniotic fluid. In both cases, cells obtained reflect the fetal genetic complement and are used to test for the disorder of interest.

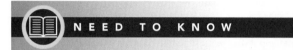

NEED TO KNOW

First Trimester Fetal Anatomy Survey

Given Ms. Sorenson's anxiety level, an early assessment of her fetus' anatomy would be very welcome. Traditionally, a transvaginal first trimester scan has been used to identify an intrauterine pregnancy and includes measurement of crown-rump length for gestational dating, fetal heart rate, number of fetuses, placentation, and uterine and ovarian anatomy. However, there has been growing interest in assessing fetal anatomy during the first trimester and increasing evidence shows that it can be done accurately, given the development of high frequency vaginal ultrasound transducers.

In a specialized setting, the first trimester examination can visualize significant portions of the fetal anatomy. Beginning at 10 weeks, one can measure the biparietal diameter, head circumference, femur length, and abdominal circumference. Also by this time the cerebral anatomy can be well visualized, revealing the lateral ventricles, choroid plexus, falx cerebri, tentorium, third ventricle, posterior fossa, foramen magnum, and cerebellar peduncles. By week 12, the physiologic midgut herniation has resolved and in 90% of cases the internal organs, such as kidneys, intestines, bladder, liver, stomach, and diaphragm, can be visualized and a four-chamber view of the heart can be obtained, as well as a view of the fetal face (Fig. 24.1). By 13 weeks the humerus, radius, ulna, and tibia can be measured and fingers and toes can be counted. A complete transvaginal fetal echocardiogram can also be performed at 13 weeks. At 14 weeks, a complete anatomy scan can be performed, including fetal gender.

The reported detection rate of fetal anomalies during first trimester and early second trimester scans ranges from 30% to 82%. This wide range of sensitivity is likely due to the operator-dependant nature of ultrasonography. In addition, many structures at this point have not fully developed and cannot be assessed during the first trimester. Taking this into consideration, there are suggestions that the traditional 18- to 20-week anatomy scan be replaced by a 12- to 14-week scan followed by a more detailed scan at 20 to 24 weeks.

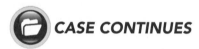

CASE CONTINUES

Ms. Sorenson decides to continue the pregnancy but does desire an early ultrasound. She is discharged from the hospital 3 days later and makes an appointment with you for prenatal care.

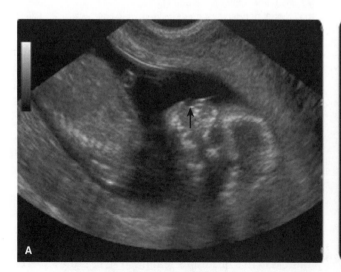

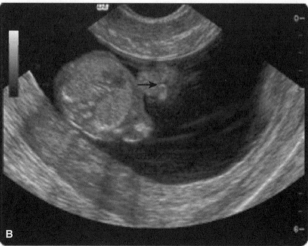

Figure 24.1 Cleft lip diagnosed at 12.5 weeks of gestation. **A:** sagittal view. **B:** transverse view, with cleft (arrow). (Reproduced with permission from Weiner Z, Goldstein I, Bombard A, Applewhite L, Itzkovits-Eldor J. Screening for structural fetal anomalies during the nuchal translucency ultrasound examination. Am J Obstet Gynecol. 2007;197(2):181.e1–5.)

At 13 weeks, an anatomy survey is performed, which shows no signs of neural tube, cerebral, or cardiac anomalies and otherwise normal anatomy. A follow-up examination at 20 weeks confirms the earlier findings.

Decision 3: Pregnancy management

Which of the following follow-up tests would be most useful given this patient's pregnancy history?

A. Nonstress testing beginning at 30 weeks
B. Fetal growth assessment
C. Fetal Doppler
D. Fetal echocardiogram

The correct answers are B and D: Fetal growth assessment and fetal echocardiogram. As previously discussed, this patient has been exposed to several potential teratogens that can often result in intrauterine growth restriction. Even though it is relatively unlikely that the fetus has suffered lasting effects from these teratogens, the fetal exposure of 4.5 rad is near the generally accepted limit of 5 rad and warrants closer observation. Similarly, the patient has been exposed to phenytoin during the period of cardiac development. As noted above, phenytoin is a known teratogen with potential cardiac effects. The detection of cardiac defects by standard fetal ultrasound examination is known to be problematic. Despite a normal early fetal anatomy survey, fetal echocardiography is probably a prudent precaution.

Although many practitioners would perform serial fetal well-being testing (nonstress test and amniotic fluid index) on this pregnancy beginning in the early third trimester, there is no evidence that this improves outcome in the absence of other signs of fetal compromise such as deficient fetal growth. Fetal umbilical artery Doppler flow velocimetry would only be indicated if the anatomy scan showed evidence of growth restriction.

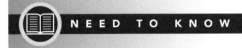

Late Risks: Neurobehavioral Alterations After Teratogen Exposure

A problem in identifying teratogenic effects is that they can be subtle or not evident until years after the exposure. This is particularly true with neurobehavioral effects given the fact that extensive neurologic and behavioral development occurs after delivery, and that infant development is also influenced by social, environmental, and hereditary factors. However, there have been certain teratogens that have been linked to decreased IQ, hyperactivity, learning disorders, and developmental delay. Teratogens have also been implicated in more subtle disorders, such as hyperactivity and autism. Of these teratogens, none is as well-known as alcohol. No safe alcohol dose has been established although its effects are known to be dose dependent. Thus pregnant women are told to abstain completely. Fetal alcohol effects include a spectrum of disorders that fall under the term "fetal alcohol spectrum disorders" or FASD, with fetal alcohol syndrome (FAS) representing the most severe diagnosis in this spectrum. The fetus is at increased risk for FAS if the mother consumes alcohol on a daily basis in large quantities throughout pregnancy. Fetal effects of alcohol exposure may include physical malformations, including microcephaly, and abnormalities of kidneys, heart, and face. In addition, alcohol use is associated with delayed motor and social skills, learning disabilities, hyperactivity, language problems, and memory deficits. Infants of women who consume smaller amounts of alcohol continue to be at risk for the neurobehavioral effects of FAS, although these infants rarely demonstrate the physical malformations. Although the exact mechanism of injury to the fetus is unclear, it is known that alcohol easily crosses the placenta and can accumulate in the amniotic fluid, thus prolonging fetal exposure.

Another well-known teratogen that can more subtly affect development is cocaine. Newborns prenatally exposed to cocaine may exhibit increased reflexes, decreased motor maturity, and an inability to control their state of attentiveness. Once in school, exposed children were reported to score lower on intelligence examinations than unexposed children and had shorter attention spans. There was also an increased rate of learning disabilities.

One teratogen receiving much attention is methylmercury contained in fish. Significant fetal exposure may cause abnormalities in neuronal cell division leading to developmental delays in attention, memory, language, and reaction time. It can also result in microcephaly and brain damage. Mercury enters the ocean from both man-made and natural sources and is converted into the more toxic methylmercury by bacteria. Methylmercury is ingested by fish and is stored in their fatty tissue. Higher doses of methylmercury are seen in older and larger fish, and fish that eat other fish, such as shark, tuna, king mackerel, and tilefish. The FDA recommends that pregnant women abstain from these types of fish during the entire pregnancy. Women may eat up to 12 ounces per week of fish that potentially contain small amounts of mercury such as shrimp, salmon, pollock, catfish, and canned light tuna. In addition, they should eat no more than 6 ounces of albacore (white) tuna per week.

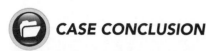

CASE CONCLUSION

The remainder of Ms. Sorenson's pregnancy is uncomplicated. A follow-up ultrasound at 24 weeks shows the estimated fetal weight to be appropriate. No further scans are performed and the patient delivers a normal appearing female infant at 39 weeks, with normal Apgar scores, weighing 3,700 g.

SUGGESTED READINGS

American College of Obstetricians and Gynecologists. Guidelines for Diagnostic Imaging during pregnancy. Committee Opinion No. 299, September 2004.

American College of Obstetricians and Gynecologists. Teratology. ACOG Educational Bulletin 236. Washington, DC: ACOG; 1997.

Bertrand J, Floyd RL, Weber MK, et al. Alcohol Syndrome: Guidelines for Referral and Diagnosis. Atlanta, GA: Centers for Disease Control and Prevention; 2004.

Brent RL. The effect of embryonic and fetal exposure to x-ray, microwaves, and ultrasound: counseling the pregnant and nonpregnant patient about these risks. Semin Oncol. 1989;16:3 47–68.

Fisher B, Rose NC, Carey JC. Principles and practice of teratology for the obstetrician. Clin Obstet Gynecol. 2008;51:106–18.

Goodsitt MM, Christodoulou EG. Diagnostic imaging in pregnancy: risks to the fetus. In: Pearlman M, Tintinalli JE, Dyne PL, editors. Obstetric and Gynecologic Emergencies: Diagnosis and Management. New York, NY: McGraw-Hill; 2003. pp. 535–48.

Lowe SA. Diagnostic radiography in pregnancy: risks and reality. Aust NZ J Obstet Gynecol. 2004;44:191–6.

Timor-Tritsch IE, Fuchs KM, Monteagudo A, D'alton ME. Performing a fetal anatomy scan at the time of first-trimester screening. Obstet Gynecol. 2009;113(2 Pt 1):402–7.

Wapner R, Thom E, Simpson JL, et al. First-trimester screening for trisomies 21 and 18. N Engl J Med. 2003;349:1405.

Cervical Incompetence

Sarah Yamaguchi

 CASE PRESENTATION

You are called to evaluate Ms. Myoto in triage. She is a 25-year-old G2 P0 at 20 0/7 weeks of gestation. She is complaining of mild, irregular uterine contractions as well as vaginal discharge for the past 2 days. She denies any gross rupture of membranes or vaginal bleeding. She says that she has not been sexually active for the past month. She denes any prior complications in this pregnancy, and reports no abdominal trauma, significant medical illness, or illicit drug use. She has been getting regular prenatal care since 10 weeks and her prenatal labs and first trimester screen are normal. She has a history of one prior pregnancy loss at 18 weeks. This loss occurred after a similar episode of mild cramping and increased vaginal discharge.

Ms. Myoto is afebrile, her pulse is 86 bpm, and her blood pressure is 110/72 mm Hg. Her cardiac and pulmonary examinations are unremarkable. Her abdomen is without evidence of trauma and her fundus is at the umbilicus. The fetal heart rate is 142 bpm. A sterile speculum examination is performed and the cervix appears closed. There is a small amount of pooling in the posterior cul de sac, but nitrazine testing is negative and there is no ferning under the microscope. A wet mount of the vaginal fluid shows only epithelial cells. A transvaginal ultrasound reveals that the cervix is 1.8 cm long. There is no funneling and there are no dynamic changes.

 Decision 1: Risk factors

What risk factors does this patient have for cervical insufficiency?

A. Maternal age
B. Gestational age
C. Prior pregnancy loss
D. Ethnicity

The correct answer is C: Prior pregnancy loss. A second trimester loss, especially with minimal perceived uterine activity, may be an indication of cervical insufficiency, and

puts the patient into a high-risk group for this condition. The patient's cervical length also increases her risk for premature delivery. Cervical insufficiency is not related to maternal age (Answer A), gestational age (Answer B), or maternal ethnicity (Answer D).

 NEED TO KNOW

Cervical Insufficiency

Cervical insufficiency, also called cervical incompetence, is characterized by the inability of the cervix to retain the pregnancy to term. Although diagnostic criteria are not standardized, the diagnosis traditionally requires a history of painless cervical dilatation. Signs and symptoms suggestive of silent cervical dilatation include an increase in vaginal discharge and a feeling of pelvic pressure. Conditions thought to predispose to failure of the cervix include developmental and traumatic injuries to the cervix, and a prior pregnancy loss characterized by painless cervical dilatation has been used to select patients for treatment. Unfortunately, many of the reported risk factors have not held up under scrutiny (Table 25.1). Formerly, cervical insufficiency was thought to be a condition distinct from preterm labor, and the occurrence of uterine contractions would negate the diagnosis. Current thinking is that cervical insufficiency and premature labor likely represent a continuum, with cervical insufficiency representing one part of the spectrum of disease. Accurate measurement of cervical length with ultrasound in the midtrimester has revealed a continuum of cervical lengths with a cervical length less than the 10th percentile (~2.5 cm) associated with a marked increase in the risk for preterm delivery (Fig. 25.1). These findings suggest that painless cervical shortening precedes most spontaneous early deliveries, whether or not uterine contractions eventually occur. The incidence of cervical insufficiency, based on hospital discharge diagnoses, is about 1 in 200 or 0.5%. The diagnosis of cervical insufficiency is thus further

TABLE 25.1

ALLEGED RISK FACTORS FOR CERVICAL INSUFFICIENCY

Risk Factor	Comment
Congenital	
Mullerian abnormalities	Limited information. Cerclage improved live birth rate from 21% to 62% in 14 selected patients
DES exposure	Increased second trimester pregnancy loss RR = 4–5. No available evidence that cerclage improves outcome
Abnormal collagen (Ehlers–Danlos syndrome)	Preterm delivery (21% if mother affected, 40% if infant affected). Cerclage commonly used but efficacy not proven
Traumatic	
Cone biopsy	Increase in preterm delivery RR = 5.3 Cerclage commonly used but efficacy not proven
LEEP	No increase in preterm delivery. Cerclage not indicated
Laceration at delivery	No effect on subsequent delivery. Cerclage not indicated
Dilatation and Curettage	Reports of increased risk of preterm delivery, RR = 1.36. Cerclage not indicated

complicated by the relative rarity of the disorder compared with preterm labor. As the incidence of preterm delivery among the 10% of patients with a midtrimester cervical length <2.5 cm may be as high as 60%, we are likely underreporting the occurrence of cervical insufficiency.

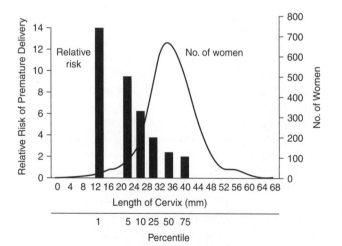

Figure 25.1 Distribution of cervical length measurements found at 24 weeks by vaginal ultrasound. The relative risks are for preterm delivery (before 35 weeks GA) for gravidas with cervical length at or below the 1st, 5th, 10th, 25th, 50th, and 75th percentile, compared with those with cervical length above the 75th percentile.

 CASE CONTINUES

Ms. Myoto is sent home on bedrest and pelvic rest. She returns at 22 weeks of gestation to your office complaining of increased vaginal pressure. She denies any uterine cramping. Transvaginal ultrasound reveals that her cervix is now 0.5 cm long and is 0.5 cm dilated. There is no evidence of bulging or hourglassing membranes on sterile speculum examination or on ultrasound. She is sent to the delivery room, where she is monitored overnight and she still shows no evidence of infection or preterm labor.

 Decision 2: Management

What management options are available?

- **A.** Cervical cerclage
- **B.** Pregnancy termination
- **C.** Progesterone
- **D.** Terbutaline

A (Cervical cerclage), **B** (pregnancy termination), or **C** (progesterone therapy) may be appropriate in this case. Cervical cerclage, or a suture placed around the cervix, is the most common treatment of cervical insufficiency and has been shown to reduce the rate of preterm delivery in patients who, like Ms. Myoto, have both a history of a prior preterm delivery and a cervix <1.5 cm in length. Even with cerclage, however, there remains a significant risk (about 20%) that Ms. Myoto will deliver by 30 weeks of gestation, leading to a significant risk of death or handicap to the fetus. If pregnancy termination is available, some patients would elect to terminate this pregnancy to avoid the risk of an extremely preterm infant, and would attempt another pregnancy. Finally, a variety of progesterone preparations have been reported to reduce the risk of preterm delivery in patients with a positive history. Some, but not all, studies have also found progesterone to be effective in preventing preterm delivery in the patient with a short cervix. Studies of the combination of progesterone and cerclage are not yet available. Terbutaline (Answer D) is incorrect because it is used as a tocolytic agent. This patient is not contracting so the use of a tocolytic would not be expected to improve her outcome.

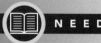 **NEED TO KNOW**

Preparation for Cerclage

Prior to performing a cerclage, the patient undergoes a workup to assess her chance of complications and her fitness for the procedure. She requires an examination to exclude any evidence of preterm labor or rupture of the membranes, which would be contraindications to the procedure. Other contraindications would be evidence of intraamniotic infection, multiple gestation, or if the patient does not consent. A sterile speculum examination is performed to evaluate the cervix and to determine whether the membranes are visible at the os. During the speculum examination, cultures may be taken for intravaginal infection. There is no consensus on which cultures should be performed, but obvious vaginitis, or known sexually transmitted infections should be treated prior to cerclage.

Given that intraamniotic infection frequently accompanies cervical shortening, some authors perform an amniocentesis to exclude infection prior to cerclage. The risk of an infection in the amniotic sac ranges from 1% to 2% in patients with simple shortening to 50% for those with advanced cervical dilatation. The recommendation has been made to perform an amniocentesis in those with dilated cervix or prolapsed membranes, and in any others with a suspicion for intraamniotic infection.

Ultrasound is performed to document fetal number and fetal life and to exclude lethal fetal anomalies. Additional prenatal testing will depend on the clinical situation and maternal preference. If time permits, and if the mother wants the information, other fetal testing, including first trimester NT screening, genetic amniocentesis, or chorionic villus sampling may be performed prior to an elective cerclage.

Finally, prior to the procedure, the patient must be informed of the risks and benefits, and must give consent. The risks and anticipated benefits of the procedure vary according to the degree of cervical change (Table 25.2).

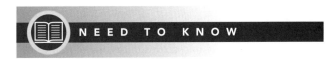

NEED TO KNOW

Cerclage Technique

General Considerations

Although antibiotics are recommended for active infection, prophylactic antibiotic use in cerclage placement has not been shown to improve outcome, and is not recommended, even in emergent cerclage. Similarly, tocolytic use is an area of controversy. Active preterm labor is a contraindication to cerclage, but many patients with an incompetent cervix will have some contractions with cervical manipulation. Many authorities use tocolytics (often indomethacin) immediately after cerclage, although this treatment has not been shown to alter outcome.

When the membranes are prolapsing into or beyond the cervix, some technique must be used to reduce the membranes into the uterus prior to performing the cerclage. When the degree of prolapse is minor, often putting the patient into a Trendelenburg position will reduce the prolapse. If the time is available, indomethacin can be used to reduce fetal urine flow and reduce the amniotic fluid volume, leading to reduction of the membranes. Indomethacin treatment will generally take 48 to 72 hours to be effective, and thus is often not an option. For acute reduction of prolapsing membranes, two alternatives are available: either amnioreduction prior to the procedure or physical reduction of the membrane during the procedure.

Amnioreduction is performed by inserting a needle into the amniotic cavity and withdrawing as much amniotic fluid as possible. This is effective in reducing membranes prolapsed into the cervix and has the advantage that there is no need to directly manipulate

TABLE 25.2

RISKS AND BENEFITS OF CERCLAGE BASED ON INDICATION CLASS

Class (ACOG, 2003)	Class (Berghella, 2007)	Risks of Procedure	Reduction in Preterm Birth
Elective (past history/ risk factors)	History-indicated	ROM: <1% Infection: 1%–2%	Reduced from 32% to 15%, *only in patients with three prior STL*
Urgent (Ultrasound shortening, cx <2.5 cm)	Ultrasound-indicated	ROM: <1% procedure-related, 15% overall. Infection: less than untreated (5% vs. 13%)	Reduced (RR = 0.6) *in patients with a history of a prior PTD or STL. Reduction may be limited to cx <1.5 cm*
Emergent (advanced cervical dilatation)	Physical examination-indicated	ROM: 13% Infection: 22%–50%	No randomized data. Cohort study suggests significant improvement from untreated (untreated: 90% PTD, 40% PND)

PND, perinatal death; PTD, preterm delivery; STL,- second trimester loss.
Reprinted by permission from Macmillan Publisher Ltd: Journal of Perinatology, Ventolini G, Genrich TJ, Roth J, et al. Pregnancy outcome after placement of `rescue' of Shirodkar cerclage, 29:276, 2009.

the prolapsing membrane. Amnioreduction may be performed after the induction of anesthesia for cerclage if desired for patient comfort. Complications of amnioreduction include rupture of the membranes, induction of contractions, and direct injury to the fetus or placenta. There are limited reports of amnioreduction prior to cerclage, but one small study reported an improved outcome in patients treated with amnioreduction as opposed to physical replacement of the membranes alone.

The membranes can also be physically reduced at the time of the cerclage procedure; amnioreduction and physical reduction are also sometimes used together. The membranes may be reduced by filling the maternal bladder. This has a low likelihood of causing harm but may obscure the operative field. The membranes may also be physically held out of the surgical field with a balloon catheter; many centers use a Foley catheter with a 30-cc balloon, overfilled to fill the lower uterine segment. The catheter is left in place until the cerclage suture is placed, deflated, and removed prior to tying the suture.

Surgical Technique

A cerclage may be placed transvaginally or transabdominally. Transvaginal placement is the more commonly performed route and is placed under either regional or general anesthesia. The two most common types of transvaginal cerclage are the McDonald and Shirodkar (Fig. 25.2).

The McDonald cerclage involves using a nonabsorbable suture to make a purse string suture at the junction of the cervix and vagina while being careful to avoid

the bladder. Starting at 12 o'clock, four bites are taken circumferentially on the cervix taking care not to enter the cervical canal. Once the ends are tied, care should be taken to leave the sutures long enough for easy identification and removal, as the McDonald cerclage is commonly removed prior to delivery. The McDonald cerclage is technically the easiest cerclage to perform and is the only feasible vaginal procedure in patients with a dilated and effaced cervix.

The Shirdokar cerclage attempts to insert the cerclage at the level of the internal os of the cervix. In this case, a transverse incision is made on the anterior and posterior cervix at the vaginal and cervical junction. The bladder and rectum are then dissected off the cervix bluntly. Doubly needled permanent suture is then used to enter the cervix at the lateral edges of the dissection and passed medial to the cervical branch of the uterine artery from anterior to posterior. The suture is then tied posteriorly. The vaginal mucosa can then be repaired over the suture. The Shirodkar suture may be removed prior to delivery, or it may be placed permanently, with Cesarean delivery required. There is no evidence of a difference in outcome between McDonald and Shirodkar cerclage procedures; however, in some cases with multiple prior procedures or past vaginal lacerations, the dissection involved in a Shirodkar cerclage may be needed to successfully place a suture.

Abdominal cerclage placement is a more morbid procedure given that it requires a laparotomy or laparoscopy to place and then a second procedure to deliver the fetus, but it allows for a more proximal placement of the cerclage and avoidance of a foreign body in the vagina that could become a nidus for infection. Abdominal cerclage is intended to be permanent and are left in place between pregnancies. Once the abdominal cavity is entered, the bladder is dissected from the uterus. Permanent suture is passed lateral to the uterus and medial to the branches of the uterine arteries at the level where the uterus and cervix meet on both sides of the uterus. The suture is then tied at the level of the insertion of the uterosacral ligaments. Abdominal cerclage tends to be reserved for patients with severe cervical anomalies, where placement of a vaginal cerclage is not possible.

 CASE CONTINUES

After discussing the treatment options as well as the risks and benefits, Ms. Myoto decides to have a cerclage placed. Her cervical cultures are all negative and she has no contraindications to cerclage placement. A McDonald cerclage is performed without complications under regional anesthesia. Postprocedure, she has no contractions and she is sent home with instructions to adhere to

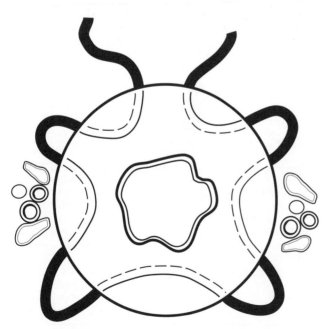

Figure 25.2 McDonald cerclage: Nonabsorbable suture is placed around the cervix, avoiding the vascular structures on the lateral cervix and the endocervix.

modified bedrest, and to return for bleeding, cramping, or rupture of membranes. She does well until 4 weeks after the procedure, at 26 weeks, when she complains of sudden loss of fluid. Her sterile speculum examination reveals an intact cerclage, but positive pooling of fluid in the vagina. The fluid tests positive for nitrazine and ferning is present, suggesting rupture of the membranes.

Decision 3: Management

What is the management at this point?

A. Remove cerclage
B. Antibiotics
C. Tocolytics
D. Steroids

The correct answers are antibiotics (Answer B) and steroids (Answer D). The fetus is now viable, and management includes standard management for a patient with preterm premature rupture of the membranes. These interventions include ampicillin and erythromycin, which have been demonstrated to increase the latency period between membrane rupture and delivery, and betamethasone, which reduced the incidence of respiratory distress in the newborn. Although neither of these interventions have been specifically tested in the patient with a cerclage in situ, their use is considered standard of care. In the absence of bleeding, uterine contractions or signs of infection, removal of the cerclage (Answer A) is generally not recommended. Despite concerns related to the risk of infection, studies have demonstrated either no difference or an improvement in outcome if the suture is left in place until delivery. Similarly, in the absence of uterine contractions there is no indication for tocolytics (Answer C).

CASE CONCLUSION

Ms. Myoto receives two doses of betamethasone 24 hours apart. She is kept hospitalized during this time and begins to have uterine contractions on her third hospital day. Her cerclage is immediately removed. She sponta-

neously progresses and has a vaginal delivery 7 hours later of a viable female infant weighing 980 g with the neonatologist in attendance. Subsequently, the baby does well with no evidence of intraventricular hemorrhage or infection and she is discharged home at 10 weeks of age.

The possibility of elective cerclage placement in subsequent pregnancies is discussed with the patient given her history and some evidence that cerclage may improve the outcome of patients with two prior episodes of cervical insufficiency. Alternatively, she is offered intensive surveillance of cervical length, with cerclage for cervical length less than 2.5 cm.

SUGGESTED READINGS

ACOG Practice Bulletin. Cervical insufficiency. Obstet Gynecol. 2003; 102:1091.

Berghella V, Odibo AO, To MS, Rust OA, Althuisius SM. Cerclage for short cervix on ultrasonography: meta-analysis of trials using individual patient-level data. Obstet Gynecol. 2005;106(1):181–9.

Berghella V, Seibel-Seamon J. Contemporary use of cervical cerclage. Clin Obstet Gynecol. 2007;50(2):468–77.

Harger JH. Cerclage and cervical insufficiency: an evidence-based analysis. Obstet Gynecol. 2002;100:1313.

Iams JD, Goldenberg RL, Meis PJ, et al. The length of the cervix and the risk of spontaneous premature delivery. National Institute of Child Health and Human Development Maternal Fetal Medicine Unit Network. N Engl J Med. 1996;334(9):567–72.

Kristensen J, Langhoff-Roos J, Kristensen FB. Increased risk of preterm birth in women with cervical conization. Obstet Gynecol. 1993;81: 1005.

Locatelli A, Vergani P, Bellini P, Strobelt N, Arreghini A, Ghidini A. Amnioreduction in emergency cerclage with prolapsed membranes: comparison of two methods for reducing the membranes. Am J Perinatol. 1999;16(2):73–7.

Nelson L, Dola T, Tran T, Carter M, Luu H, Dola C. Pregnancy outcomes following placement of elective, urgent and emergent cerclage. J Matern Fetal Neonatal Med. 2009;22(3):269–73.

Owen J, Hankins G, Iams JD, et al. Multicenter randomized trial of cerclage for preterm birth prevention in high-risk women with shortened midtrimester cervical length. Am J Obstet Gynecol. 2009; 201(4):375.e1–8.

Shirodkar VN. A new method of operative treatment for the habitual abortions in the second trimester of pregnancy. Antiseptic. 1955; 52:299.

To MS, Alfirevic Z, Heath VC, et al. Cervical cerclage for prevention of preterm delivery in women with short cervix: a randomized controlled trial. Lancet. 2004;363:1849.

Vyas NA, Vink JS, Ghidini A, et al. Risk factors for cervical insufficiency after term delivery. Am J Obstet Gynecol. 2006;195:787.

Ventolini G, Genrich TJ, Roth J, Neiger R. Pregnancy outcome after placement of 'rescue' Shirodkar cerclage. J Perinatol. 2009;29: 276–9; doi:10.1038/jp.2008.221; published online 22 January 2009.

Preterm Labor

Roy Z. Mansano

CASE PRESENTATION

Ms. Primo, a 24-year-old African-American female G2 P0100 presents to your office for prenatal care. She is transferring prenatal care as she has recently moved, and she is currently at 23 weeks of gestational age based on an early ultrasound that is consistent with her last menstrual period.

Ms. Primo reports that she has had no difficulties with her pregnancy up to this point. She denies significant past medical or surgical history. Her past Ob history is significant for a premature delivery. During that pregnancy, Ms. Primo started having uterine contractions at 27 weeks of gestation, which she confused for food poisoning and did not seek medical attention. When she finally started having vaginal spotting, she went to the hospital. On the way to the hospital, she began to feel vaginal pressure and delivered her baby in the parking lot of the hospital. This baby did not survive. She is a smoker, using 20 to 25 cigarettes daily. She recently moved in with her parents as her husband was deployed overseas with the military. She reports that her previous Ob was giving her weekly injections with the current pregnancy; she thinks that these were vitamin shots. She denies other medication use except for prenatal vitamins. The patient reports that she has been seen regularly by her Ob/Gyn during this pregnancy and he has even sent her to a high-risk obstetrician because of her history. With this pregnancy, her physician was performing regular vaginal ultrasounds and when she felt vaginal pressure at a specific visit, he "performed a test using a swab of my cervix." The patient reported that these tests were all normal. She last saw her Ob/Gyn approximately 2 weeks ago.

On physical examination, this is a slender woman who is in no distress. Her blood pressure is 140/75 mm Hg, her present weight is 140 lb (prepregnancy weight was 130 lb), and she is 67 inches tall. The remainder of her physical examination is within normal limits, and her fundal height is 22 cm above the pubic symphysis.

NEED TO KNOW

Preterm Labor and Delivery

Preterm delivery is defined as delivery prior to 37 completed weeks of gestation. Preterm delivery accounts for approximately 13% of all deliveries in the United States. Of those approximately 40% are due to spontaneous preterm labor (PTL), 35% are secondary to preterm premature rupture of the membranes, and 25% are obstetrically indicated. Preterm delivery also accounts for almost 70% of infant deaths (Fig. 26.1). In addition to death, the risk of long-term morbidity increases with increasing prematurity, with infants born <2,500 g having a 10-fold higher risk of neurologic impairment as compared with infants weighing more than 2,500 g. Although the majority of preterm deliveries occur near term (i.e., late preterm delivery), most of the morbidity and mortality associated with preterm delivery is experienced by those babies born before 34 weeks of gestation.

PTL is defined as labor prior to 37 weeks of gestation. PTL is a major contributor to preterm delivery, and it may be associated with an otherwise normal pregnancy. Given these facts, it appears that finding ways to reduce the risk of PTL would substantially reduce perinatal mortality.

Decision 1: Risk management

Which is a modifiable risk factor for PTL in this patient?

  A. African-American race
  B. Smoking
  C. Living situation
  D. Underweight

The correct answer is B: Smoking. Smoking is a risk factor for PTL, and smoking cessation may help to reduce her risk. African-American race (Answer A) is a risk factor;

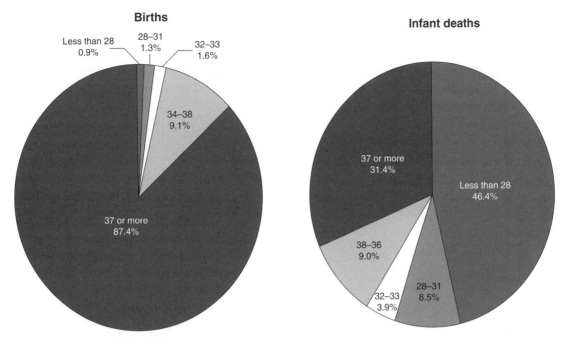

Figure 26.1 Perinatal mortality versus gestational age at delivery. Although infants born at <28 weeks of gestation are only 0.8% of total births in the United States, they account for almost half of infant deaths. (Adapted from 2005. National Vital Statistics Reports. 2006;57:2.)

however, it is not modifiable. The patient's living situation (Answer C) may be a cause of stress, which, in some studies, may be associated with PTL. Being underweight (Answer D) is a risk factor for PTL, but this patient is not underweight by body mass index (BMI) criteria, having a prepregnant BMI of 20.4.

Although much research effort has been devoted to decreasing the rates of preterm delivery, rates have not changed over the last 40 years. This is partially because of a failure to identify modifiable risk factors for PTL and to develop and institute interventions. Table 26.1 lists a number of risk factors (modifiable and not) that have been identified.

Several studies have evaluated methods of risk assessment in the hope of identifying women at higher risk of preterm delivery and thus potentially utilizing preventative measures. Studies have evaluated such parameters as history, physical examination, uterine activity monitoring, biochemical tests, and ultrasound. Unfortunately these studies were able to conclude that history, physical examination, and uterine activity monitoring are not sufficiently sensitive for the identification of the majority of at-risk women.

Modification of risk factors has, in general, been disappointing. Of the factors listed in Table 26.1, infection has been identified as an etiology of PTL that could be treated. For example, bacterial vaginosis (BV) increases the risk of preterm delivery approximately twofold. Treatment of symptomatic BV may be of value, though treatment of asymptomatic BV may paradoxically increase the rate of preterm delivery. Similarly, periodontal disease is associated with an

increased risk of preterm delivery, but prophylactic treatment of periodontal disease during pregnancy had no effect on the rate of preterm birth.

A history of preterm delivery does provide one instance in which prophylactic treatment has been shown to affect outcome. In women with such a history, treatment with progesterone has shown to decrease the recurrence of preterm delivery. Specifically, 17 hydroxy progesterone caproate has been shown to decrease the rate of PTL by approximately 37% in patients with prior preterm delivery, as shown by two large randomized trials. Other progesterone preparations have also shown an effect in smaller trials. The therapy starts at 16 to 24 weeks and continues until 36 weeks. Progesterone is not a treatment of PTL, but a preventative measure. However, once PTL occurs and is inhibited with tocolytic therapy, progesterone supplementation may reduce the rate of cervical shortening.

 CASE CONTINUES

At 27 weeks of gestation, Ms. Primo presents to labor and delivery complaining of uterine contractions. The patient reports that since she woke up in the morning she feels contractions that are very painful (8/10) and are occurring regularly every 5 to 10 minutes. She denies leakage of fluid and reports that the baby is frequently moving; however, she does report that she noticed minimal vaginal spotting when she used the

TABLE 26.1

RISK FACTORS FOR PRETERM DELIVERY. THE CATEGORIZATION OF MATERNAL RISK FACTORS IS ARBITRARY IN SOME CASES, FOR EXAMPLE, AFRICAN-AMERICAN RACE IS KNOWN TO BE ASSOCIATED WITH AN INCREASED RISK OF PRETERM LABOR/DELIVERY; HOWEVER, THE REASON FOR THIS IS UNKNOWN. SOME HAVE HYPOTHESIZED THAT SOCIAL PRESSURES ARE INCREASED ON WOMEN OF COLOR, LEADING TO AN INCREASE IN PTL

- Previous preterm delivery
- Maternal factors
  - Stress
- Anxiety
- Depression
- Life events (divorce, separation, death)
  - Social or economic stress
- Single women
- Low socioeconomic status
- African-American race
- Low level of educational achievement
- Maternal age (<18 or >40)
- Inadequate prenatal care
  - Fatigue
- Work standing
- Use of industrial machines
- Physical exertion
  - Inflammation
- Sexually transmitted infections
- Urinary tract infection
- Systemic infection
- Abdominal surgery during pregnancy
- Periodontal disease
  - Nutritional

- Poor nutrition and low body mass index
- Anemia (hemoglobin <10 g/dL)
  - Other/unexplained
- Substance abuse or smoking
- Maternal hypoxemia
- Anatomic factors
  - Cervical
- History of second trimester abortion
- History of cervical surgery
- Premature cervical dilatation or effacement
  - Uterine
- Uterine distention
- Multiple gestation
- Polyhydramnios
- Uterine anomaly
- Diethylstilbestrol
- Leiomyomata
  - Placental
- Placenta previa
- Placental abruption
- Vaginal bleeding
- Fetal factors
  - Congenital anomaly
  - Growth restriction

bathroom. She is very concerned that she will lose this pregnancy as she did the last one. Her manual cervical examination is 1 cm dilated and 50% effaced with the fetal vertex at −2 station.

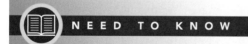 **N E E D   T O   K N O W**

Screening for Preterm Labor

Fetal fibronectin, a component of extracellular matrix between the chorion and decidua, is increased in cervicovaginal secretions of women who delivered early. Clinical trials have demonstrated that the negative predictive value (if negative, the patient will not go into labor) was the most significant utility of the test. Thus, if a patient has a negative fetal fibronectin, she has a 99% chance that she will not deliver within 14 days. If the test is positive, she has an increased chance of delivering early. The absolute risk depends on her a priori risk, but is <50% for most patients.

Vaginal ultrasound is also an effective tool in identifying those gravid patients at risk for preterm delivery. The vaginal ultrasound allows for a more objective approach to the examination of the cervix than the physical examination, and a quantification of the cervical length (Fig. 26.2). Ultrasound also provides a view of entire cervical canal including the internal os. This allows for visualization of funneling. In funneling, the membranes protrude past the internal os, giving a funnel appearance. On physical examination, the cervix may appear normal, although it is truly shortened with membranes funneling down as low as the external os. A short cervix has been defined as one that is below the 10th percentile for gestational age, or less than ~2.5 cm for the pregnancy less than 30 weeks gestation. The negative predictive value of this examination is similar to that of fetal fibronectin, and thus it has a similar utility in identifying those women not at risk for a premature delivery. Cervical length has been utilized primarily in asymptomatic women while fibronectin is currently best utilized in patients presenting with preterm uterine contractions.

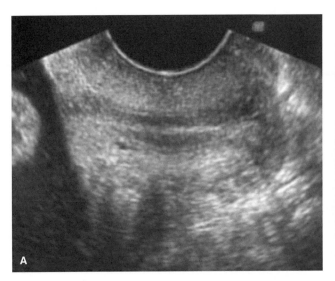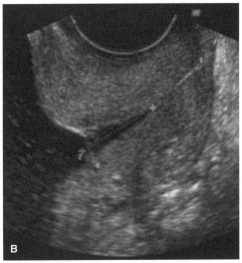

Figure 26.2 Ultrasound transvaginal examination of the cervix. A: Normal cervix at 23 weeks, measuring 38 mm. B: Short cervix at 16 weeks measuring 12 mm (also note the presence of a funnel). White arrow = functional internal os, black arrow = external os, arrowheads = cervical canal. (Reproduced with permission from Mella MT, Berghella V. Prediction of preterm birth: cervical sonography. Semin Perinatol. 2009;33(5):317–24. Review.)

In many centers, ultrasound-determined cervical length and fetal fibronectin are used together to predict the risk of preterm delivery among symptomatic patients. One such scheme is described in Figure 26.3. With a normal cervical length, the risk of preterm delivery is small and the patient can safely be discharged (Fig. 26.4). If the cervix is short (<1.5 cm) and uterine contractions present, the patient is generally admitted. For cervical lengths in the midrange (e.g., 1.5–3 cm), the fetal fibronectin test is sent; if this is negative there is a very high negative predictive value for delivery within 7 days. The patient can once again be managed conservatively, assuming contractions abate.

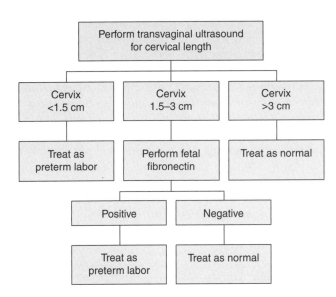

Figure 26.3 Triage of the symptomatic patient presenting in possible preterm labor. Initial triage is by the transvaginal ultrasound cervical length. For patients with intermediate cervical length values, fetal fibronectin is used to clarify risk status.

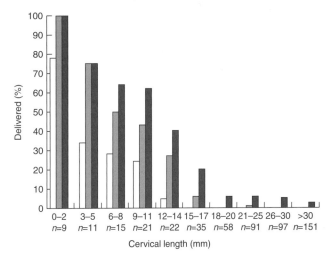

Figure 26.4 Risk of delivery within 48 hours (open bars), within 7 days (gray bars) and before 35 weeks of gestation (black bars) based on cervical length at presentation among women presenting with threatened premature labor. (Adapted from Tsoi E, Fuchs IB, Rane S, et al. Sonographic measurement of cervical length in threatened preterm labor in singleton pregnancies with intact membranes. Ultrasound Obstet Gynecol. 2005;25:353–6.)

Decision 2: Diagnosis

What criteria must be met to diagnose PTL?

A. Positive fetal fibronectin
B. Transvaginal cervical length <2.5 cm
C. Cervical dilatation of 1 cm
D. Regular uterine contractions and evidence of cervical change

The correct answer is D: Regular uterine contractions and evidence of cervical change. A positive fetal fibronectin (Answer A) and a cervical length <2.5 cm (Answer B) increase the risk that the patient will have PTL and delivery, but they are not diagnostic criteria for actual PTL. A cervical dilatation of 1 cm (Answer C) may be normal in this multigravid patient, although it may also be due to PTL.

Once a patient presents complaining of preterm uterine contractions, an evaluation must to be made to diagnose PTL. This diagnosis, as outlined by the American College of Obstetrics and Gynecology is confirmed by either

1. Regular uterine contractions associated with cervical change or
2. A cervix that is dilated on presentation.

 CASE CONTINUES

Ms. Primo has a cervical length of 1 cm and a positive fetal fibronectin. After 2 hours of observation she is contracting every 5 minutes and her cervical examination is 2 cm dilated, 80% effaced with the fetal vertex at −2 station.

 Decision 3: Treatment

How should the patient be managed at this time?

A. Continued observation
B. Cervical cerclage
C. Magnesium sulfate tocolysis
D. Betamethasone intramuscular (IM) only

The correct answer is C: Magnesium sulfate tocolysis. The patient has met criteria for PTL, and should be treated with tocolytic medications. Continued observation (Answer A) would be inappropriate given the presumed PTL. Cervical cerclage (Answer B) is not appropriate in a patient with contractions. Betamethasone (Answer D) is administered to induce pulmonary maturity in a patient expected to deliver. Betamethasone is not expected to reduce uterine contractions. In addition, the effect of steroids wanes after 1 week, while multiple doses are associated with decreased fetal size. Many practitioners would refrain from adminis-

tering steroids until the delivery seemed likely to occur within the next one to two weeks. These practitioners might wait to assess the effect of tocolytic medication before administering steroids for pulmonary maturity.

 NEED TO KNOW

Treatment of Preterm Labor

Once PTL is diagnosed, treatment is initiated. Treatment efforts are aimed at preventing newborn complications secondary to early delivery and are thus based on three main concepts.

- First tocolytics are used to try to stop or slow down the progress of labor in an attempt to administer corticosteroids and allow possible transfer to a center with experienced neonatal intensive care unit (NICU).
- Corticosteroids are administered to accelerate the maturation of the fetus, anticipating an early delivery.
- Antibiotics are used as prophylaxis against possible fetal/neonatal group B streptococcus infection.

In addition, it is customary to have the patient at bedrest, although there is no evidence that this is an effective intervention.

After extensive research, the effectiveness of tocolytics for the treatment of PTL remains controversial. Most tocolytics have significant adverse side effects while evidence showing effectiveness is limited, and such evidence is often limited to prolongation of the pregnancy for 48 hours. In studies with a placebo treatment arm, 40% to 60% of patients with "PTL" responded to placebo, suggesting that in many patients treatment is not necessary. Significantly, there is no clear evidence in the data that tocolysis improves perinatal outcome, with the exception of permitting 48 hours for the administration of corticosteroids. Based on this information, most experts do not recommend the use of tocolytics at or after 34 weeks of gestation, as steroids are not used routinely after 34 weeks. In addition, tocolysis should not be initiated if there is a contraindication to continued pregnancy, such as intrauterine infection or fetal demise. There are four commonly used tocolytics, which are also the best studied. These are magnesium sulfate, indomethacin, nifedipine, and terbutaline.

Magnesium Sulfate

Magnesium sulfate is the most commonly used tocolytic in the United States. It is no better than other commonly used tocolytics; its widespread use can be attributed to its ease of administration with intravenous drip and its familiarity on the delivery floor. Magnesium appears to act by inhibiting voltage-dependent calcium channels, thus reducing calcium-dependent myometrial contraction. There are several common maternal side effects including nausea, dry mouth, maternal flushing, drowsiness, blurred vision, and headache. Magnesium toxicity is the most concerning side effect, with such outcomes as loss of deep tendon reflexes, mental status changes, respiratory depression, pulmonary edema, severe hypotension, and ultimately cardiac arrhythmias and cardiac arrest. Magnesium sulfate is also of concern for the fetus since it easily crosses the placenta and thus may result in depression (both motor and respiratory) of the newborn. Alternatively, magnesium has also been reported to benefit the newborn; one study reported a 45% reduction in cerebral palsy when the infant had been exposed to magnesium in utero.

Magnesium is cleared through the kidney. Prior to using magnesium the physician should be aware of the patient's renal status to reduce the risk of magnesium overload. In addition, the evaluation of the patient should include a baseline mental status examination, pulmonary evaluation, and normal deep tendon reflexes. Once the above is established, magnesium is usually started with a 6-g loading dose over 20 to 30 minutes, followed by 1 to 3 g/hr for maintenance. In many centers, the infusion is begun at 2 g/hr IV. The magnesium drip may be adjusted upward if the patient continues to contract, to a maximum of 3 g/hr. Conversely, the dose may be adjusted down if the patient begins to have intolerable symptoms. To exclude signs of magnesium toxicity, the patient is regularly evaluated for deep tendon reflexes and for mental status changes. If either of these evaluations is abnormal, the magnesium drip should be discontinued or slowed, followed by an emergent assessment of serum magnesium levels. If the patient is experiencing life-threatening symptoms, such as respiratory depression, calcium gluconate may be administered intravenously to reverse the effects of the magnesium. This should rarely occur. The therapeutic range of magnesium is 5 to 8 mg/dL. In general, serum magnesium levels of 9 to 13 mg/dL are associated with loss of the deep tendon reflexes, while levels of >14 mg/dL are associated with respiratory depression. Most patients will experience loss of the reflexes and other symptoms (blurry vision, lethargy) significantly before the onset of respiratory depression. Magnesium therapy has been shown to be delay delivery for 48 hours. However, efficacy beyond the 48-hour window is unproven.

Indomethacin

Indomethacin, a nonselective cyclooxygenase (COX)-2 inhibitor, works by inhibiting prostaglandin synthesis at the level of the decidua. It is an effective tocolytic perhaps because the mechanism of PTL is often inflammatory and ultimately involves prostaglandin synthesis. The side effects of indomethacin can be divided into maternal and fetal. Maternal toxicity with indomethacin is uncommon and consists primarily of allergic reactions, stomach upset and gastrointestinal bleeding. The fetal side effects are more problematic, as they include constriction or premature closure of the ductus arteriosus and oligohydramnios. Closure of the ductus appears to be more likely in the fetus above 32 weeks of gestation. There has also been concern for an increased risk of intraventricular hemorrhage, although this risk has not been demonstrated in randomized trials. Contraindications to the use of indomethacin include allergy to aspirin or other nonsteroidal anti-inflammatory medications, maternal coronary artery disease or renal failure, fetal cardiac lesions or oligohydramnios, and gestational age >32 weeks.

The most common indomethacin dosage is a 100 mg loading dose followed by 50 mg four times daily for up to 48 hours. Indomethacin is usually limited to a 48-hour course because of the risk of ductal constriction and oligohydramnios. To monitor for fetal side effects during treatment, a periodic evaluation of amniotic fluid index is often performed. If oligohydramnios occurs, stopping the medication will usually result in reaccumulation of the amniotic fluid.

Nifedipine

Nifedipine is a calcium channel blocker. It causes smooth muscle relaxation by decreasing calcium influx into the cell. Several recent studies have demonstrated that nifedipine is also effective for the standard 48-hour time period required for the administration of steroids. As compared with other tocolytics, nifedipine is associated with fewer side effects. Maternal side effects are headache, nausea, flushing, hypotension, tachycardia, and hepatotoxicity. The fetal side effects are not known. It appears that nifedipine is well tolerated by the human fetus. A possible concern is that nifedipine is associated with fetal acidosis and hypoxemia in some animal studies, perhaps due to reduction in uteroplacental perfusion. When compared with other tocolytic agents, nifedipine demonstrated a similar effect with fewer side effects. One current dosing scheme for nifedipine is 10 mg PO every 20 minutes for a total of three doses, followed by 10 to 20 mg every 4 to 6 hours.

Terbutaline

Subcutaneous terbutaline (0.25 mg) is used in some centers to quiet uterine contractions in a patient who is not thought to be in PTL, or who has excess uterine activity. Repeated doses may be administered, though it is not utilized for long-term tocolysis. As a betamimetic, intravenous terbutaline therapy was associated with a high risk of maternal tachycardia, hypotension, hypokalemia, hyperglycemia, and pulmonary edema. Accordingly, intravenous terbutaline is rarely used for tocolysis.

Corticosteroids

Steroids currently provide the only evidence-based rational for administration of tocolytics. With properly administered steroids, the risk of neonatal respiratory distress syndrome and intraventricular hemorrhage is decreased by approximately 50%. The risk of necrotizing enterocolitis and nonpulmonary neonatal death are also decreased. A decrease in neonatal death is not consistently seen in fetuses born after 34 weeks of gestation. Given this timeline, tocolysis and steroids are not recommended after a gestational age of 34 weeks. Current dosing recommendations are two IM doses of 12 mg betamethasone, 24 hours apart. Full benefit is reached only 24 hours after the second dose. Four IM 6 mg dexamethasone doses 12 hours apart is an acceptable alternative to betamethasone. The difference in mortality with steroids only persists for 1 to 2 weeks, and there is considerable controversy as to the best response to recurrent PTL after 7 days. One study found that a single repeat dose of steroids improved outcome, while others have found that multiple repeat doses were associated with reduced fetal growth and birth weight. Concerns have also been raised about the long-term effect of steroids on the health of the child into adulthood due to the presumed role of steroids in the phenomenon of fetal programming. This information has led some authorities to recommend that steroids be reserved for the fetus that is very clearly going to deliver within the next week.

Antibiotics

Antibiotics are used prophylactically to prevent group B beta-streptococcus (GBS) infection in the neonate. All patients in PTL are considered at high risk for neonatal GBS and thus should receive prophylactic antibiotics if they are known carriers or if they are of unknown GBS status. The recommended treatment is penicillin is 5 million units loading dose followed by 2.5 million units every 4 hours. Penicillin allergic patients should get a culture and sensitivity of the GBS if possible.

Although antibiotic use can increase the latency interval in patients with ruptured membranes, large trials have failed to show that antibiotics increase the time to delivery in PTL with intact membranes. In one large study, children treated in utero with antibiotics to prevent preterm delivery had an increased risk of cerebral palsy. Therefore, prophylactic antibiotic use is contraindicated other than for GBS.

CASE CONCLUSION

You administer nifedipine for tocolysis. After an additional 2 hours, the patient continues to have contractions every 10 to 15 minutes, and you administer the first dose of betamethasone for fetal lung maturity. Uterine contractions eventually abate, and Ms. Primo is transferred to the ward with the cervix 2 to 3 cm dilated and 80% effaced after completion of her steroid course. On the fifth hospital day, she experiences premature rupture of the membranes. She is returned to labor and delivery, where she is found to be in active labor. Two hours later she delivers a viable female infant weighing 1,076 g with the NICU team in attendance. She does well after the delivery and is discharged on postpartum day two. The baby remains in the NICU for intensive care due to prematurity.

SUGGESTED READINGS

ACOG practice bulletin number 43, May 2003: Management of preterm labor.

Blumenfeld YJ, Lyell DJ. Prematurity prevention: the role of acute tocolysis. Curr Opin Obstet Gynecol. 2009;21(2):136–41. Review.

Elliott JP, Lewis DF, Morrison JC, Garite TJ. In defense of magnesium sulfate. Obstet Gynecol. 2009;113(6):1341–8. Review.

Mella MT, Berghella V. Prediction of preterm birth: cervical sonography. Semin Perinatol. 2009;33(5):317–24. Review.

Mercer BM, Merlino AA, Society for maternal-fetal medicine. Magnesium sulfate for preterm labor and preterm birth. Obstet Gynecol. 2009;114(3):650–68. Review.

Ness A. Prevention of preterm birth based on short cervix: symptomatic women with preterm labor or premature prelabor rupture of membranes. Semin Perinatol. 2009;33(5):343–51. Review.

Offenbacher S, Beck JD, Jared HL, et al. Effects of periodontal therapy on rate of preterm delivery: a randomized controlled trial. Obstet Gynecol. 2009;114(3):551–9.

Rode L, Langhoff-Roos J, Andersson C, et al. Systematic review of progesterone for the prevention of preterm birth in singleton pregnancies. Acta Obstet Gynecol Scand. 2009;88(11):1180–9. Review.

Uterine Anomalies

Tasmia Q. Henry

CASE PRESENTATION

Your are asked to see Ms. Price, a 24-year-old G1 P0 at 19 6/7 weeks of gestation, who presents to the emergency department complaining of 2 days of uterine cramping and 1 day of vaginal bleeding. She has recently moved to town but reports that she had prenatal care with a midwife from 12 weeks of gestation. She denies any significant past medical history and has never had a surgical procedure. She denies the use of alcohol, tobacco, or illicit drugs. Her medications are prenatal vitamins and iron. Examination in the emergency department reveals a thin anxious woman in moderate distress from uterine contractions. Her pulse is 100 bpm, blood pressure is 110/63 mm Hg, and she is afebrile. Her physical examination is unremarkable except for her pelvic examination: on speculum examination the cervix is 5 cm dilated with membranes protruding from the cervical os. Twenty minutes after the speculum examination, Ms. Price delivers a nonviable infant weighing 186 g. Shortly thereafter, she delivers the placenta, and is admitted to the hospital overnight for observation.

Ms. Price is devastated that she has lost her baby and asks you what could have gone wrong.

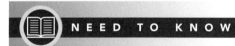

Etiologies of Second Trimester Loss

The factors associated with spontaneous second trimester pregnancy loss are similar to those associated with first trimester losses (Table 27.1), although the proportions of patients in the various categories is different. Second trimester losses represent a small fraction (about 2%) of all miscarriages. About 15% of second trimester losses may be associated with uterine anomalies, and 30% to 50% (depending on the population studied) are associated with signs of placental inflammation and presumed infection. A minority of second trimester losses are due to fetal chromosomal abnormalities. The etiology of second trimester loss is of concern, as about 25% of patients will experience another second trimester loss in the subsequent pregnancy.

CASE CONTINUES

The fetus appears normal on physical examination, and pathologic examination of the placenta does not suggest an infectious cause.

Decision 1: Workup

Which of the following is the best approach to screen for a uterine anomaly?

- **A.** Ultrasound
- **B.** Computed tomography (CT) scan
- **C.** Hysteroscopy
- **D.** Laparoscopy

The correct answer is A: Ultrasound. An ultrasound (US) (Answer A), can effectively evaluate the internal and external uterine contour, can detect a pelvic mass, hematometra, or hematocolpos, and can confirm the presence of ovaries. It is also useful for detection of noncommunicating or obstructed uterine horns that are not visualized by hysterosalpingogram (HSG) (Fig. 27.1).

An addition to the ultrasound examination, a sonohysterogram, can be performed to evaluate the uterine cavity only. This procedure involves injection of saline into the uterine cavity and permits further delineation of the intracavitary space. This may give more detailed information regarding filling defects caused by either endometrial polyps or uterine synechiae (adhesions).

An HSG, which is not listed, is often the first diagnostic modality used to screen for a uterine anomaly. Using this technique, a radiopaque dye is injected into the uterine cavity. A radiograph of the uterine cavity is then taken. An HSG can help evaluate tubal patency along with internal structure of the uterus. HSG, however, will not be able to identify obstructed, atretic, or noncommunicating uterine horns.

Hysteroscopy (Answer C) and laparoscopy (Answer D) are often used in combination to further evaluate and to treat uterine anomalies. Hysteroscopy allows direct visualization of the inside of the uterine cavity. Laparoscopy can

TABLE 27.1
FACTORS ASSOCIATED WITH SECOND TRIMESTER LOSS. THESE FACTORS REPRESENT ASSOCIATIONS; A CAUSAL RELATIONSHIP HAS NOT BEEN PROVEN. THE RELATIONSHIP OF INHERITED THROMBOPHILIAS AND PREGNANCY LOSS HAS BEEN CALLED INTO QUESTION

a. Fetal
   i. Chromosomal abnormalities
   ii. Congenital anomalies
b. Maternal
   iii. Anatomic factors (e.g., incompetent cervix, intrauterine adhesions, leiomyomata, uterine anomalies)
   iv. Immunologic factors (e.g., antiphospholipid antibodies [anticardiolipin antibody and lupus anticoagulant])
   v. Infection (e.g., bacterial vaginosis, intra-amniotic infection)
   vi. Placental problems (e.g., hematoma, retained intrauterine device, placental abruption, placenta previa)
   vii. Severe acute illness
   viii. Thrombophilia (e.g., factor V Leiden, protein S deficiency, prothrombin *G202 10 A* mutation)
   ix. Uncontrolled chronic illness (e.g., diabetes, hypertension)
   x. Other: Drug use, preterm premature rupture of membranes, smoking, teratogen exposure, trauma (e.g., physical abuse)

From Michels TC, Tiu AY. Second trimester pregnancy loss. Am Fam Physician. 2007;76:1341–6, 1347–8.

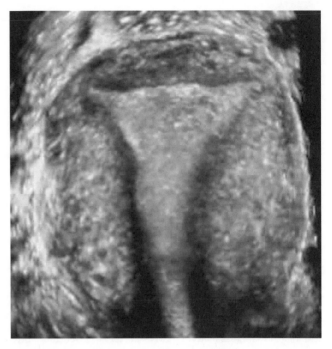

Figure 27.1 Ultrasound of normal uterus. This type of image is typically obtained by manipulation of a 3D volume. The exterior of the uterus is globular; the internal cavity is triangular. The cervix is at the bottom of the image. (Reproduced with permission from: http://www.advancedfertility.com/uterus.htm.)

then be employed to directly visualize the outer surface of the uterus. This may be necessary to differentiate a uterine septum (a division within the cavity) from a divided uterus.

Urinary tract abnormalities are often seen in conjunction with uterine anomalies. These include horseshoe or pelvic kidney, renal agenesis, duplication of the collecting system, and ectopic ureters. The preferred imaging modalities to evaluate the renal system are intravenous pyelogram, renal ultrasound, or a CT scan (Answer B).

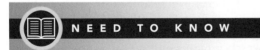

N E E D   T O   K N O W

Types of Developmental Abnormalities of the Female Genital Tract

The uterus, cervix, and upper vagina are formed by fusion of the paramesonephric (Mullerian) ducts in embryonic life; the fallopian tubes represent the more proximal, unfused ends of these ducts. Developmental abnormalities of the female genitalia (Mullerian abnormalities) can result from failure to complete bilateral duct elongation, fusion, canalization, or septal resorption. The overall incidence varies from 0.02% to 74%,

depending on classification used and populations studied. Mullerian anomalies may be associated with pregnancy loss as a result of reduced uterine size and/or abnormalities of vascularization.

The American Society for Reproductive Medicine developed a seven-part classification system for Mullerian anomalies (Table 27.2). As a simplification, Mullerian anomalies can be classified into three major categories: agenesis and hypoplasia, lateral fusion defects, and vertical fusion defects. Lateral fusion defects may be amenable to surgical correction and are further discussed here. Lateral fusion defects may occur due to failure of migration of one Mullerian duct, fusion of the Mullerian ducts, or absorption of the intervening septum between the ducts.

Unicornuate Uterus

Embryologic Defect
Failure of one Mullerian duct to complete bilateral duct elongation. This is an asymmetrical lateral fusion defect that usually results in a functional uterus with a normal cervix and unilateral fallopian tube, and varying configurations of abnormal Mullerian development on the contralateral side.

Didelphic Uterus

Embryologic Defect
Failure of fusion of the two Mullerian ducts, resulting in duplication of Mullerian structures. There are two uteri,

TABLE 27.2

CLASSIFICATION OF MULLERIAN ABNORMALITIES

Class I: Hypoplasia/uterine agenesis.

Class II: Unicornuate uterus:
   a) Has a functioning endometrium and communication with the main uterine cavity. ☐
   b) Also has an endometrial structure that responds to hormonal stimulus; however, there is no communication with the external genital tract. ☐
   c) Has a rudimentary structure with no activity, attached to a more fully developed uterine horn. ☐
   d) Results from the development of only one Müllerian duct, with complete agenesis of the contralateral duct.

Class III: Uterus didelphys.

Class IV: Bicornuate uterus:
   a) Complete: when the indentation produced in the fundic region is deep, thus indicating that fusion failed from the level of the cervical region. ☐
   b) Incomplete: when the division is higher, not extending to the level of the cervix, indicated by the shallower indentation in the contour of the region of the uterine fundus.

Class V: Septate uterus:
   a) When the septum extends into the internal cervical ostium, possibly including the cervical canal, and divides the cervix into two tunneled cavities. A vaginal septum is often also present. ☐
   b) When the septum does not divide the uterine cavity along its entire length, and circulation exists between the two chambers.

Class VI: Arcuate uterus: This anomaly involves a protrusion into the fundal endometrial cavity, without a change in the uterine contour. It has the lowest association with reproductive complications, and is sometimes treated as a normal variant.

Class VII: T-shaped uterus resulting from the use of DES.

From Ribeiro SC, Tormena RA, Peterson TV, et al. Müllerian duct anomalies: review of current management. Sao Paulo Med J. 2009;127(2):92–6. Review.

endometrial cavities, and cervices. Approximately 75% of cases will also have a longitudinal vaginal septum. These women have a high fetal loss rate. Women who present with a history of recurrent pregnancy loss or preterm delivery may be candidates for surgical correction. A live birth rate of up to 80% has been reported following this procedure.

Bicornuate Uterus

Embryologic Defect

Incomplete fusion of two Mullerian ducts at the level of the fundus, extending a variable distance into the endometrial cavity, with a single cervix. The external contour of the uterus is indented, defined as more than 1 cm.

Septate Uterus

Embryologic Defect

A defect in resorption of midline septum between the two Mullerian ducts, resulting in a fibromuscular uterine septum. The extent of septation varies, however, the external contour of the uterus is normal appearing. A longitudinal vaginal septum is found most frequently with this anomaly.

The septate uterus is the most common Mullerian anomaly and has the poorest reproductive outcome, depending upon the size of the septum. The poor obstetrical outcome is believed to be due to poorly vas-

cularized fibromuscular tissue in the septum. This may compromise decidual and placental growth. Another proposed mechanism is impaired fetal growth due to the reduced endometrial capacity and distorted cavity.

 CASE CONTINUES

Six weeks following her delivery, Ms. Price is referred for an ultrasound. Ultrasound is suggestive of a bicornuate uterus.

 Decision 2: Workup

What additional diagnostic testing is desirable?

   A. Magnetic resonance imaging (MRI)
   B. Serum estrogen levels
   C. Renal ultrasound
   D. Laparoscopy

MRI (Answer A), is considered the gold standard for imaging uterine anomalies. It is less operator dependant than ultrasound, and may be more accurate. It may more readily outline the uterine contour, and therefore can distinguish between a bicornuate, didelphic, and septate uterus.

TABLE 27.3

PREGNANCY OUTCOMES WITH VARIOUS MULLERIAN ANOMALIES. THESE OUTCOMES MAY BE EXAGGERATED, DUE TO PUBLICATION BIAS

	Miscarriage (%)	Premature Delivery (%)	Fetal Survival (%)
Septate uterus	>60	–	6–28
Unicornuate uterus	43.8	25	43.7
Uterus didelphys	35	19	60
Bicornuate uterus	40	–	62

From Ribeiro SC, Tormena RA, Peterson TV, et al. Müllerian duct anomalies: review of current management. Sao Paulo Med J. 2009;127(2): 92–6. Review.

Many specialists also consider laparoscopy (Answer D) to be an ideal method for detection, especially when, as in this case, the uterine contour is a primary concern. If a uterine anomaly is confirmed, a renal ultrasound (Answer C) should also be performed due to the high association of coexisting renal abnormalities. Estrogen (Answer B) is an ovarian hormone, and would not be helpful in the diagnosis of uterine abnormalities.

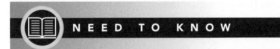

Pregnancy Outcomes with Uterine Anomalies

Pregnancy outcomes with Mullerian anomalies have been reported to be poor (Table 27.3). However, the

true fetal loss rate with these anomalies is likely lower, as the uterine anomaly is more likely to be diagnosed in a patient who has experienced a loss. In patients who have a history of pregnancy loss, surgical treatment may improve outcome in patients with a uterine septum or with a bicornuate uterus/uterus didelphys. Surgery on a unicornuate uterus does not appear to improve reproductive outcome (Table 27.4).

 CASE CONTINUES

MRI reveals that Ms. Price has a septate uterus. She states that she would like to attempt another pregnancy as soon as possible.

 Decision 3: Management

Which management options are appropriate?

- **A.** Hysteroscopy with septoplasty
- **B.** D&C
- **C.** Cerclage
- **D.** Uterine reunification procedure

Answer A: Hysteroscopy with septoplasty (resection of the septum) is correct. If there was any doubt as to the exact diagnosis, this might be combined with a laparoscopy to ensure that the patient did not have a bicornuate/didelphic uterus that would lead to a uterine perforation if septostomy were attempted. D&C (Answer B) would be unlikely to fully remove the septum. Although a patient with a Mullerian anomaly may be at increased risk for cervical insufficiency, cerclage (Answer C) would be inappropriate in this patient unless asymptomatic cervical shortening were seen in a subsequent

TABLE 27.4

PREGNANCY OUTCOMES WITH A SEPTATE UTERUS. THERE IS A WIDE RANGE OF REPORTED OUTCOMES; HOWEVER, AN AVERAGE FULL-TERM BIRTH RATE OF ONLY 14% IS FELT TO JUSTIFY ATTEMPTS TO CORRECT THE UTERINE SEPTUM

References	No. of Patients	No. of Pregnancies	Abortion Rate (%)	Premature Birth Rate (%)	Full-Term Rate (%)	Fetal Survival (%)
Maneschi (1915)	12	31	32	10	58	65
Gray (1984)	30	65	94	1	5	6
Buttram (1983)	72	208	67	33	0	28
Daly (1983)	17	40	85	13	2	10
Heinonen (1982)	41	81	26	9	68	75
Total	172	425	65	21	14	32

From Propst AM, Hill JA. Anatomic factors associated with recurrent pregnancy loss. Semin Reprod Med. 2000;18(4).

pregnancy. Uterine reunification (Strassman) procedures (Answer D) are used in cases with a double uterus (bicornuate or didelphic).

 CASE CONCLUSION

After discussion of the options, Ms. Price undergoes a hysteroscopy with resection of her septum. Six months following the resection, an intrauterine pregnancy at 12 weeks is confirmed. The patient is followed closely during her pregnancy, and eventually delivers a healthy female infant at 38 weeks.

SUGGESTED READINGS

Cooney MJ, Benson CB, Doubilet PM. Outcome of pregnancies in women with uterine duplication anomalies. J Clin Ultrasound. 1998;26:3–6.

Michels TC, Tiu AY. Second trimester pregnancy loss. Am Fam Physician. 2007;76:1341–6, 1347–8.

Propst AM, Hill JA. Anatomic factors associated with recurrent pregnancy loss. Semin Reprod Med. 2000;18(4).

Rackow BW. Arici A. Reproductive performance of women with Mullerian anomalies. Curr Opin Obstet Gynecol. 2007;19: 229–37.

Ribeiro SC, Tormena RA, Peterson TV, et al. Müllerian duct anomalies: review of current management. Sao Paulo Med J. 2009;127(2): 92–6. Review.

Zlopasa G, Skrablin S, Kalafatic D, Banovic V. Uterine anomalies and pregnancy outcome following resectoscope metroplasty. Int J Gynecol Obstet. 2007;98:129–33.

Premature Rupture of Membranes and Chorioamnionitis

28

Carol L. Archie

 CASE PRESENTATION

You have been covering labor and delivery on a quiet evening when you are called by the triage nurse to evaluate Mrs. Hsu. When you enter triage you find an anxious appearing woman in no obvious physical distress. The triage nurse's note reports that she is a 30-year-old G3 P2 at 30 weeks of gestational age by last menstrual period. She is concerned that she is leaking fluid. You confirm that she has had two prior vaginal deliveries at term. Her current pregnancy had been uncomplicated, and her pregnancy dating is confirmed by first and second trimester ultrasounds. The patient reports that she awakened from a deep sleep feeling wet. She first she thought she had urinated on herself so she went to the bathroom, cleaned herself and returned to bed. She became concerned when she continued to feel wet. She denies any contractions or bleeding and reports good fetal movement.

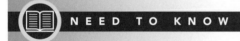 **NEED TO KNOW**

Defining Rupture of Membranes

A. Spontaneous Rupture of Membranes (SROM) is a normal component of labor and delivery. In most cases, SROM occurs when the membranes rupture prior to vaginal delivery but after labor commences.

B. Premature Rupture of Membranes (PROM) is the loss of amniotic fluid from the uterine cavity of a pregnancy at or beyond 37 weeks prior to the onset of labor. When PROM occurs at term labor usually begins spontaneously or is induced within 12 to 24 hours.

C. Preterm Premature Rupture of Membranes (PPROM) is the loss of amniotic fluid from the uterine cavity of a pregnancy prior to 37 weeks. This complication of pregnancy occurs in 2% to 4% of singleton deliveries and is associated with 18% to 20% of perinatal deaths.

The management of PPROM is dependent upon the gestational age at which it occurs. Management demands balancing the risks of prematurity against the risks of infection for the fetus while considering the impact of prolonging gestation on the risks to the mother for infection or delivery complications. The timely and accurate diagnosis of PPROM is vital to provide gestational age–specific interventions that will optimize pregnancy outcomes, while preventing unnecessary and dangerous interventions in unaffected pregnancies.

? **Decision 1:** Diagnosis of preterm premature rupture of membranes

All of the following findings are reliably confirmatory of the diagnosis of PPROM except

A. Vaginal pooling and ferning
B. Ultrasound for amniotic fluid volume assessment
C. Vaginal pH
D. Placental alpha-microglobulin 1 (PAMG-1) immunoassay

The correct answer is B: Ultrasound examination of amniotic fluid volume may be suggestive of membrane rupture by documenting oligohydramnios, but it is not diagnostic. All of the other tests can be used in the diagnosis of premature rupture of the membranes, with varying degrees of sensitivity and specificity described in Table 28.1.

The diagnosis of PPROM is traditionally made clinically via sterile speculum examination. The Guidelines for Perinatal Care of the American Congress of Obstetricians and Gynecologists call for the diagnosis to be made on the basis of history, physical examination, including a sterile speculum examination for pooling of fluid, and confirmatory laboratory tests. The most common confirmatory tests include the pH of the cervicovaginal discharge (alkaline, turning yellow nitrazine paper blue) and/or microscopic ferning of the cervicovaginal discharge on drying as seen in Figure 28.1. Each of these clinical signs is of limited diagnostic accuracy, and these diagnostic limitations are exaggerated as time from

TABLE 28.1

PERFORMANCE OF NONINVASIVE TESTS TO DIAGNOSE RUPTURE OF THE FETAL MEMBRANES

Test/Reference	Commercial Name	Cutoff	Sensitivity (%)	Specificity (%)
Nitrazine (pH)	—	Positive/negative	90–97	16–70
Ferning and/or pooling	—	Positive/negative	51–98	70–88
Commercial tests for ROM				
PAMG-1	AmniSure® ROM test	>5.0 ng/mL	98–99	88–100
IGFBP-1 (not approved in the United States)	PROM-TEST® AMNI Check®	>3 μg/L	74–97	74–97

IGFBP-1, insulin-like growth factor binding protein 1; PAMG-1, placental alpha-microglobulin 1.
Adapted from Caughey AB, Robinson JN, Norwitz ER. Contemporary diagnosis and management of preterm premature rupture of membranes. Rev Obstet Gynecol. 2008;1(1):11–22.

the rupture of membranes increases. The reliance on clinical findings alone leads to both false-positive and false-negative results. For example, the nitrazine test is designed to discriminate between alkaline cervicovaginal secretions (pH 4.5–6.0) and amniotic fluid (pH 7.1–7.3). It can give false-positive results in the presence of cervicitis, bacterial vaginosis, blood, urine, or semen. The fern test refers to the microscopic observation of crystallization of amniotic fluid when allowed to dry on a slide. False-positive results may be observed due to contamination with semen or cervical mucus or even the presence of fingerprints. False-negative results can be associated with sample collection errors, contamination with blood, or minimal residual fluid after prolonged leakage.

If the clinical history or physical findings are unclear, especially remote from term when an erroneous diagnosis could lead to significant harm, a dye such as indigo carmine can be instilled into the amniotic sac and the patient observed for the leakage of blue-stained fluid vaginally. Leakage of blue fluid within an hour (which stains a vaginal tampon) is diagnostic of PROM. There are, clearly, significant limitations to the use of this test. The amniotic injection is invasive and uncomfortable for the patient. It requires advanced skills, and it may not be technically possible in the face of anhydramnios. Risks include infection, iatrogenic PROM, and fetal trauma.

In the face of the limitations of the currently available diagnostic tools, investigators have searched for alternative methods that would be more reliable and objective. One test that has been approved in the United States by the Food and Drug Administration (FDA) is a bedside immunoassay, which identifies PAMG-1, a placental glycoprotein found in large amounts in amniotic fluid. Levels of PAMG-1 in amniotic fluid are 2,000 to 25,000 ng/mL as compared with 5 to 25 ng/mL in maternal blood and 0.05 to 0.2 ng/mL in cervicovaginal secretions. Thus leakage of amniotic fluid into the vagina can be easily detected. This assay can reportedly be used in gestations from 15 to 42 weeks and remains specific in the face of semen, urine, blood, and vaginal infections. A test for insulin-like growth factor receptor in the vaginal secretions has also been reported to be accurate for the diagnosis of PROM; however, this test is not available in the United States.

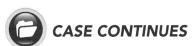

CASE CONTINUES

After a sterile speculum examination, the diagnosis of ruptured membranes is confirmed. Ultrasound demonstrates a single male fetus in cephalic presentation. The

Figure 28.1 Ferning of amniotic fluid. (Reproduced with permission from Creative Commons Attribution ShareAlike 2.0.)

fetal weight is 1,530 g (47th percentile for 30 weeks) and the amniotic fluid is clearly decreased (amniotic fluid index [AFI] is 4.3 cm). The fetal heart rate pattern shows no evidence of compromise. The maternal status is also reassuring. Mrs. Hsu denies any contractions, and feels the baby moving. She has no fever and no uterine tenderness. Her white blood cell count is 10.2/mm³ with no left shift. Taken all together these findings reassure you that Mrs. Hsu is not in labor and does not appear to have an active infection. These conclusions are critical as you prepare to counsel your patient on how to proceed.

 Decision 2: Delivery planning

Which of the following is not a critical factor in determining when delivery of this pregnancy should be initiated?

A. Fetal gestational age
B. Fetal presentation
C. Evidence of maternal intrauterine infection
D. Prior cesarean delivery

The correct answers are B and D: Fetal presentation and prior cesarean delivery. The fetal presentation is an important factor in *how* rather than *when* the fetus is delivered. A noncephalic presentation would typically require a cesarean section. Similarly, a patient with a prior cesarean delivery may be considered for either a repeat cesarean or a vaginal delivery, but delivery timing is unchanged.

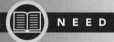 **N E E D   T O   K N O W**

Clinical Decision Making and Patient Counseling

The fetal membranes serve as a barrier to ascending infection. The management of PPROM is based on balancing the risks of prematurity versus the risks of infection for the fetus while also avoiding serious adverse maternal consequences. Major immediate risks of prematurity include respiratory distress syndrome, necrotizing enterocolitis, intraventricular hemorrhage, sepsis, and death. Premature infants also have an increased risk of long-term sequelae including sensory deficits, impaired intellectual development, and cerebral palsy. The incidence and severity of these outcomes are lessened as gestational age increases. This knowledge drives the desire to avoid delivery for as long as possible. Unfortunately, the introduction of infection into the setting of PPROM worsens both the frequency and severity of these outcomes significantly. Overall polymicrobial

intra-amniotic infection, which occurs in 15% to 30% of women with PPROM, is associated with a fourfold increase in neonatal death and a threefold increase in intraventricular hemorrhage over what would be expected for gestational age. These findings suggest that the optimum outcome involves avoiding fetal infectious sequelae.

The majority (50%–75%) of pregnancies with PPROM will deliver within a week of membrane rupture. Given the high likelihood of a preterm delivery, it is important that, whenever possible, the pregnancy complicated with PPROM be managed in a hospital where the neonatal nursery is capable of managing the anticipated level of prematurity. It has been shown that neonatal outcomes are generally better when babies are transferred prior to birth than when they are transferred after delivery. Therefore, one of the first decisions to be made is whether or not the hospital can offer the appropriate level of care and, if not, whether the patient is stable for transfer. If there is evidence of acute fetal or maternal distress, advanced active labor or any other indication that maternal transport would be contraindicated, then transfer of the baby after delivery may be required.

Once the setting of ongoing care is determined, the patient should be informed of the management options including the risks, benefits, and alternatives to proposed care plans. In addition to the maternal–fetal medicine specialist, it is often helpful to have a pediatrician–neonatologist counsel the patient. The basic choice that must be made is between active management (delivery) and expectant management (continuing pregnancy with maternal and fetal surveillance). The patient needs to know the risks of prematurity associated with delivery at her current gestational age and estimated fetal weight (EFW) as well as how those risks would be expected to change with time (one published table is seen in Table 28.2). She must also know the risks to herself and her child of expectant management, including intrauterine infection, placental abruption, cord prolapse, and fetal demise. Fetal pulmonary hypoplasia complicates 26% of PPROM that occurs prior to 22 weeks, and skeletal deformities such as club foot are related to the severity and duration of oligohydramnios. Maternal risks include chorioamnionitis and postpartum endometritis, which are seen more commonly in women with prolonged PPROM, severe oligohydramnios, PPROM at an early gestational age, and following multiple digital vaginal examinations. The mother is also at an increased risk of cesarean section due to malpresentation or fetal heart rate changes associated with decreased amniotic fluid. Taking all these factors into consideration, the management of PPROM suggested by the American Congress of Obstetricians and Gynecologists (ACOG) is based on gestational age as summarized in Table 28.3.

TABLE 28.2

OUTCOMES OF DELIVERY AT DIFFERENT GESTATIONAL AGES

Outcomes	Gestation (Weeks)								
	23	**24**	**25**	**26**	**27**	**28**	**29**	**30**	**31**
Total number of births	138	182	150	150	223	268	300	377	487
Stillbirth (%)	55	35	25	25	20	10	10	<5	<5
Deaths prior to NICU admission (%)	20	15	10	<1	<1	<1	<1	<1	<1
Admitted to nursery (%)	25	50	65	75	80	90	90	>95	>95
Number admitted to NICU	32	94	101	149	173	250	260	320	418
Mean birthweight (gram)	600	650	750	900	1,000	1,100	1,300	1,500	1,600
Discharged alive (%)	30	50	60	80	90	90	95	>95	>95
RDS (%)	95	95	95	90	85	80	70	50	40
PDA treated (%)	>70	70	45	45	40	25	15	10	5
NEC (%)	>20	20	5	5	5	5	5	3	2
Sepsis	>60	60	50	40	40	25	20	10	5
IVH (%) grades 3–4	30	15	15	10	10	5	5	1	1
PVL (%)	—	5	1	1	1	1	1	1	1
Moderate to severe disability (%)	60	40	15	10	10	10			

Modified from Bolisetty S, Bajuk B, Abdel-Latif ME, Vincent T, Sutton L, Lui K. Preterm outcome table (POT): a simple tool to aid counselling parents of very preterm infants. Aust N Z J Obstet Gynaecol. 2006;46(3):189–92. NICU, neonatal intensive care unit; RDS, respiratory distress syndrome; PDA, patent ductus arteriosus; NEC, necrotizing enterocolitis; IVH, intraventricular hemorrhage; PVL, periventricular leukomalacia.

TABLE 28.3

RECOMMENDED MANAGEMENT OF PREMATURE RUPTURE OF THE FETAL MEMBRANES BASED ON GESTATIONAL AGE

Gastational Age	Management
Term (37 wk or more)	■ Proceed to delivery, usually by induction of labor ■ Group B streptococcal propyhloids recommended
Near term (34 wk to 36 completed weeks)	■ Same as for term
Preterm (32 wk to 33 completed weeks)	■ Expectant management, unless fetal pulmonary maturity is documented ■ Group B streptococcal prophylasis recommended ■ Corticosteroid—no consensus, but some experts recommend ■ Antiboitics recommended to prolong latency if there are no contraindications
Preterm (24 wk to 31 completed weeks)	■ Expectant management ■ Group B streptococcal prophylasis recommended ■ Single-course conticosteroid use rcommended ■ Tocolytics—no consensus ■ Antibiotics recommended to prolong latency if there are no contraindications
Less than 24 wk[a]	■ Patient counseling ■ Expectant management or induction of labor ■ Group B streptococcal prophyloids is not recommended ■ Corticosteroids are not recommended ■ Antibiotics—there are incomplete data on use in prolonging latency

[a]The combination of birth weight gestational age and sex provide the best estimate of chances of arrival and should be considered in individual cases.
From ACOG Committee on Practice Bulletins-Obstetrics. ACOG Practice Bulletin No. 80: premature rupture of membranes. Clinical management guidelines for obstetrician-gynecologists. Obstet Gynecol. 2007 Apr;109(4):1007–19, used with permission.

TABLE 28.4

CONTRAINDICATIONS TO EXPECTANT MANAGEMENT OF PPROM

Absolute contraindications
   Gestational age >37 weeks
   Documented fetal lung maturity
   Evidence of fetal hypoxia
   Active labor
   Clinically evident intra-amniotic infection
   Nonviable anomalous fetus
   Acute abruption
Relative contraindications (delivery strongly considered)
   Gestational age of >34 weeks
   Gestational age >32 weeks status post completed course of
      steroids
   Previable fetus
   Maternal immune compromise
   Chronic abruption

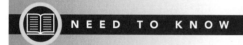 **NEED TO KNOW**

Interventions to Prolong Latent Period

Prior to undertaking interventions to prolong the latent period (the time from PROM to delivery), contraindications to expectant management must be considered (Table 28.4). In general, expectant management is contraindicated when the fetus is not expected to benefit from the delay in delivery or when the risk of delay is greater for mother or fetus than the risk of immediate delivery.

A major focus of the management of PPROM is delay of delivery and early detection of chorioamnionitis. The diagnosis of chorioamnionitis is primarily a clinical diagnosis evidenced by fetal tachycardia, maternal tachycardia, fever (temperature ≥100.4°F), and/or uterine tenderness. The diagnosis may also be supported by visualization of purulent discharge from cervix on speculum examination. Amniocentesis is not universally recommended in all women presenting with PPROM, although some centers perform amniocentesis on all patients who are candidates for expectant management. In addition to providing the opportunity to evaluate fetal lung maturity, amniocentesis may confirm intra-amniotic infection with a positive amniotic fluid culture. An infection is strongly suggested when the fluid has an elevated white blood cell count, elevated lactate dehydrogenase, positive Gram stain or decreased glucose, although none of these tests is highly sensitive.

Specific interventions

a. Antibiotics.
   The latency period in PPROM may be extended by a
   2-day intravenous course of ampicillin and ery-

thromycin followed by 5 days of oral amoxicillin and erythromycin. This regimen has been shown to decrease both infectious- and gestational age–dependent morbidity in cases of PPROM. While receiving the 7-day course, patients are adequately covered for group B streptococcus (GBS). Specific treatment for GBS prophylaxis will again be required for delivery if a patient is either GBS positive or has unknown GBS status and delivery occurs after the 7-day course is complete.

b. Antenatal corticosteroids.
   A single course of steroids for fetal lung maturity should be administered to women with PROM at <32 weeks of gestational age and >24 weeks to decrease the risks of respiratory distress syndrome, perinatal mortality, and other morbidities. Benefits of corticosteroids for patients > 32 weeks are not as well documented; however, several clinicians advocate their use on a case by case basis.

C. Tocolytics.
   There is little evidence to support the long-term use of tocolytics in the setting of PPROM. Indeed, such use has not shown to improve perinatal morbidity or mortality long term. Short-term use of tocolysis may be justified to allow administration of corticosteroids for fetal lung maturity or to facilitate transfer of the patient to a tertiary care center.

 CASE CONTINUES

You and your colleague in pediatrics have counseled Mrs. Hsu thoroughly about the management risks, benefits, and alternative options and you have decided to proceed with expectant management. Mrs. Hsu is given a course of antenatal corticosteroids. Over the following weeks, periodic antenatal testing has been reassuring with a fetal heart rate baseline between 150 and 155 bpm, and the AFI has remained 3 to 7 cm. Mrs. Hsu's temperature and heart rate have remained normal, and she has reported continued minimal leakage of fluid, which did not significantly increase as she increased her activity level with bathroom privileges and a biweekly shower. One night, 2 weeks after you admitted her (at gestational age of 32 weeks), you are called to Mrs. Hsu's bedside. She is complaining of abdominal pain. Upon evaluation you note that she has no uterine tenderness, but contractions are palpable. Your ultrasound confirms cephalic presentation, AFI 4 cm and EFW now 1,940 g. With external fetal monitor placement, you note contractions every 5 to 8 minutes and a fetal heart rate pattern consistent with fetal wellbeing. Mrs. Hsu asks if you will stop her labor.

Decision 3: Delivery timing

What would be an indication for delivery at this time?

A. Gestational age
B. Uterine contractions
C. Worsening oligohydramnios
D. Maternal desire to leave the hospital

The correct answers are A and B: Gestational age and/or uterine contractions. The patient is now 32 weeks with an EFW of nearly 2,000 g. The risks of complications of prematurity have diminished greatly while the risks of intrauterine infection and other complications persist, with the advent of uterine contractions representing a possible early infection. ACOG recommends that delivery be considered after 32 weeks if pulmonary maturity can be documented, and that pregnancies not be continued after 34 weeks in any case.

Each of the other possible answers may represent softer indications to reevaluate management. They are among the many possible clinical scenarios for which there are insufficient evidence to guide management definitively. Hospitalization until delivery is the standard in PPROM because it is not possible to predict accurately which pregnancy might develop complications such as cord prolapse, cord compression, or placental abruption. In addition, the earliest signs of development of infection may be subtle and there is some evidence it is more likely to present nocturnally. Despite these unknowns, in very rare cases, outpatient management may be considered. Such a case who require a highly compliant patient who had been stable in-house for 48 to 72 hours, who lives near the hospital with 24-hour availability of immediate transportation and is able to maintain bedrest and pelvic rest at home. This patient would have to be willing and able to accurately take and record her temperature at home and to be seen weekly by a practitioner either in the office or at home. Very few fulfill all these criteria and, given the potential risks to mother and fetus, it is unclear that such an approach would be cost-effective.

The management of uterine contractions, especially in pregnancies otherwise stable and distant from term is uncertain. It is certainly possible to attempt brief tocolysis to avoid delivery of a very immature fetus in such a setting, but a benefit of doing so is unproven. It is also unclear how much isolated oligohydramnios should influence management in PPROM, especially after 26 to 28 weeks. It is clear that severe oligohydramnios is associated with a reduced latency period and an increased risk of cord compression, but generally oligohydramnios alone is not an indication for delivery in cases of PPROM in the absence of other factors.

CASE CONCLUSION

You discuss with Mrs. Hsu that you do not feel that she is a candidate for tocolysis, and you review with her your reasons. You discuss augmentation versus expectant management, and Mrs. Hsu requests expectant management for now, at least until her husband can arrive. After several hours her husband is with her and Mrs. Hsu appears to enter active labor. When checked she is 7 cm dilated. She requests and receives an epidural, and 2 hours later she delivers a 2,030-g male infant with Apgar score of 9 and 9 at one and five minutes. Mother and baby leave the hospital together on postpartum day 3.

SUGGESTED READINGS

ACOG Committee on Practice Bulletins-Obstetrics. ACOG Practice Bulletin No. 80: premature rupture of membranes. Clinical management guidelines for obstetrician-gynecologists. Obstet Gynecol. 2007;109(4):1007–19.

Bolisetty S, Bajuk B, Abdel-Latif ME, Vincent T, Sutton L, Lui K. Preterm outcome table (POT): a simple tool to aid counselling parents of very preterm infants. Aust N Z J Obstet Gynaecol. 2006;46(3):189–92.

Caughey AB, Robinson JN, Norwitz ER. Contemporary diagnosis and management of preterm premature rupture of membranes. Rev Obstet Gynecol. 2008;1(1):11–22.

Mercer BM, Arheart KL. Antimicrobial therapy in expectant management of preterm premature rupture of membranes. Lancet. 1995; 346:1271–9.

Mercer M, Sabai BM. Maternal and perinatal outcome of expectant management in premature rupture of membranes with mature amniotic fluid at 32 to 36 weeks: a randomized trial. Am J Obstet Gynecol. 1990;162:46–52.

Neerhof MG, Cravello C, Haney EI, Silver RK. Timing of labor induction after premature rupture of membranes between 32 and 36 weeks gestation. Am J Obstet Gynecol. 1999;180:349–52.

Shumway J, Al-Malt A, Amon E, et al. Impact of oligohydramnios on maternal and perinatal outcomes of spontaneous premature rupture of membranes at 18–28 weeks. J Matern Fetal Med. 1999; 8:20–3.

Breech Presentation

Tasmia Q. Henry

 CASE PRESENTATION

Your patient, in the office, is Ms. Ahmed, a 42-year-old G6 P5 who has been referred by the midwife for the suspicion of a breech presentation at 33 weeks of gestation. You review the records sent with Ms. Ahmed, which reveal that she has had an unremarkable prenatal course to this point. She declined prenatal screening as she would not have an abortion. She had an early dating ultrasound at 7 weeks, but missed her appointment for second trimester scan because her youngest child was ill. She has had five prior vaginal deliveries without incident; her largest prior infant weighed 3,720 g and her last pregnancy was 10 years ago. You perform a brief ultrasound that reveals that her fetus is in a frank breech presentation.

 Decision 1: Diagnosis

Which condition is associated with breech presentation?

- **A.** Anencephaly
- **B.** Cystic fibrosis
- **C.** Preeclampsia
- **D.** Maternal diabetes

The answer is A: Anencephaly. The other answers are not specifically associated with breech presentation. In general, most fetuses adopt the head-down cephalic presentation during the third trimester. About 25% of fetuses are still breech at 32 weeks of gestation, but only 3% to 5% remain breech by term. Breech presentations are therefore more common in premature pregnancies and whenever maternal or fetal factors interfere with either fetal movement or positioning of the fetal head in the maternal pelvis. Table 29.1 lists some common risk factors for breech presentation at term.

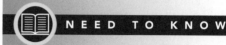 **NEED TO KNOW**

Definition and Types of Breech

The fetal position is described as breech when the fetus lies longitudinally with the buttocks and or feet presenting nearest the cervix. By convention the relation of the breech fetus to the maternal pelvis is described with reference to the fetal sacrum. A fetus presenting as a breech with the spine toward the mother's left would be described as being left sacrum transverse.

Breech presentations are further classified by the position of the legs and feet as shown in Figure 29.1. In a frank breech, the buttocks present first with flexed hips and legs extended on the abdomen; only the buttocks are palpated vaginally. A complete breech involves flexion at both the fetal knees and hips, with feet and buttocks presenting. If one foot presents with the buttocks, this is referred to as an incomplete breech. Finally, if neither hips nor knees are fully flexed, one or both feet may present without the buttocks; this is called a footling breech. Footling breech presentation is of concern in a laboring patient, as it is more likely to be associated with prolapse of the umbilical cord and potentially with entrapment of the fetal head, both life-threatening complications for the fetus.

 CASE CONTINUES

You discuss with Ms. Ahmed that her baby is in the breech position, that this is not currently a problem, but that it will complicate her delivery if her baby is still breech when she goes into labor. You schedule her for a fetal anatomy survey to exclude obvious fetal abnormalities, and you ask her to return at 37 weeks of gestation for a follow-up ultrasound for fetal position. She asks if there is anything she can do to help her fetus to turn to vertex.

TABLE 29.1

FACTORS ASSOCIATED WITH BREECH PRESENTATION IN A TERM INFANT. BREECH PRESENTATION IS ALSO MORE COMMON IN PREMATURE FETUSES

Factor	Comment
Maternal Factors	
Interfere with fetal turning	
Uterine anomalies	Bicornuate, unicornuate, or septate uterus
Space occupying lesions	Myomas distorting the cavity
Placental location	Cornual implantation
Oligohydramnios	
Interfere with descent of head into pelvis	
Contracted pelvis	
Space occupying lesions	Lower segment myomas, ovarian masses
Placental location	Placenta previa
Polyhydramnios	
Grand multiparity	With poorly contractile uterus
Fetal Factors	
Interfere with fetal turning	
Fetal movement disorders	
Other fetal disorders	Anencephaly
Fetal death	
Interfere with descent of head into pelvis	
Enlarged fetal head	Hydrocephalus, tumors
Multiple gestation	

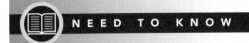

Variations of the breech presentation

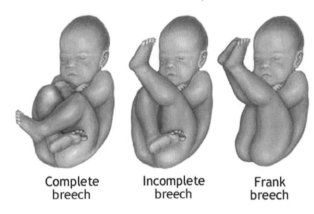

Complete breech   Incomplete breech   Frank breech

✸A.D.A.M.

Figure 29.1 Types of breech. In a complete breech, the legs are completely flexed, with buttocks and feet presenting. In a frank breech, the knees are extended, with buttocks only presenting. Presentations with one knee flexed and one extended are called "incomplete." A fetus may also present with extension at both hips and knees, so that only the feet are presenting, this is called a footling breech (not shown). (Reproduced with permission. Copyright 1997–2011, A.D.A.M., Inc.)

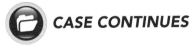

NEED TO KNOW

Patient Advice with a Breech

A patient with a breech fetus has traditionally been counseled to adopt a knee-chest position to prevent descent of the fetal breech into the pelvis and enhance the chance that her fetus will turn to vertex. A randomized controlled trial of this intervention, however, did not indicate any effect of knee-chest positioning. Moxibustion, or burning herbs at an acupuncture point on the fifth toe, has been reported in randomized controlled trials to decrease the risk of breech presentation at term. Despite this information, moxibustion is not generally felt to be an established therapy, and it is not often used in clinical practice.

CASE CONTINUES

Ms. Ahmed's fetal anatomy survey is read as normal. She returns at 37 weeks of gestation, and ultrasound reveals a frank breech presentation.

Decision 2: Management

What are the possible management options?

A. Cesarean section at 39 weeks
B. Immediate cesarean section
C. Vaginal breech delivery at 39 weeks
D. External cephalic version (ECV)

The best answer is either **A:** Cesarean section at 39 weeks or **D:** ECV. The choice between these options ultimately depends on the clinical picture and the patient's wishes, along with physician expertise. An immediate cesarean section would only be indicated for fetal or maternal complications. For example, if the patient were in labor or if there were signs of fetal distress. A vaginal breech delivery is typically not recommended, following the publication of the results of the Term Breech Trial in 2000. This was a large, international multicenter randomized clinical trial conducted to compare planned cesarean delivery with planned vaginal delivery for term singleton fetuses in breech presentation. Perinatal mortality, neonatal mortality, and serious neonatal morbidity were significantly lower with planned cesarean delivery compared with planned vaginal delivery. Vaginal breech delivery also requires a significant degree of physician skill and experience. For both of these reasons, vaginal breech delivery is generally reserved for emergency situations, or for situations not covered by the Term Breech Trial, such as delivery of the second twin.

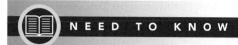

External Cephalic Version

ECV is the procedure used to turn the fetal presenting part from breech to cephalic. It may be utilized in the management of singleton breech presentations or, after delivery of the first twin, for a nonvertex second twin. The goal for a singleton breech is to increase the proportion of vertex presentations near term, thus increasing the chance for a vaginal delivery. ECV is performed in patients who are at least 37 weeks of gestation so that the risk of spontaneous reversion is decreased, and, if complications arise, delivery of a term infant can be accomplished. Reported success rates for ECV range from 35% to 85% (mean 60%).

Prior to attempting ECV, fetal well-being is documented, usually with a reactive NST, and the amniotic fluid volume is assessed. ECV is performed using manual pressure by the practitioner on the mother's abdomen as shown in Figure 29.2. Some practitioners use a tocolytic agent prior to the procedure, and some practitioners prefer to initiate epidural anesthesia prior to ECV; there is no evidence to support these interventions. The breech is elevated out of the maternal pelvis and then the fetus is gently guided in either direction to a vertex presentation. Fetal heart motion is documented after every attempt, and after the procedure, whether successful or not, the pregnancy is typically monitored for both uterine activity and fetal heart rate.

Relative contraindications to ECV include active labor, engagement of the presenting part in the pelvis, oligohydramnios, uterine anomalies, presence of nuchal cord, multiple gestation, premature rupture of membranes,

contraindications to vaginal delivery such as placenta previa or previous uterine surgery (including myomectomy or metroplasty), and suspected or documented congenital malformations or abnormalities (including intrauterine growth retardation).

Complications following ECV are rare, occurring in only 1% to 2% of all procedures and may include fetal heart rate deceleration and fetomaternal hemorrhage. Other reported though uncommon complications include placental abruption, uterine rupture, rupture of membranes with resultant umbilical cord prolapse, amniotic fluid embolism, and fetal demise. Because of the potential for catastrophic outcome, ECV should be performed in a facility where immediate access to cesarean delivery is available. Patients require counseling regarding the version procedure, with disclosure of pertinent risks, benefits, and alternatives so that an informed consent can be obtained.

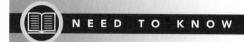

Breech Delivery Technique

Although vaginal delivery is seldom used in a singleton breech, the maneuvers used in vaginal breech delivery are also useful in delivering the singleton breech at cesarean or in delivering the second twin who presents as a breech. The technique of vaginal breech delivery is described here, with the understanding that the maneuvers may be used on the breech being delivered abdominally as well.

Breech deliveries are described as spontaneous if the fetus delivers completely through the mother's expulsive efforts only. Although some preterm fetuses can

External version

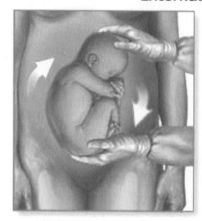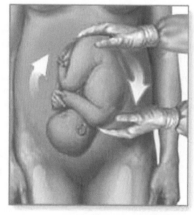

Figure 29.2 External cephalic version. Using manual pressure on the maternal abdomen, the fetus is rotated from a breech to a cephalic presentation. (Reproduced with permission. Copyright 1997–2011, A.D.A.M., Inc.)

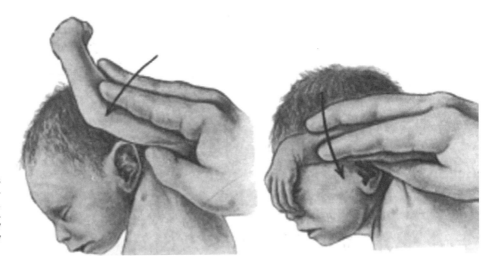

Figure 29.3 Delivery of the arms of the breech. The arms are delivered while the head is in the vagina, not shown in this illustration. (Reproduced with permission from http://latina.obgyn.net/pr/articles/pelvico/index.htm.)

deliver spontaneously, most breech fetuses require some assistance from the practitioner for a safe delivery. The most common type of breech delivery is the assisted breech delivery.

At an assisted breech delivery, the fetus delivers spontaneously to the level of the umbilicus. At this point, the delivery practitioner exerts gentle traction on the fetus by placing the index fingers in the inguinal crease and pulling until the scapulae are seen. The legs are delivered via a Pinard maneuver if they have not already delivered. The arms are delivered by sweeping the humerus across the fetal chest and out as shown in Figure 29.3. Finally, the fetal head is delivered via the Mauriceau maneuver shown in Figure 29.4. In this maneuver, the operator exerts pressure on the fetal maxillae to maintain flexion of the head while the head is delivered via a combination of maternal pushing and extension of the fetal body around the maternal

symphysis. Fetal head delivery can also be accomplished by the use of Piper forceps if traction on the head is necessary.

Finally, a breech birth may take place by breech extraction. This maneuver is used for the delivery of a breech second twin, and sometimes for deliveries at the time of cesarean. In a breech extraction, the operator reaches into the uterus and grasps the fetal feet. The fetus is pulled into the birth canal and delivered to the level of the umbilicus; the remainder of the delivery is as for an assisted breech delivery.

 CASE CONTINUES

You review her options with Ms. Ahmed. Although you feel that she would be a good candidate for an ECV, she opts for a scheduled cesarean delivery at 39 weeks. At 38 weeks and 5 days of gestation, she returns to labor and delivery in labor. The nurse examines her, and describes the cervix as 5 cm dilated, but she is unable to palpate a presenting part. A brief ultrasound reveals that the fetus is now in a transverse position, back down (Fig. 29.5). The estimated fetal weight is 3,200 g, and the fetal status is reassuring at this time.

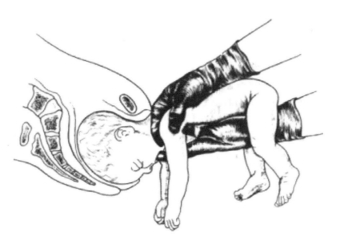

Figure 29.4 Mauriceau maneuver for delivery of the head at breech birth. (Reproduced with permission from http://latina.obgyn.net/pr/articles/pelvico/index.htm.)

 Decision 3: Management

What are the options for delivery with a back-down transverse lie?

A. Low transverse cesarean section
B. Vaginal delivery
C. Breech extraction
D. Low vertical cesarean section

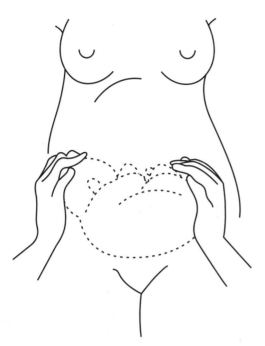

Figure 29.5 Back down transverse lie. (Reproduced with permission from http://who.int/reproductive-health/impac/Symptoms/table_S12.html.)

The best answer is D: Low vertical cesarean section. A low transverse uterine incision may not allow the surgeon to grasp the baby during the delivery with this presentation. In practice, many surgeons may attempt to exert pressure on the uterus after the abdomen is open to turn the fetus into a polar (vertex or breech) lie, so as to avoid the risk to the mother of a vertical incision. If this does not work, a low vertical or classical cesarean is the preferred method of delivery.

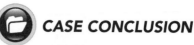 **CASE CONCLUSION**

Given her advanced cervical dilatation, you take Ms. Ahmed for urgent cesarean delivery. At surgery, there is a large myoma in the lower uterine segment that prevents you from turning the fetus and you perform a classical cesarean delivery. Mother and baby do well, and are discharged from the hospital together. You remind Ms. Ahmed that she should not labor in a future pregnancy due to the risk of rupture of her classical uterine scar. She understands this information and states that she will consult with her family about permanent sterilization in the future.

SUGGESTED READINGS

ACOG Committee Opinion. Mode of term singleton breech delivery. Obstet Gynecol. 2006;108(1):235–7.

Coyle ME, Smith CA, Peat B. Cephalic version by moxibustion for breech presentation. Cochrane Database Syst Rev. 2005;(2):CD003928.

External Cephalic Version for Breech Presentation. ACOG Practice Bulletin 2000;13.

Hannah ME, Hannah WJ, Hewson SA, Hodnett ED, Saigal S, Willlan AR. Planned caesarean section versus vaginal birth from: breech presentation at term: a randomized multicentre trial. Term Breech trial Collaborative group. Lancet. 2000;356(9239):1375–83.

Hofmeyr GJ, Kulier R. External cephalic version for breech presentation at term. Cochrane Database Syst Rev. 1996:(1):CD000083.

Oats J, Abraham S. Llewellyn-Jones Fundamentals of Obstetrics and Gynaecology. 8th ed. Elsevier Mosby: Edinburgh; 2005. pp. 168–71.

Smith C, Crowther C, Wilkinson C, Pridmore B, Robinson J. Knee-chest postural management for breech at term: a randomized controlled trial. Birth. 1999;26(2):71–5.

van den Berg I, Bosch JL, Jacobs B, Bouman I, Duvekot JJ, Hunink MG. Effectiveness of acupuncture-type interventions versus expectant management to correct breech presentation: a systematic review. Complement Ther Med. 2008;16(2):92–100.

Witkop CT, Zhang J, Sun W. Natural history of fetal position during pregnancy and risk of nonvertex delivery. Obstet Gynecol. 2008; 111:875–80.

Placenta Accreta

30

Richard H. Lee   Jeotsna Grover

 CASE PRESENTATION

You are asked to evaluate Ms. Perkins, a 38-year-old G5 P3 at 33 weeks of gestation with a chief complaint of vaginal spotting. She has recently initiated care with your practice; the ultrasound report from her previous provider indicates that she was found to have a placenta previa at 18 weeks of gestation. Her prenatal labs were normal, and her diabetes screen was negative. Her past obstetrical history is significant for three prior term cesarean births and one spontaneous pregnancy loss at 8 weeks for which she had a D&C. Otherwise she denies significant past medical history. She takes no drugs other than prenatal vitamins, and she denies the use of tobacco, alcohol, or recreational drugs.

On physical examination, she is a slender anxious Caucasian female. Her blood pressure is 130/70 mm Hg, and her pulse is 90 bpm. She is afebrile. She has uterine contractions every 6 to 8 minutes that are mildly uncomfortable; her uterus relaxes and is nontender between contractions. The remainder of her physical examination is unremarkable.

You perform a bedside ultrasound. The fetus is growing appropriately; however, the placenta is an anterior complete previa. You cannot visualize the lower uterine segment well, and you are concerned about the possibility of placenta accreta.

 Decision 1: Diagnosis

What factors put this patient at highest risk for a placenta accreta?

A. Age and multiparity
B. Prior cesarean section and placenta previa
C. Gestational age
D. Prior D&C and maternal age.

The correct answer is B: Prior cesarean section and placenta previa. Several risk factors for placenta accreta have been identified. Two of the most important appear to be prior cesarean delivery and placenta previa, and these risks are additive. Clark et al. reported a 5% incidence of placenta accreta among women with placenta previa and no previous cesarean sections. The incidence increased to 24% with one previous cesarean section and to 45% with two or more. Similarly, among 723 women with prior cesarean delivery and previa, Silver et al. reported the risk for accreta to be 3%, 11%, 40%, 61%, and 67% for one, two, three, four, and five or more cesarean deliveries. Cesarean section alone is a risk factor for placenta accreta, but the risk is much less dramatic. Among 29,409 women with cesarean delivery and no previa the risk for accreta was 0.03%, 0.2%, 0.1%, 0.8%, 0.8%, and 4.7% for one, two, three, four, five, and six or more cesarean deliveries.

Advanced maternal age (Answers A and D) has also been reported to be an independent risk factor for placenta accreta among women with placenta previa. Miller reported on the incidence of accreta in women with placenta previa but no prior cesarean. Those who were younger than 25 years of age had a 3.2% risk of accreta, while those who were aged 35 years and older had a 14.6% risk. In this group of patients, multiparity (Answer A) conferred no additional risk. A prior surgical abortion by D&C (Answer D) has been associated with an increased risk of placental complications in a subsequent pregnancy in some, but not all, studies. One study found a minimal relative risk of 1.17 for a retained placenta in the subsequent pregnancy of a patient with a prior abortion. Pregnancies complicated by placenta accreta deliver earlier, but gestational age (Answer C) per se is not a risk factor for accreta.

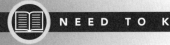 **NEED TO KNOW**

Incidence and Types of Placenta Accreta

Over the past two decades, the reported incidence of placenta accreta ranged from 1 in 533 to 1 in 2,510 deliveries. The majority of placenta accretas (75+%) invade a short distance into the myometrium. If the invasion is deep into the myometrium (17% of cases) the condition is placenta increta. Invasion through the uterine wall and serosa (and often into other structures) is placenta percreta (5%–7% of cases) (Fig. 30.1).

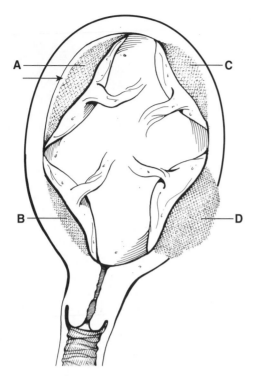

Figure 30.1 Forms of placenta accreta. **A:** normal placenta. Nitabuch's layer is the clear space indicated by the *arrow*. **B:** placenta accreta—note the lack of the Nitabuch's layer. **C:** Placenta increta, with deeper invasion into the myometrium. **D:** Placenta percreta, penetrating the uterine serosa.

Retained placenta, or a placenta that does not spontaneously separate from the uterine wall at delivery, may be a very mild form of placenta accreta, but this is not included in these totals.

 CASE CONTINUES

Ms. Perkins' contractions abate with hydration and you consult a maternal fetal medicine specialist for further evaluation of the placenta by ultrasound. The specialist describes the placenta as having lacunar lakes and absence of the retroplacental hypoechoic layer. Color Doppler reveals turbulent lacunar flow. The consultant advises that these findings are highly suspect for placenta accreta (Fig. 30.2).

?   Decision 2: Diagnosis

How accurate is the diagnosis of placenta accreta by ultrasound?

A. Sensitivity 20%, specificity 90%
B. Sensitivity 50%, specificity 95%
C. Sensitivity 70%, specificity 90%
D. Sensitivity 80%, specificity 95%

The answer is D: In experienced hands, ultrasound has an 80% sensitivity and a 95% specificity for the diagnosis of placenta accreta in the third trimester. There are no studies evaluating the diagnosis of accreta in the first half of pregnancy. With an anterior placenta, ultrasound and magnetic resonance imaging (MRI) are equivalent in their ability to diagnose accrete. However, MRI is the only modality capable of making the diagnosis with a posterior placenta.

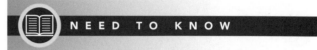

Pathophysiology of Placenta Accreta

As ultrasound demonstrates, placenta accreta is characterized pathologically by partial or complete absence of the deciduas basalis and Nitabuch's layer between the chorionic villi and the myometrium (Fig. 30.3). It also is characterized by deeper, but less complete remodeling of the uterine vessels and by direct contact between the chorionic villi and the muscle. Theories about the cause of placenta accreta include the presence of a defect in the decidua or increased invasion of the trophoblast. Factors supporting the theory that placenta accreta is caused by a decidual defect include the finding that the incidence of accreta is greatly increased when the placenta is implanted in the lower uterine segment or over a uterine scar; both areas where the decidual layer is disrupted. Excessive invasiveness of the trophoblast is suspected in cases where accreta occurs in an area of normal decidua. It seems most likely that the ultimate defect is in communication between the decidua and the trophoblast. Under normal conditions, the trophoblast is an invasive tissue; this invasiveness is modulated by the decidua so as to limit the depth and extent of trophoblast invasion. Either a defect in the decidua or a defect in trophoblast responsiveness to decidual signaling would lead to enhanced trophoblast invasion. This occurs early in gestation; at approximately 7 weeks of gestation in the absence of a normal Nitabuch's layer in the decidua basalis, there is pathologic invasion by chorionic villi into the myometrium leading to placenta accreta. A number of cases in the literature have confirmed the first trimester origin of placenta accreta with the finding of invasive placenta in first trimester hysterectomy specimens.

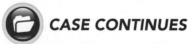 **CASE CONTINUES**

You observe Ms. Perkins overnight, and she remains stable after prolonged observation. You discuss with her your concern that she may have extensive bleeding at the

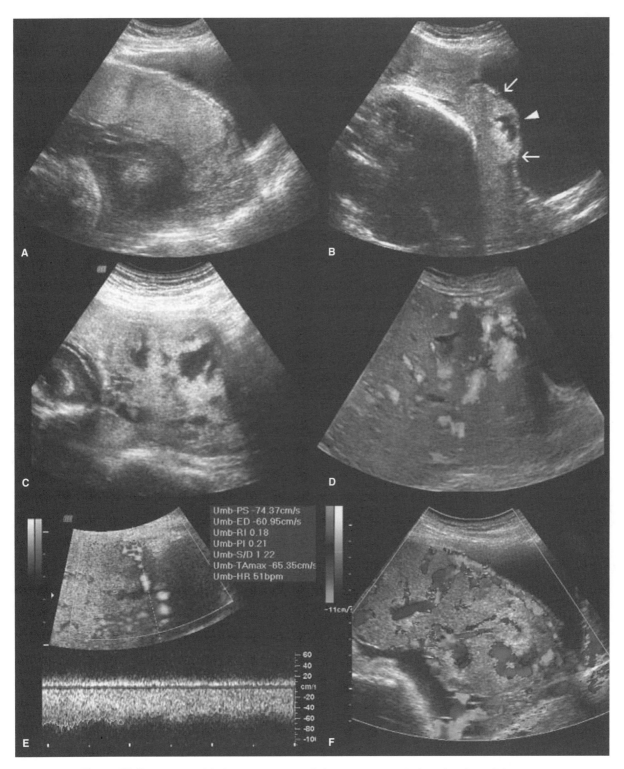

Figure 30.2 Ultrasound findings suggestive of placenta accreta. **A:** Complete loss of the retroplacental sonolucent zone. **B:** Focal disruption of hyperechoic bladder mucosa (*arrows*) and the presence of an exophytic placenta invading the bladder (*arrowhead*). **C:** Appearance of placental lacunae. **D:** Pattern of diffuse lacunar flow visualized by color Doppler. **E:** Multiple vascular lakes with low-resistance turbulent flow. **F:** Hypervascularity of serosa–bladder interface. (Reproduced with permission from Shih JC, Palacios Jaraquemada JM, Su YN, et al. Role of three-dimensional power Doppler in the antenatal diagnosis of placenta accreta: comparison with gray-scale and color Doppler techniques. Ultrasound Obstet Gynecol. 2009;33(2):193–203.)

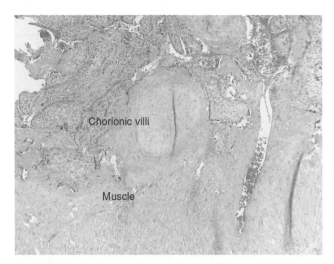

Figure 30.3 Placenta accreta (pathology specimen). Note the chorionic villi directly apposed to the myometrial muscle, without a decidual layer.

time of delivery, will likely require hysterectomy and may require blood transfusion. In order to avoid the patient going into labor, you and Ms. Perkins agree to perform an amniocentesis at 36 weeks and to deliver her as soon as the fetal lungs are predicted to be mature. She is distressed at the idea of a hysterectomy, and asks if there are not other options for her.

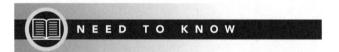

Surgical Options with Placenta Accreta

In women who are considered to be at high risk for placenta accreta, cesarean delivery may be performed electively prior to 37 weeks after confirming fetal pulmonary maturity. The patient should be counseled preoperatively regarding the risks of hemorrhage, transfusion, and hysterectomy. The operating room should be staffed by experienced personnel, equipped with appropriate hysterectomy instruments, and blood products/blood salvage equipment should be available if their use is planned. The placement of prophylactic intravascular balloon catheters for placenta accreta is not recommended, as it has failed to produce any substantial decrease in maternal morbidity.

Hysterectomy remains the definitive procedure, and the procedure of choice. The uterine incision is made away from the suspected placental location. The fetus is delivered and the placenta is allowed to spontaneously deliver with only gentle traction on the cord. Attempts to manually deliver the placenta can cause massive hemorrhage if there is indeed a placenta accreta. If placental

delivery is unsuccessful or if uncontrollable hemorrhage ensues, the surgeon should leave the placenta in place and proceed with hysterectomy.

Control of potentially life-threatening hemorrhage is the first priority; however, in the absence of an emergency the patient's desire for future fertility must be taken into consideration. If the patient is hemodynamically stable and strongly desires future fertility conservative management may be cautiously considered – keeping in mind that the literature regarding conservative management is based on case series or reports and is therefore of unproven safety. If the patient is unstable, conservative management is generally not an option. The risks of conservative management include delayed hemorrhage (requiring reoperation) and infection.

Conservative techniques include those applied in the setting when a focal accreta is encountered after attempted removal of the placenta. These include curettage and/or oversewing the placental bed, or wedge resection of the area of accreta with subsequent repair of the myometrium. In addition to these techniques for managing a focal accreta, planned conservative management has been described in which a placenta accreta diagnosed before delivery is left in situ without attempts to deliver the placenta. Thereafter adjunctive therapy is administered either with uterine artery embolization, methotrexate, or delayed placental removal. These methods of management have not been subject to randomized controlled trials and should be considered investigational.

Conservative approaches generally should be considered only in patients who strongly desire future fertility and who understand and accept the risks of delayed hemorrhage, infection, and death. The patient should be counseled that this approach cannot be used if she has profuse bleeding or is hemodynamically unstable. Timmermans et al. reviewed 60 pregnancies managed conservatively. The most common complication consisted of vaginal bleeding (21/60). The timing of blood loss ranged from immediately postpartum up to 3 months after delivery. Treatment failure due to vaginal bleeding occurred in 15% of case (9/60). Fever occurred in 21/60 cases, 11/60 had endomyometritis, and 2/60 required hysterectomy for definitive treatment. Importantly, the authors caution that the number of complications in the literature may be underrepresented due to publication bias of reported successful cases.

 ## CASE CONTINUES

At 36 weeks Ms. Perkins undergoes another ultrasound and amniocentesis for fetal lung maturity. The MFM calls you to report that he now sees a defect in the bladder mucosa under the placenta suggestive of a percreta with extension into the bladder wall.

Decision 3: Management

How do you respond to this additional finding?

A. Perform a cesarean hysterectomy as scheduled.
B. Ask the urologist to perform cystoscopy prior to the procedure.
C. Plan to leave the placenta in situ.
D. Place catheters for embolization in the uterine artery.

The correct answer is B: Ask the urologist to perform cystoscopy prior to the procedure. The urologist may be able to more accurately assess the involvement of the bladder wall and will also be able to place ureteral stents, which may aid in the dissection to be performed. If a cesarean hysterectomy is performed without this assessment (Answer A), formation of the bladder flap may involve a rent in the bladder, with the risk that ureteral reimplantation will become necessary if the trigone of the bladder is involved. Although one response to this situation is to plan to leave the placenta in situ (Answer C) so as to avoid trauma to the bladder, this should be done after the best possible assessment of the situation (i.e., cystoscopy). Catheters for embolization of the uterine artery (Answer D) will have no effect on bleeding from the bladder and are not indicated in this situation.

CASE CONCLUSION

The urologist performs cystoscopy at the time of the planned cesarean. There is evidence of possible invasion of a small area of the dome of the bladder without involvement of the mucosa. She feels that this amount of bladder wall can be sacrificed if necessary. With this information, you perform a classical uterine incision and deliver a 2,970-g female infant with Apgar score of 8/9.

The placenta does not deliver. To limit blood loss you place O'Leary sutures around the uterine arteries, and then you and the urologist carefully dissect the bladder off the lower uterine segment. A 1 × 2 cm area of bladder wall is densely adherent to the lower segment, and bleeds profusely when you try to dissect it off. You proceed with a total hysterectomy, and the urologist closes the bladder defect after ascertaining that there is urine coming from both ureters. The estimated blood loss is 2,500 cc, and Ms. Perkins receives three units of packed red blood cells intraoperatively. She subsequently does well and is discharged with an indwelling urinary catheter with the plan to remove it 10 days after the surgery.

SUGGESTED READINGS

Chou MM, Ho ES, Lee YH. Prenatal diagnosis of placenta previa accreta by transabdominal color Doppler ultrasound. Ultrasound Obstet Gynecol. 2000;15:28–35.

Clark SL, Koonings PP, Phelan JP. Placenta previa/accreta and prior cesarean section. Obstet Gynecol. 1985;66:89–92.

Comstock CH, Love JJ Jr, Bronsteen RA, et al. Sonographic detection of placenta accreta in the second and third trimesters of pregnancy. Am J Obstet Gynecol. 2004;190:1135–40.

Miller DA, Chollet JA, Goodwin TM. Clinical risk factors for placenta previa-placenta accreta. Am J Obstet Gynecol. 1997;177:210–4.

Shih JC, Palacios Jaraquemada JM, Su YN, et al. Role of three-dimensional power Doppler in the antenatal diagnosis of placenta accreta: comparison with gray-scale and color Doppler techniques. Ultrasound Obstet Gynecol. 2009;33(2):193–203.

Shrivastava V, Nageotte M, Major C, Haydon M, Wing D. Case-control comparison of cesarean hysterectomy with and without prophylactic placement of intravascular balloon catheters for placenta accreta. Am J Obstet Gynecol. 2007;197:402 e1–5.

Silver RM, Landon MB, Rouse DJ, et al. Maternal morbidity associated with multiple repeat cesarean deliveries. Obstet Gynecol. 2006;107:1226–32.

Timmermans S, van Hof AC, Duvekot JJ. Conservative management of abnormally invasive placentation. Obstet Gynecol Surv. 2007;62:529–39.

Twickler DM, Lucas MJ, Balis AB, et al. Color flow mapping for myometrial invasion in women with a prior cesarean delivery. J Matern Fetal Med. 2000;9:330–5.

Wu S, Kocherginsky M, Hibbard JU. Abnormal placentation: twenty-year analysis. Am J Obstet Gynecol. 2005;192:1458–61.

Placenta Previa

31

Racine N. Edwards-Silva

 CASE PRESENTATION

Ms. Rouge is a 22-year-old G1 P0 at 25 0/7 weeks of gestation who presents to OB triage complaining of painless vaginal bleeding. The patient states that she was watching TV on the couch when she felt some wetness. When she went to the bathroom she noted bright red blood in her underwear and on the toilet paper. She did not feel any contractions or back pain. Ms. Rouge reports that she has soaked a total of three perineal pads prior to arriving to the hospital. She denies previous problems in this pregnancy. Her past medical history is remarkable only for iron deficiency anemia. She is a smoker. Today, patient admits that she has been unable to stop smoking or to cut back on her cigarettes. She continues to smoke 8 to 10 cigarettes per day.

On physical examination, she is a thin Caucasian female who appears anxious. Her blood pressure is 110/60 mm Hg, and her pulse is 95 bpm. She is afebrile. Her general physical examination is unremarkable.

 N E E D   T O   K N O W

Differential Diagnosis of Third Trimester Bleeding

Third trimester vaginal bleeding is classically associated with placenta previa, placental abruption, and vasa previa. Other causes of vaginal bleeding in pregnancy (not confined to the third trimester) include cervical lesions, including ectropion, polyps, cancer, and cervicitis. The patient may also have experienced trauma to the cervix or vagina. Finally, nonvaginal bleeding may be mistakenly described as coming from the vagina; sources include rectal bleeding and hematuria. Placental abruption and placenta previa can lead to major hemorrhage and are life-threatening for the mother and fetus. Notably, as the fetal blood approximates 80 to 110 mL/kg fetal body weight, the fetal blood volume at term averages ~300 mL. Thus, significant maternal bleeding

exceeding this amount represents primarily maternal blood. Accordingly, vasa previa can lead to rapid fetal exsanguination and death but does not affect the mother hemodynamically.

Placenta previa is found when the placenta implants in the lower uterine segment in advance of the fetal presenting part. The classic presentation of placenta previa is painless, bright-red vaginal bleeding. Placenta previa is a common incidental finding on second trimester obstetric ultrasonography, and more than 90% of previas found in the second trimester will resolve prior to delivery. Previa complicates approximately 1 out of 200 of pregnancies in the third trimester, although the incidence is increasing, potentially a consequence of the increased rate of cesarean sections. Risk factors for placenta previa include multiparity, advanced maternal age, prior placenta previa, prior cesarean delivery, male fetus, smoking, and multiple uterine curettages for spontaneous or elective abortions (Table 31.1). Maternal morbidities include antepartum bleeding, placenta accreta, intrapartum hemorrhage, hysterectomy, postpartum hemorrhage, blood transfusion, and thrombophlebitis. Women with a history of cesarean delivery who present with a placenta previa are at an especially high risk for placenta accreta, and may benefit from a focused evaluation for an accreta. Fetal conditions associated with previa include malpresentation, intrauterine growth restriction, and velamentous cord insertion.

Placental abruption occurs when there is separation of the placenta from the uterine wall prior to delivery of the fetus. The classic presentation of acute placental abruption is vaginal bleeding with painful uterine contractions and abdominal tenderness, which may be associated with a nonreassuring fetal heart rate tracing (FHT). Abruption is seen in approximately 1% of pregnancies, although there may be a higher incidence of minor, partial abruptions. In complete abruption cases, there is a significant risk of maternal mortality due to massive obstetric hemorrhage and risk of fetal demise due to fetal hypoxia. Disseminated intravascular coagulation due to release of thromboplastin into the maternal circulation occurs in about 10% of acute placental abruptions.

Chronic placental abruption manifests as recurrent episodic vaginal bleeding with pain and contractions.

TABLE 31.1
RISK FACTORS FOR MAJOR CAUSES OF THIRD TRIMESTER VAGINAL BLEEDING

Placenta Previa	Placental Abruption	Vasa Previa
Chronic hypertension	Chronic hypertension	In vitro fertilization
Multiparity	Multiparity	Second trimester placenta previa
Multiple gestation	Preeclampsia	Low-lying placenta
Advanced maternal age	Previous abruption	Marginal cord insertion
Previous cesarean delivery	Sudden decompression of an overdistended uterus	Multiple gestation
Tobacco use	Tobacco, cocaine, or methamphetamine use	Succenturiate-lobed and bilobed placenta
Uterine curettage	Trauma	
Male fetus	Uterine fibroids	
	Thrombophilias	
	Unexplained elevated maternal serum alpha-fetoprotein level	
	Short umbilical cord	

Because of the reduction in the area available for maternal–fetal exchange, there is a potential for uteroplacental insufficiency and fetal growth restriction, although it is generally believed that abruptions involving <50% of placental area can be tolerated by the fetus. In cases of significant chronic abruption, consideration should be given to performing serial ultrasounds for fetal growth along with antenatal surveillance in the third trimester. Risk factors for placental abruption include chronic hypertension, preeclampsia, prior placental abruption, abdominal trauma, smoking, cocaine use, multiple gestation, polyhydramnios, uterine anomaly, thrombophilias, prolonged premature rupture of membranes, and antepartum anticoagulant use.

Vasa previa occurs when fetal vessels, unprotected by placenta or umbilical cord, traverse the membranes in the lower uterine segment in advance of the presenting fetal part. Vasa previa results either from velamentous insertion of the cord into the membranes (type 1) or from vessels running between lobes of a placenta with one or more accessory lobes (type 2). Fetal exsanguination can occur with artificial rupture of membranes or with spontaneous rupture of the membranes in labor, while the apparent blood loss may appear small. The estimated incidence of vasa previa is approximately 1 in 2,500 deliveries. Risk factors include a second-trimester low-lying placenta, pregnancies in which the placenta has accessory lobes, multiple gestation, and pregnancies resulting from in vitro fertilization. In some cases, vasa previa may be diagnosed prenatally when, using transvaginal ultrasonography with color Doppler, the fetal vessels can be seen overlying the internal os of the cervix. However, this examination is not a part of standard obstetric care. Should vasa previa be diagnosed, a planned cesarean delivery between 35 and 36 weeks of gestational age prior to rupture of the membranes minimizes perinatal mortality.

 Decision 1: Evaluation

What workup should be done on admission?

A. Bimanual examination
B. Ultrasound examination
C. NST
D. Magnetic resonance imaging (MRI)

The correct answers are B: Ultrasound examination and **C:** NST. Ultrasound is the most useful modality for evaluation of vaginal bleeding in the gravid patient. Transvaginal sonography (TVS) is the gold standard for identifying a placenta previa. TVS most accurately demonstrates the relationship of the placental edge to the internal cervical os. If a vaginal probe is unavailable, one can use translabial imaging with excellent visualization of the relationship between the placenta and cervix. The NST or fetal monitoring will assess the condition of the fetus and is advisable in a situation in which fetal well-being may be compromised. A bimanual examination (Answer A) is contraindicated in a gravid patient presenting with vaginal bleeding, until evaluation for placenta previa is completed, as the bimanual examination may provoke profuse vaginal bleeding in the patient with a previa. An MRI (Answer D) is most useful for the diagnosis of placenta accreta and can assist in delineating the extent of placental invasion into the myometrium or bladder; it is not necessary for the diagnosis of placenta previa.

 CASE CONTINUES

Both transabdominal and TVS are performed and a complete placenta previa is found by sonographic evaluation. The cervical length is 3.8 cm; no cervical dilatation or funneling is seen. There is a male fetus seen in a vertex presentation. The estimated gestational age is 24⁵/₇ weeks, the estimated fetal weight is 700 g, and adequate amniotic fluid is noted. A careful sterile speculum examination is performed: there is no evidence of active bleeding or cervical pathology, and the cervix appears closed by visualization. The FHT is appropriate for gestational age and no contractions are visible on the monitor. Laboratory examination reveals that Ms. Rouge's hemoglobin is 8 g/dL, and her hematocrit is 24%.

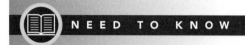

N E E D   T O   K N O W

Definition/Types of Placenta Previa

The placenta previa is classified as complete, partial, or marginal depending on the proximity of the placental edge to the internal cervical os (Fig. 31.1).

Complete **Placenta Previa**—the placenta completely covers the internal os of the cervix.
Partial **Placenta Previa**—the placental edge partially covers the internal cervical os.
Marginal **Placenta Previa**—the placental edge just reaches the internal os but does not cover it.
Low-lying **Placenta**—the placenta lies in the lower uterine segment and the placental edge is near, but not overlying, the internal os.

Previas and low-lying placentas identified early in pregnancy tend to migrate away from the cervix and out of the lower uterine segment. This was originally thought

to be an artifact due to the development of the lower uterine segment, but it is now thought that the placenta grows preferentially toward a better-vascularized area such as the fundus (trophotropism).

Decision 2: Management

What should be considered next in this preterm patient?

- **A.** Blood transfusion
- **B.** Cesarean section
- **C.** Betamethasone
- **D.** Tocolysis

The correct answer is A: Blood transfusion. Laboratory studies showed a hematocrit (hct) of 24%. Given the constant threat of a catastrophic bleed with placenta previa, preparations should be made for maternal fluid resuscitation if needed. A prudent course of action might be to prophylactically administer packed red blood cells (PRBCs) to a hct of 30%, so as to provide a "buffer" in the event of further bleeding. With the lack of ongoing bleeding, and with a stable mother and fetus, immediate cesarean section (Answer B) would be contraindicated with this very premature fetus. Similarly, without uterine contractions, tocolysis (Answer D) is probably not beneficial. The use of steroids for fetal lung maturation (Answer C) is controversial when there is a low expectation of delivery within 7 to 14 days. However, this patient may well be expected to deliver during this period.

Because of the high risk of maternal bleeding, it is usual to admit the patient with an episode of bleeding from a previa to labor and delivery for close maternal and fetal surveillance. If the bleeding is ongoing, two large bore intravenous lines may be established and crystalloid

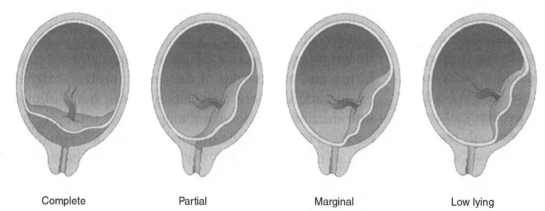

Complete   Partial   Marginal   Low lying

Figure 31.1 Types of placenta previa. Placenta previa is categorized by the relationship of the placenta to the internal cervical os. Complete previa: the placenta completely covers the internal os. The placenta in the illustration might also be called a central previa, indicating that the middle of the placenta covers the os. Partial previa: the placental edge partially covers the os. Marginal previa: the placental edge extends to the cervical os. The risk of bleeding relates to the uncertainty in diagnosis and to the possibility that the placental marginal sinus covers the os. Low-lying placenta: the placental edge extends near the os. Again, the risk of bleeding is related to the uncertainty in diagnosis. (Adapted from www.womenshealthsection.com.)

administration initiated to maintain hemodynamic stability and for adequate urine output. Laboratory studies should be reviewed to assess for appropriate blood product replacement. Management of an acute bleed should take into account the gestational age and the risks of prematurity. If the fetus is extremely premature, an attempt may be made to defer delivery and stabilize the mother and fetus with aggressive resuscitation measures. Ultimately, however, cesarean section is the delivery route of choice and is necessary in most cases of placenta previa to prevent critical maternal bleeding. Exceptions are patients with low-lying placentae where the margin does not approach the os. In the absence of any emergency, an elective cesarean section is usually recommended for a complete placenta previa at 36 to 37 weeks. Some authorities perform amniocentesis to document fetal lung maturity, whereas others believe that the small chance of fetal breathing difficulties at 36 weeks is offset by the risk of maternal bleeding with further delay in the delivery. Patients who must deliver earlier may benefit from a course of steroids as for other preterm deliveries.

Tocolysis in the setting of obstetric hemorrhage from placenta previa tends to be controversial. There is concern for concealment of the signs of continued bleeding, especially with the use of beta-mimetics, such as terbutaline that may, themselves, cause tachycardia and hypotension. However, tocolysis may be utilized to break the vicious cycle of vaginal bleeding, which may cause uterine contractions which then incites more bleeding and contractions that may exacerbate placental detachment. Therefore, it is reasonable to use tocolytics cautiously in women with placenta previa who are having contractions after maternal and fetal stabilization to administer a course of antenatal steroids and to attempt to prolong the pregnancy. In some studies, tocolytic therapy has been shown to prolong the pregnancy and result in an increased infant birth weight.

The location of patient care after initial stabilization is controversial. Many centers will send a patient home after a resolved first bleed, if she can remain at rest and if she has reliable transportation back to the hospital in case of recurrent bleeding. Many centers will keep a mother hospitalized

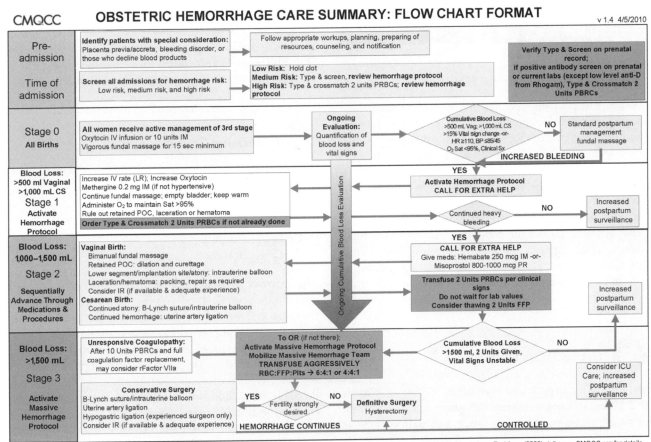

Figure 31.2   Flow diagram for the management of obstetrical hemorrhage, developed by the California Maternal Quality Care Collaborative. Especially in emergent situations, quality care requires that every member of the team knows their role and knows the procedure to be followed. This document can be posted on the wall of the delivery room and structures the response to obstetrical bleeding from minor spotting to massive hemorrhage.

TABLE 31.2

BLOOD COMPONENTS USED IN RESUSCITATION

Component	Indication	Notes
Packed red blood cells	To improve O$_2$ carrying capacity	Raise Hb 1 g/dL
Fresh-frozen plasma	Replace clotting factors PT and /or PTT >1.5 × upper normal	Start with 2 U FFP or 15–20 mL/kg ideal body weight
Cryoprecipitate	Fibrinogen <75–100 μg	1 U/10-kg body weight with fibrinogen <75
Platelets	Platelets <50,000	Increase platelets 5,000–10,000/mm^3 per unit
Albumin	Volume replacement bind bilirubin in newborns albumin <1.0 g/dL (total protein <4.0)	Use 5% albumin

PT, prothrombin time; PTT, partial thromboplastin time; Hb, hemoglobin; FFP, fresh frozen plasma.
Santoso JT, Saunders BA, Grosshart K. Massive blood loss and transfusion in obstetrics and gynecology. Obstet Gynecol Surv. 2005;60(12):827–37. Review.

until delivery after the second or third bleed. This form of management is unproven; limited data suggest that hospitalization does not improve outcome.

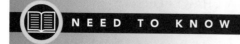 **NEED TO KNOW**

Approach to Obstetrical Hemorrhage

A major hemorrhage requires the patient management team to work in concert (Fig. 31.2). A maternal blood sample is sent for immediate type and crossmatch for 4 to 6 units of PRBCs. The need for transfusion of blood products should be guided by the rate of vaginal bleeding, stability of maternal vital signs, urine output, and laboratory values (complete blood cell count, and coagulation profile of fibrinogen, prothrombin time [PT], and activated partial thromboplastin time [PTT]) and based on the expected effect of the various blood components available (Table 31.2). RhD-immune globulin should be considered in RhD negative women at the initial bleeding episode.

 CASE CONTINUES

Ms. Rouge receives 2 L of crystalloid, 2 units of PRBCs, and 12 mg of betamethasone 24 hours apart for a total of two injections. While on labor and delivery she is noted to have contractions and is started on magnesium sulfate tocolysis to administer the full course of antenatal steroids. The FHT remains reassuring throughout this time. The patient is ultimately stabilized and transferred to the antepartum unit where she remains for 4 days

without any further vaginal bleeding or contractions. After 4 days on the antepartum unit, Ms. Rouge is discharged home with instructions to maintain bedrest and close proximity to the hospital, ensure reliable transportation, and return immediately to the hospital if any further vaginal bleeding occurs.

Ms. Rouge remains in home for 3 weeks and returns again with acute heavy vaginal bleeding at 28 4/7 weeks gestation. Laboratory values on admission are Hct = 18%, fibrinogen = 150 mg/dL, PT = 16 seconds, and PTT = 46 second, and she has minimal vaginal bleeding.

 Decision 3: Management

What are options for immediate management of a recurrent acute bleed?

A. Immediate IV access and crystalloids
B. Tocolysis
C. Fetal monitoring
D. Cesarean section

The correct answers are A: Immediate IV access and crystalloids and *C:* Fetal monitoring. Without ongoing bleeding, if maternal and fetal resuscitation and stabilization can be accomplished at this gestational age, the prolongation of the pregnancy would allow for further fetal maturation and decrease the morbidities of prematurity. In addition, resuscitation and stabilization of the mother is desirable, if possible, prior to a surgical delivery. Immediate cesarean section (Answer D) is indicated with placenta previa if there is uncontrollable excessive vaginal bleeding, nonreassuring fetal heart rate, or worsening maternal hemodynamic instability despite aggressive resuscitation measures. Tocolysis (Answer B) is not utilized in the setting of acute severe vaginal bleeding.

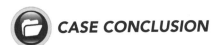

CASE CONCLUSION

Ms. Rouge is successfully resuscitated with 3 L of crystalloid, 4 units of PRBCs, and 2 units of fresh frozen plasma. Maternal vital signs improve from a blood pressure of 90/50 to 120/60 mm Hg, a pulse of 130 to 100 bpm, and O_2 saturation varied from 92% to 95%. The FHT initially has a baseline of 110 bpm with decreased variability and occasional late decelerations. With aggressive resuscitation, the tracing improves to a baseline of 120 bpm with moderate variability, accelerations, and resolution of late decelerations.

Because of the severity of this second episode of bleeding and the unpredictability of further bleeding episodes, the patient is hospitalized until delivery. The patient remains for an additional 3 weeks without further heavy bleeding. However, she continues to have occasional episodes of scant-to-mild vaginal bleeding.

Adequate interval fetal growth is confirmed with a repeat sonogram for fetal biometry, amniotic fluid volume. At 32 2/7 weeks, the FHT becomes nonreassuring with decreased variability and fetal tachycardia with a rate of 175 bpm. Also, the patient reports an increasing amount of vaginal bleeding with the passage of clots when she urinates. An urgent cesarean section is performed with delivery of a male infant weighing 1,750 g with Apgar score of 4/8, at 1 and 5 minutes, respectively. The cesarean section was complicated by an intrapartum blood loss of 1,500 cc for which the patient received another 2 units of PRBCs and 2 L of crystalloid. After delivery, Ms. Rouge's recovery was uneventful, and she was discharged home on the fourth postpartum day. Her baby did well in nursery, and was discharged on the 12th day of life.

SUGGESTED READINGS

Creasy, et al. Chapter 37. Placenta previa, placenta accreta, abruptio placentae, and vasa previa. In: Creasy & Resnik's Maternal-Fetal Medicine Principles and Practice. 6th ed.

Cunningham, et al. Chapter 25. Obstetrical Hemorrhage. In: Williams Obstetrics. 21st ed. 2001. pp. 619–35.

Demissie K, Breckenridge MB, Joseph L, et al. Placenta previa: preponderance of male sex at birth. Am J Epidemiol. 1999;149: 824–30.

Fox MC, Hayes JL. Cervical preparation for second trimester surgical abortion prior to 20 weeks gestation. Society of Family Planning. Contraception. 2007;76:486–95.

Halperin R, Vaknin Z, Langer R, Bukovsky I, Schneider D. Late midtrimester pregnancy termination in the presence of placenta previa. J Reprod Med. 2003;48(3):175–8.

Kuo PL, Guo HR. Nucleated red blood cells in maternal blood during pregnancy. Obstet Gynecol. 1999;94:464–8.

Oyelese KO, Turner M, Lees C, Campbell S. Vasa previa: an avoidable obstetric tragedy. Obstet Gynecol Survey. 1999;54(2):138–45.

Oyelese Y, Smulian JC. Placenta previa, placenta accreta, and vasa previa. Obstet Gynecol. 2006;107:927–41.

Oyelese Y, Catanzarite V, Prefumo F, et al. Vasa previa: the impact of prenatal diagnosis on outcomes. Obstet Gynecol. 2004;103: 937–42.

Russo-Stieglitz K, Lockwood CJ. Placenta previa and vasa previa. UpToDate. 2005. Version 13.2.

Russo-Stieglitz K, Lockwood CJ. Management of placenta previa. UpToDate. 2009. Version 17.1.

Sakornbut E, Leeman L, Fontaine P. Late pregnancy bleeding. Am Fame Physician. 2007;75:1199–206.

Santoso JT, Saunders BA, Grosshart K. Massive blood loss and transfusion in obstetrics and gynecology. Obstet Gynecol Surv. 2005; 60(12):827–37. Review.

Placental Abruption

Matthew Kim

32

CASE PRESENTATION

You are paged to the emergency department for a pregnant trauma victim. Upon arrival, a nurse informs you that the patient is Ms. Franklin, a 40-year-old nullipara who has just arrived by ambulance. After introducing yourself to the patient, you obtain a history and learn that she is 36 weeks pregnant and has just experienced trauma as a restrained passenger in a car that ran into another car. She reports that since the accident, she is not feeling fetal movement but has felt continuous and worsening abdominal pain. Her previous medical and obstetrical history is unremarkable. Although she denies loss of consciousness or head trauma, the patient appears drowsy and is difficult to engage.

On physical examination, vital signs are pulse 120 bpm, blood pressure 90/60 mm Hg, respirations 16/min, and temperature 36.5°C. Positive findings on physical examination include a diagonal contusion across the chest and abdomen, generalized abdominal tenderness, and a hard, painful uterine fundus. There is a blood clot at the vaginal introitus. Doppler fetal heart tones by a handheld device are approximately 140 bpm. Fetal ultrasound has been ordered.

Decision 1: Workup

What is the next step in your evaluation of this patient?

A. Sterile speculum and digital vaginal examination
B. Wait for the abdominal ultrasound results
C. Initiation of intravenous (IV) access and fluid resuscitation
D. Immediate cesarean delivery

The correct answer is C: Initiation of IV access and fluid resuscitation. Since the clinical presentation is suggestive of developing hypovolemic shock with tachycardia and hypotension, physiologic support of the mother is the primary focus in the initial or acute management of this pregnant woman. A vaginal examination (Answer A) is ill advised as localization of the placenta should precede vaginal examination in the bleeding obstetric patient. Waiting

for the ultrasound (Answer B) is partially correct, but patient resuscitation should be initiated without delay, prior to completing the diagnostic evaluation. Although cesarean delivery (Answer D) may eventually be required, the initial response is maternal resuscitation. There is presently no indication for performing major surgery on a potentially unstable patient.

NEED TO KNOW

Initial Evaluation of Vaginal Bleeding

The obstetrician must be prepared for all contingencies when called to the emergency department. Although in this case a history and physical examination were able to be obtained, the opportunity to perform such an evaluation cannot be assumed. Thus, it is important for a physician to clearly understand not only the differential diagnosis of typical presenting signs and symptoms but also the clinical priority of response that should occur in an acute setting. In a significant trauma with concerning vital signs, the first priority is resuscitation and stabilization of the patient. Resuscitation should not be delayed unduly for diagnostic testing, but rather resuscitation and testing are done concurrently.

Resuscitation

Obstetric hemorrhage is a critical emergency for both mother and fetus. Given the substantial volume of blood flow to the uterus during pregnancy, any significant disruption of the uterine vasculature may result in a rapid destabilization of mother and fetus. The initial response to hypovolemic shock is similar whatever the cause of the hypovolemia. The first task is to provide volume intravenously. Establishing peripheral venous access is a critical initial step in the management of hemorrhage patients and should occur at first presentation or concern as, due to the physiologic response to hemorrhage, peripheral access for intravenous fluids is difficult once blood loss has become severe. It should also be noted that for rapid and massive volume replacement, large bore peripheral access is superior to central line access due to the direct physical relationship between resistance to flow and length of tubing. Once intravenous access is established in the patient with evidence of hypovolemia, crystalloid is infused with the goal of providing two to three times the estimated volume lost. At the same time, specimens are sent to the laboratory for clotting studies (to evaluate for consumptive coagulopathy and to assess the need for clotting factor replacement) and for blood to be crossmatched. In a true emergency, the patient can be transfused with type-specific uncrossmatched blood, or even O negative blood.

Diagnosis

Vaginal bleeding is a common presenting complaint in the pregnant woman. Although the passage of blood is not necessarily alarming, the circumstances surrounding the bleeding as well as the findings on history and physical examination can establish a more likely diagnosis amongst several very different etiologies and levels of urgency. To begin with, the medical history is an important opportunity to establish a differential diag-

nosis. The nature of the bleeding should be clarified. In particular, quantity (spotting or number of menstrual pads), quality (color, constant or intermittent), and any associated symptoms such as contractions, pain, or rupture of membranes should be elicited. Although the history may be invaluable in establishing the differential, establishing a firm diagnosis based only on the history is a common error. Every effort should be made to maintain an open mind throughout the evaluation and care of the inpatient. Sources of vaginal bleeding in the third trimester of pregnancy that may be considered are seen in Table 32.1.

The obstetric physical examination is typically focused on the maternal abdomen, vagina/cervix, and an evaluation of fetal status. However, in the case of a presentation for vaginal bleeding, no attempts at direct vaginal examination should occur prior to the determination of placental location, as exacerbation of bleeding from a placenta previa may result. Placental location is definitively established by ultrasound. Although prior ultrasound reports may be reliable, a new presentation for significant vaginal bleeding should prompt a complete reevaluation of the patient, including ultrasound for placental position. Vaginal bleeding, especially from an abruption or vasa previa, confers a significant risk of

TABLE 32.1

DIFFERENTIAL DIAGNOSIS: COMMON SOURCES OF SIGNIFICANT VAGINAL BLEEDING IN THE THIRD TRIMESTER OF PREGNANCY

Source of Bleeding		Characteristic History
Pregnancy	Placental abruption	Painful bleeding
		May have history of trauma or other predisposing factors
		May have evidence of coagulopathy
	Placenta previa	Painless bleeding
	Vasa previa	Severe fetal distress or death in the absence of significant maternal symptoms
	Labor: "bloody show"	History suggestive of active labor
Vagina/cervix	Cervical polyp	Painless or minimally painful bleeding, often after intercourse
	Cervical cancer	Painless or minimally painful bleeding, often after intercourse
		May have a history of abnormal Pap smears
	Vaginal trauma (especially sexual assault)	History of recent traumatic intercourse or other vaginal penetration
Nongynecologic	Rectal bleeding	May be asymptomatic, or may have symptoms of diarrhea or constipation
	Hematuria	Blood seen with urination

fetal compromise. Thus, it is important not only to establish normal fetal heart tones (definitively identified separate from the maternal heart rate) but also to assess fetal oxygenation status by external fetal monitoring.

After a placenta previa is excluded, a sterile speculum examination followed by digital examination may further help to determine the source and nature of bleeding. In particular, the volume of flow as well as the potential that active labor is occurring can be assessed. The examination should assess the presence of lacerations, cervical tumors, or nongynecologic sources of bleeding such as anorectal hemorrhoids. A final consideration is the presence of ruptured membranes. Although bloody or blood-tinged amniotic fluid is usually lighter than frank blood, blood-stained amniotic fluid may mimic frank hemorrhage in some circumstances.

 CASE CONTINUES

A large-bore IV is inserted, and lactated Ringer's solution is infused at 200 cc/hr after a 1 L bolus. Ms. Franklin's vital signs stabilize with a pulse of 120 bpm and a blood pressure of 100/60 mm Hg. You observe that there is noticeable urine output. Laboratory testing for complete blood cell count, fibrinogen and D-dimer, and a toxicology screen are sent and pending. A specimen has been sent for type and crossmatch.

A bedside ultrasound is performed and it demonstrates a 36-week singleton gestation with size equal to dates. The amniotic fluid index (AFI) is 15 cm. The placenta is clearly visualized as it is anterior and fundal. However, there appears to be a hypoechoic layer between a portion of the placenta and the uterus (see Fig. 32.1).

 Decision 2: Diagnosis

What is the diagnosis?

A. Placenta previa
B. Friable cervix
C. Placental abruption
D. Rupture of membranes

The correct answer is C: Placental abruption. Placenta previa (Answer A) is incorrect as the placenta is fundal, well away from the os. In a placenta previa, the placenta overrides the endocervical os. Although vaginal bleeding can present from a friable cervix, it is unlikely to result in hemorrhage or symptomatic blood loss (Answer B). Rupture of membranes (Answer D) is not associated with the ultrasound findings, or the normal AFI.

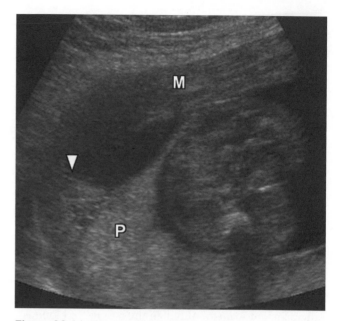

Figure 32.1 Ultrasound of the placenta. M is the myometrium, P the placenta. There is a hypoechoic area between the edge of the placenta and the myometrium. (Reproduced with permission from Elsayes KM, Trout AT, Friedkin AM, et al. Imaging of the placenta: a multimodality pictorial review. Radiographics. 2009;29(5):1371–91.)

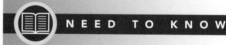 **N E E D   T O   K N O W**

Placental Abruption

Placental abruption is the premature separation of the placenta from the uterine wall, prior to delivery of the fetus. The incidence of clinically significant abruption is about 1%; however, there are many small placental separations that do not become evident in labor; the total incidence of abruption appears to be closer to 4%. Although vaginal bleeding with abdominal pain occurs in 70% to 80% of cases of abruption, occasionally the bleeding will be hidden or contained in the uterus, most often between the placenta and the uterus as a retroplacental bleed or clot. With greater degrees of placental separation comes a greater risk for maternal consumptive coagulopathy and hypovolemic shock, and a greater risk for fetal hypoxia and death. A particularly severe form of abruption involves extravasation of blood into the myometrium; this is known as a Couvelaire uterus. A Couvelaire uterus may exhibit atony after delivery requiring hysterectomy and is associated with a higher risk of maternal hypovolemic shock and fetal asphyxia. Some authors use a grading system for abruption based on the maternal and fetal status (Table 32.2).

Abruption is associated with a number of conditions, including infection, maternal hypertension, and trauma (Table 32.3). The common factor in many of these

TABLE 32.2
ABRUPTION CLASSIFICATION

Sher's classification:
1—Minimal or no bleeding with viable fetus
2—Viable fetus with bleeding and uterine tenderness
3a—Dead fetus, no bleeding problems (70% of grade 3)
3b—Dead fetus, coagulopathy (30% of grade 3)

[a]Sher (1985) proposed the classification system most often used for placental abruption in 1985. At that time, coagulopathy was most often diagnosed by abnormal bleeding and most pregnancies with coagulopathy were characterized by a fetal demise. With more sensitive testing, coagulopathy is more often diagnosed in the patient with a live fetus.

appears to be disruption of the decidual–placental interface with extravasation of blood. Blood collects between the placenta and deciduas basalis, interrupting the flow of maternal blood to the placenta. Maternal clotting factors are consumed both locally in the uterus and throughout the body, perhaps due to the release of thromboplastins from the placenta. If unabated, the final result may be fetal death, maternal coagulopathy, and shock and finally maternal death.

The classic presentation of placental abruption is unrelenting abdominal/uterine pain accompanied by vaginal bleeding. The pain is due to the uterine tetany that accompanies abruption, due either to a direct irritating effect of the blood on the myometrium or to the release of prostaglandins. Monitoring of uterine contractions in abruption reveals an increased baseline uterine tonus,

with frequent uterine contractions of low amplitude. The uterine contractions further reduce blood flow to the placenta, with resulting fetal hypoxia and abnormalities of fetal heart rate. After delivery, a clot may be found adherent to the placenta in the area of the abruption. Some or all of these signs may be absent. Bleeding may be absent if the blood is retained in the uterus. The pain may not be constant, or may be minimal. The fetus may tolerate the reduction in placental blood flow, and the fetal heart rate may remain normal throughout. If the abruption is very recent, the retroplacental clot may not be seen.

The diagnosis of abruption is made clinically, as there is no specific laboratory test. Laboratory testing for coagulopathy may be of benefit; the most sensitive and commonly used tests are measures of fibrin degradation products (which also may be elevated under basal conditions of pregnancy), followed by the total fibrinogen. Ultrasound may identify the abruption, but the absence of ultrasound findings does not rule out the diagnosis.

The peak incidence of abruption is early in the third trimester, between 24 and 27 weeks of gestation. Given this timing, there is often a consideration for conservative management of the abruption patient. In some cases, small, self-limited abruptions can be closely monitored and the pregnancy allowed to continue. In many cases, however, the risk of temporizing is judged to be too high. The risk is not negligible; as up to 1% of mothers and 11% of fetuses with clinically significant abruption die.

TABLE 32.3
FACTORS ASSOCIATED WITH ABRUPTION[a]

Risk Factor	Relative Risk
Maternal Health Risks	
Maternal age and parity	1.1–3.7
Chronic hypertension	1.8–5.1
Chronic hypertension with preeclampsia	7.8
Maternal smoking	1.4–2.5
Cocaine and amphetamine use	5.0–10.0
Trauma	—
Pregnancy Complications	
Multiple gestation	1.5–3.0
Premature rupture of membranes	1.8–5.1
Oligohydramnios	2.5–10.0
Chorioamnionitis	2.0–2.5
Prior abruption	11–25

[a]The most significant prognostic factor is a prior abruption. Trauma is associated with abruption, but relative risks were not available, in part due to the variability in traumatic episodes. Other factors, including male fetus, mild preeclampsia, and nutritional deficiencies have a nonsignificant association with abruption.
Adapted from Oyelese Y, Ananth CV. Placental abruption. Obstet Gynecol. 2006;108(4):1005–16.

 ## CASE CONTINUES

On fetal heart rate monitoring after the ultrasound, Ms. Franklin has uterine contractions occurring every minute. The fetal heart rate baseline is 160 bpm with absent variability and late decelerations. Manual examination reveals the cervix to be 2 cm dilated and 80% effaced with the presenting part at −1 station. The decision is made to proceed with an immediate cesarean delivery. Initial laboratory tests demonstrate a hematocrit of 25% and a platelet count of 90×10^9/L. In addition, the coagulation profile shows a fibrinogen of 90 mg/dL (nonpregnant normal 150–300 mg/dL), PT of 14 seconds (nonpregnant normal 10–13 seconds), PTT of 35 seconds (nonpregnant normal 25–35 seconds), and D-dimer strongly positive.

 Decision 3: Diagnosis

What is the diagnosis at this point?

  A. Pancytopenia
  B. Coagulopathy
  C. Hemorrhage (alone)
  D. Thrombophilia

TABLE 32.4

SCORING SYSTEM FOR THE DIAGNOSIS OF DISSEMINATED INTRAVASCULAR COAGULATION (DIC)[a]

1. Risk assessment: Does the patient have an underlying disorder known to be associated with overt DIC?
   If yes: proceed; If no: do not use this algorithm;
2. Order global coagulation tests (platelet count, prothrombin time [PT], fibrinogen, soluble fibrin monomers, or fibrin degradation products).
3. Score global coagulation test results:
   - Platelet count (>100–0; <100–1; <50–2)
   - Elevated fibrin-related marker (e.g., soluble fibrin monomers, fibrin degradation products) (no increase-0, moderate increase-2, strong increase-3)
   - Prolonged prothrombin time (<3 sec–0; >3 sec but <6 sec–1; >6 sec–2)
   - Fibrinogen level (>1.0 g/l (100 mg/dL) –0; <1.0 g/l–1)
4. Calculate score
5. If ≥5: compatible with overt DIC

[a]Developed by the scientific subcommittee on disseminated intravascular coagulation of the international society on thrombosis and hemostasis. The system is intended for use in all patients, there is no provision for adjustment of the cutoff values in pregnancy, although pregnancy is known to alter the normal values of many clotting parameters.
Adapted from Taylor FB Jr, Toh CH, Hoots WK, Wada H, Levi M; Scientific Subcommittee on Disseminated Intravascular Coagulation (DIC) of the International Society on Thrombosis and Haemostasis (ISTH). Towards definition, clinical and laboratory criteria, and a scoring system for disseminated intravascular coagulation. Thromb Haemost. 2001 Nov;86(5):1327–30.

The correct answer is B: Coagulopathy. There is no single laboratory test to confirm the diagnosis of coagulopathy; however, the combination of low platelets and fibrinogen and elevated PT are strongly suggestive (Table 32.4). In pregnancy, the fibrinogen level is increased to as much as twice normal levels, while the platelet count is decreased. The PT and PTT are also both somewhat decreased, suggesting that the levels seen in this patient are likely abnormal for pregnancy. These findings would all support a diagnosis of early coagulopathy.

The low hematocrit and platelet count are likely due to bleeding and a consumptive coagulopathy and not

pancytopenia (Answer A). Although hemorrhage alone (Answer C) would explain the anemia and possibly the thrombocytopenia, it would not explain this degree of coagulopathy. Thrombophilia (Answer D) might explain clotting abnormalities, but would not explain the anemia.

 CASE CONTINUES

You make a diagnosis of early coagulopathy and call for blood products to be delivered to the operating room.

 NEED TO KNOW

Blood Replacement in DIC

Although surgery in a patient with a coagulopathy is counterintuitive, the coagulopathy will not likely resolve with an abruption unless uterine evacuation and tone are achieved. Thus in the presentation of massive placental abruption, surgery may not only be indicated but potentially life saving to the mother. During the surgery, blood and clotting factors must be provided so as to allow hemostasis during and after the procedure and to replace anticipated blood loss.

For the patient with coagulopathy alone, recommendations are to reverse the cause. Blood product replacement is not recommended unless bleeding ensues or is anticipated. In the case of a patient with abruption, reversal of the coagulopathy involves removing the placenta; whether this is done vaginally or abdominally bleeding can certainly be anticipated. General guidelines would then support replacement of red blood cells to support the hemoglobin/hematocrit, and reversal of coagulopathy sufficient to allow operative hemostasis (Table 32.5).

TABLE 32.5

BLOOD PRODUCT MANAGEMENT FOR DELIVERY IN THE PATIENT WITH COAGULOPATHY[a]

Product	Minimum Level	Notes
Packed red blood cells	Hemoglobin 10 g/dL (hematocrit 30%)	Each unit increases the hemoglobin by 1 g/dL
Fresh frozen plasma	N/A	Replaces multiple clotting factors. May be given empirically
Cryoprecipitate	50–100 mg/dL (0.5–1 g/L)	One bag is expected to increase blood levels by 10 mg/dL
Platelets	50 × 10⁹/L	Each platelet pack should increase blood levels by 10 × 10⁹/L

[a]Patients with levels below the minimum are given blood product to achieve the minimum level. Fresh frozen plasma may be given in a ratio with packed red cells; a 1:1 ratio is recommended, as it has been shown to give better results than a 1:4 ratio.

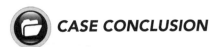

CASE CONCLUSION

Ms. Franklin is taken to the operating room and a transfusion of packed red blood cells is started. You deliver a 2,600-g female infant with Apgar score of 2 and 6 at 1 and 5 minutes. The pediatricians resuscitate the baby and she does well thereafter. On delivery of the placenta, a 1,000-cc clot is discovered behind the placenta. There is continued uterine bleeding, and 5 minutes after placental delivery the anesthesiologist reports that there is blood oozing from the IV sites. The anesthesiologist obtains another set of coagulation studies, and calls for 2 units of fresh frozen plasma. You quickly close the uterus and call for oxytocin and methylergonovine to assist with uterine contraction. You then close the abdomen, leaving a drain in the subcutaneous layer due to continued slow oozing that you conclude is due to coagulopathy. Estimated blood loss from the surgery is 1,500 cc, in addition to the clot found below the placenta. Ms. Franklin is taken to the ICU for the night, where she is given a total of 5 units of packed red blood cells and 4 units of fresh frozen plasma. By the next morning, her hematocrit is 28%, her platelet count is 57×10^9/L, her fibrinogen is 65 g/dL, and her PT is 13. She has appropriate lochia and is not bleeding from her incision or IV sites. Her drain reveals 100 cc of drainage in 12 hours. You send her to the OB floor, where she is able to be with her baby, and both she and the baby subsequently do well. They are discharged on the fifth postoperative day.

SUGGESTED READINGS

ACOG educational bulletin. Obstetric aspects of trauma management. Number 251, September 1998. American College of Obstetricians and Gynecologists. Int J Gynaecol Obstet. 1999;64(1):87–94.

Elsayes KM, Trout AT, Friedkin AM, et al. Imaging of the placenta: a multimodality pictorial review. Radiographics. 2009;29(5):1371–91.

Hall DR. Abruptio placentae and disseminated intravascular coagulopathy. Semin Perinatol. 2009;33(3):189–95.

Levi M, Toh CH, Thachil J, Watson HG. Guidelines for the diagnosis and management of disseminated intravascular coagulation. British Committee for Standards in Haematology. Br J Haematol. 2009;145(1):24–33.

Neilson JP. Interventions for treating placental abruption. Cochrane Database Syst Rev. 2003;(1):CD003247.

Oyelese Y, Ananth CV. Placental abruption. Obstet Gynecol. 2006;108(4):1005–16.

Papp Z. Massive obstetric hemorrhage. J Perinat Med. 2003;31(5):408–14.

Sher G, Statland BE. Abruptio placentae with coagulopathy: a rational basis for management. Clin Obstet Gynecol. 1985;28(1):15–23.

Thachil J, Toh CH. Disseminated intravascular coagulation in obstetric disorders and its acute haematological management. Blood Rev. 2009;23(4):167–76. Epub 2009 May 12.

Postdated Pregnancy

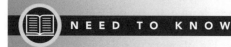

Robert Eden

 CASE PRESENTATION

You are called to labor and delivery to evaluate Ms. Jordan, a 21-year-old G1 P0 Caucasian female at 42⁵⁄₇ weeks of gestation by reported last menstrual period (LMP) who has presented because she thinks that the baby should be coming. She reports that she has recently moved to town and has not yet established prenatal care; records from her previous provider are not immediately available. Ms. Jordan denies any medical or obstetrical complications during this pregnancy. She also denies vaginal bleeding, rupture of membranes, or signs or symptoms of preeclampsia. Her physical examination is within normal limits. The fundal height is 39 cm, the estimated fetal weight (EFW) by manual palpation is 2,500 g, and the fetus is in the vertex presentation. A pelvic examination reveals that the cervix is not dilated or effaced, and that the presenting part is ballotable. The fetal heart rate (FHR) is reactive, with a baseline of 140 bpm, average variability, no decelerations, and no uterine contractions.

 Decision 1: Management

Management of this patient may include everything except:

- **A.** Amniotic fluid index (AFI) and biophysical profile (BPP)
- **B.** Ultrasound evaluation of fetal size and estimated gestational age (GA)
- **C.** Review of prenatal records
- **D.** Admission and induction of labor

The answer is D: Admission and induction of labor. At this point, the cervix is not favorable for induction, the dating is unsure, and the prenatal testing is normal. Fetal size by EFW suggests that the true GA may be less than stated. There is no indication for labor induction, and reason to be concerned that an attempted induction may either cause an iatrogenic premature delivery or an unnecessary cesarean section. Confirmation of dating is the most important task at this point. This is most conveniently done by review of the patient's prenatal records (Answer C), as dating is most accurately established early in the pregnancy. However, ultrasound for fetal

size and estimated GA (Answer B) may also be of value. AFI and BPP (Answer A) may be of benefit in assessing fetal status at the present time, and is therefore a possible management; however, these tests will not be of use in assessing GA.

NEED TO KNOW

Pregnancy Dating

By convention, in obstetrics, pregnancies are dated from the first day of the LMP. By this convention, obstetrical dates are 2 weeks more than the actual fetal age, as conception is assumed to have occurred 2 weeks after the last menses. This convention may have to be explained to a patient who knows exactly when her conception occurred and who questions why her GA differs by 2 weeks. Accurate dating of the pregnancy is critical for a number of reasons, including timing of testing for fetal anomalies, timing of elective delivery, and identification of patients who are either pre- or postterm. Pregnancy dating may be determined by

1. Sure knowledge of the date of conception (as for a patient undergoing assisted reproduction).
2. Ultrasound in the first trimester, or in the first half of the second trimester (Table 33.1) is accurate to within about 1 week.
3. Later ultrasound accuracy is reduced to 2 to 3 weeks.
4. "Certain" LMP may be incorrect in a significant number of cases and is used to guide treatment only in the absence of ultrasound dating. Menstrual dating alone is generally not used to guide invasive treatments, such as elective delivery.
5. A minimum GA can be inferred from the finding of a positive pregnancy test (indicating a minimum GA of 3 weeks) or auscultation of fetal heart tones with a Doppler stethoscope (minimum GA of 9 weeks). These findings do not indicate an upper limit for GA.
6. Other dating criteria are mentioned only for historic interest: early bimanual examination, auscultation of fetal heart tones by Delee stethoscope, or maternal perception of "quickening" are not currently recommended as pregnancy dating methods.

TABLE 33.1		
ACCURACY OF GESTATIONAL AGE ASSESSMENT BY VARIOUS TECHNIQUES		
Technique	**Gestational Age (wk)**	**95% CL (d)**
Fetal crown-rump length	7–11	2–3
	11–13	3–5
Multiple measurements (BPD, HC, AC, FL)	14–22	7

It will be apparent that, although the convention uses the terminology of menstrual dating, menstrual dating is not to be regarded as the most accurate or satisfactory method. In nearly every case, ultrasound dating in the first trimester will be more accurate; and consideration should be given to using ultrasound dates when available, even when the difference is relatively small. In addition, the first ultrasound fetal measurement is the most accurate, and a firm due date should be assigned early in pregnancy. This should not be changed based on additional examinations except in the rare instance when an early examination is clearly in error.

CASE CONTINUES

Ms. Jordan's partner is able to find some paperwork from her prior doctor and brings it to the hospital. By LMP, Ms. Jordan is at 42⁶/₇ weeks GA, but her documents include an ultrasound at 11 weeks consistent with 38²/₇ weeks of gestation today. Review of her other records reveals no medical, surgical, family, or social history that is contributory. You perform an ultrasound and the measurements of the fetus are consistent with a normally grown fetus at approximately 36⁵/₇ weeks of gestation with an EFW of 2,650 g. The fetus is in vertex presentation, the placenta is fundal and grade II, the AFI is 15.6 cm, and the BPP is 10/10.

Ms. Jordan is discharged home to be followed weekly in your office. She is instructed regarding fetal kick counts, and told to return to the hospital if she feels rupture of membranes, experiences contractions consistent with labor, vaginal bleeding, or any other medical problem.

Ms. Jordan follows up with you in the office. At 41²/₇ weeks of gestation by her early ultrasound, she still has not delivered. She has no signs and symptoms of labor, and a cervical examination reveals that she is long, closed, and the vertex is at −2 station. The fetus is in the vertex presentation and is 3,100 g by manual palpation. You discuss with her the risks of a postterm pregnancy.

Decision 2: Counseling

What are the risks of postterm pregnancy?

A. Stillbirth
B. Maternal laceration at delivery
C. Uterine rupture
D. Fetal anomalies

The correct answers are A and B: Stillbirth and maternal laceration at delivery. Uterine rupture (Answer C) is not specifically a risk of postterm pregnancy, and fetal anomalies (Answer D) are most likely the result of the fetal genetic complement or of exposures in the first trimester.

Continuation of the pregnancy postterm results in risks to both the fetus and mother. For the fetus, the risk of death, either pre- or postdelivery increases after 39 weeks, and increases sharply after 41 weeks of gestation (Fig. 33.1). These

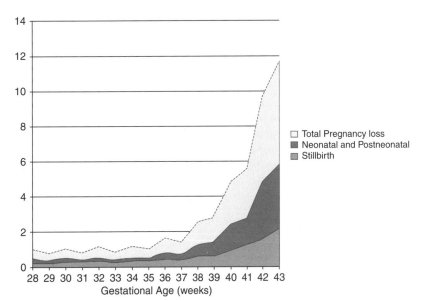

Figure 33.1 Pregnancy loss rates for deliveries at specified gestational ages. Losses are calculated compared with all ongoing pregnancies at that GA, therefore represent the risk of loss for all pregnancies achieving that gestational age. (Redrawn from Hilder L. Prolonged pregnancy: evaluating gestation-specific risks of fetal and infant mortality. BJOB. 1998;105:169–73.)

fetuses are at risk for hypoxemia at delivery, oligohydramnios, and meconium passage. In addition, the risk of fetal macrosomia increases with increasing GA, presumably due to continued fetal growth.

The mother with a postterm pregnancy incurs an increased risk of cesarean section, postpartum hemorrhage, and perineal trauma, possibly due to the relatively increased fetal size and the greater likelihood of labor induction. The increased incidence of cesarean section may be responsible for an increased incidence of infection and an increased hospital stay in these mothers.

Because of the risks to mother and baby, many practitioners will offer labor induction beginning at 41 weeks of gestation. When induction is not performed, most practitioners will follow the pregnancy with some form of fetal testing to assure fetal well-being.

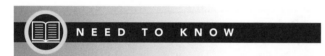

Postterm Pregnancy

The normal duration of human pregnancy is 280 days, or 10 lunar months from LMP, or 266 days of actual pregnancy. By definition, a postterm pregnancy is one extending to 42 completed weeks of gestation (or 294 days), although as noted above many practitioners will intervene in a pregnancy lasting beyond 41 weeks. In published studies, 2% to 8% of pregnancies have persisted beyond 42 weeks of gestation; accurate estimation of the naturally occurring rate is complicated both by dating inaccuracies and by the tendency to induce labor prior to 42 weeks.

Most cases of apparent postterm pregnancy are due to dating inaccuracies. Among confirmed cases, twin studies indicate that as much as 30% of postterm pregnancies are due to familial or genetic conditions. Maternal obesity, nulliparity, and male fetus are all associated with an increased risk for prolonged pregnancy. These risks are not large, however. For a maternal body mass index of ≥35, the odds ratio for postterm pregnancy was 1.5. Finally, in most mammals the timing of parturition is determined, in part, by the activation of the fetal hypothalamic/pituitary/adrenal axis and by placental steroid synthesis. In humans, fetal adrenal hypoplasia (as in anencephaly) or placental sulfatase deficiency may be associated with prolonged pregnancy.

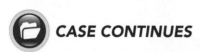

CASE CONTINUES

You offer Ms. Jordan the option of labor induction, but you acknowledge that the likelihood of a vaginal delivery is relatively low given her cervical examination. She asks

TABLE 33.2

ANTENATAL TESTING METHODS: PREDICTIVE VALUE[a]

Test	Fetal Death In Utero Within 1 Week of a Negative Test (Corrected)
NST	1.9/1,000
CST	0.3/1,000
BPP	0.8/1,000
Modified BPP (NST and AFI only)	0.8/1,000

[a]Fetal loss rates are corrected for lethal congenital anomalies and unpredictable causes of fetal death.
AFI, amniotic fluid index; BPP, biophysical profile; CST, contraction stress test; NST, nonstress test.

to wait for one more week for spontaneous labor. You agree, and initiate twice weekly modified BPP testing, with the plan to induce labor in 1 week, or earlier if the fetal status is not reassuring.

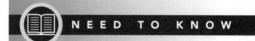

Antenatal Testing

Antenatal testing is the performance of one of a number of studies to reassure the practitioner that the fetus is unlikely to die in utero in the near future. Postterm pregnancy is one of the accepted indications for prenatal testing, although studies demonstrating a benefit of this type of testing are not available. Four testing modalities are commonly used (their relative performance is addressed in Table 33.2):

1. Nonstress test (NST). FHR is recorded in the absence of maternal contractions. A reactive (reassuring) test has two accelerations of at least 15 bpm lasting at least 15 seconds in 20 minutes (Fig. 33.2). A nonreactive test does not have two qualifying accelerations in 20 minutes in a 40-minute study. NST is easily performed and noninvasive. However, it has a high false-positive rate of nonreactive tests (up to 90% of nonreactive studies are false positives) with nonreactive tests are usually followed by another testing method, which confirms reassuring fetal status. To reduce the false-negative rate, NST is also often combined with an amniotic fluid assessment (AFI, see Chapter xx).

2. Contraction stress test (CST). FHR is recorded during maternal contractions. Contractions may be spontaneous or induced, but must total three in 10 minutes and each be ~40 seconds in duration. A negative

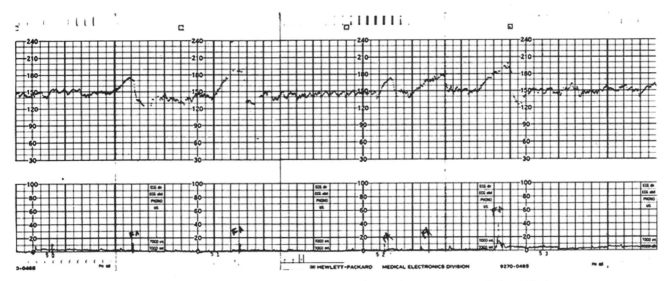

Figure 33.2 Fetal heart rate acceleration. (Adapted from Cabaniss ML, Ross MG. Fetal Monitoring Interpretation, 2nd edition. Lippincott Williams & Wilkins. 2010.)

(reassuring) test occurs when there are no late FHR decelerations (Fig. 33.3). A positive test has late decelerations following more than 50% of contractions. There is a possibility of equivocal tests, when there are fewer late decelerations, or when decelerations follow excessive contractions. In addition, the test may be unsatisfactory if sufficient contractions cannot be induced. The CST requires more time and effort to perform than does the NST. Once begun, contractions may not abate, and CST testing cannot be done in situations where uterine contractions are contraindicated, as with a placenta previa. CST is highly sensitive but has a predictive value of a positive test (PPV) of <35%.

3. BPP. The BPP is a fetal score, analogous to the Apgar newborn score, describing the fetal condition using information from the NST and fetal ultrasound. The components of the BPP are described in Table 33.3. In general, a BPP of 8 or 10 is regarded as normal. A BPP of 6 is equivocal, and a BPP of 4 or less is positive. The fetal risk associated with the different BPP scores is given in Table 33.4. The BPP is not invasive, but it does require trained staff and ultrasound equipment.

4. Modified BPP (NST and AFI). The modified BPP combines the predictive value of the BPP with much of the ease and safety of the NST. In most centers, an AFI of ≥5, plus a reactive NST constitutes a reassuring test.

In addition to the tests above, patients are often instructed in fetal movement surveillance or "kick counts." There are various protocols in use. For example, the patient is instructed to record the time taken to sense 10 fetal movements. If 10 movements are not felt in 2 hours, or if the time to "count to 10" increases dramatically, the patient is instructed to call the practitioner.

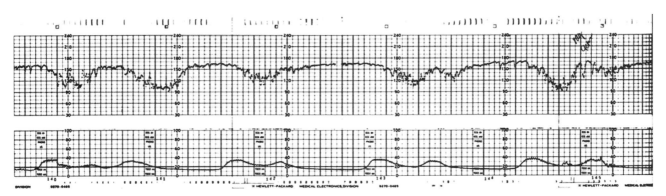

Figure 33.3 Fetal heart rate: late deceleration. The upper trace represents fetal heart rate, the lower uterine contractions. A late deceleration occurs when the nadir of the deceleration occurs after the peak of the contraction, and they usually persist after the contraction returns to baseline. (Adapted from Cabaniss ML, Ross MG. Fetal Monitoring Interpretation, 2nd edition. Lippincott Williams & Wilkins. 2010.)

TABLE 33.3

BIOPHYSICAL PROFILE: EACH ELEMENT IS GIVEN A SCORE OF "0" OR "2"

Element	Required for a Score of 2	Notes
NST	Reactive	May be omitted if remainder of the score is 8 without compromising the predictive value of the test
Amniotic fluid	Normal volume: A single pocket of at least 2 cm *or* an AFI of at least 5 cm	Many practitioners will give a score of "0" for polyhydramnios
Fetal movement	At least three discrete fetal movements in 30 min	
Fetal tone	Extension and flexion of a fetal extremity *or* opening and closing of the fetal hand	
Fetal breathing	At least one episode of fetal breathing lasting 30 sec in 30 min	

AFI, amniotic fluid index.

 CASE CONTINUES

Two days prior to the planned induction, Ms. Jordan is admitted at 42 0/7 weeks in early labor in which contractions began 5 to 6 hours earlier. She denies rupture of membranes or vaginal bleeding. She relates that the baby has been moving normally, and you note that her initial fetal testing was normal, but that she failed her last appointment. Physical examination reveals normal vital signs, a fundal height of 33 cm, an EFW of 3,100 g, and a vertex presentation. Pelvic examination reveals that the cervix is 1 to 2 cm dilated and 80% effaced with the vertex at −1 station. Ultrasound reveals a vertex presentation, marked oligohydramnios with an AFI of 2 cm, and a grade III placenta. The FHR is 150 bpm, with average variability, no accelerations are seen.

TABLE 33.4

PERINATAL MORTALITY AND THE BIOPHYSICAL PROFILE SCORE

Score	Perinatal Mortality/1,000
8–10	1.86[a]
6	9.76
4	26.3
2	94.0
0	285.7
	0.8/1,000[a] for structurally normal fetuses with a normal test within 7 d

Adapted from Manning FA, et al. Am J Obstet Gynecol. 1990;162:703. Manning FA, et al. Am J Obstet Gynecol. 1985;151:343. Manning FA, editor. Fetal Assessment: Principles and Practices. Norwalk, CT: Appleton and Lange; 1995. p. 221. http://www.iame.com/learning/bio/bio.html.

 Decision 3: Diagnosis

The likely diagnosis at this time is

A. Fetal acidosis
B. Fetal renal failure
C. Postmaturity syndrome
D. Small for GA fetus

The correct answer is C: Postmaturity syndrome. About 20% of postterm fetuses will develop the syndrome of fetal wasting with meconium passage and oligohydramnios. This syndrome is thought to be due to placental malfunction, with chronic fetal hypoxia, fetal growth restriction, and, ultimately, fetal distress. These fetuses can progress to develop meconium aspiration syndrome, pulmonary hypertension, hypoglycemia, and neurologic damage if not carefully managed. Although the fetus is likely affected, it is unlikely to be acidotic at this time (Answer A), given the normal FHR variability. The most likely cause of oligohydramnios in this case is poor urine output due to decreased renal perfusion, rather than fetal renal failure. Although fetal growth is likely impaired, the fetal size of 3,100 g is not consistent with the diagnosis of small for GA (Answer D).

 CASE CONCLUSION

After discussion with the patient describing the risks of umbilical cord compression, nonreassuring FHR tracing, and meconium aspiration, it is agreed that an attempt at vaginal delivery will be undertaken. Because of inadequate uterine activity, oxytocin augmentation is begun at 2 mU and increased per protocol. Within 2 hours the FHR demonstrates decreased variability and some late decelerations. At this time, her cervix is 2 cm dilated. Given that she appears to be remote from delivery, with a concern for her fetal status, you recommend a cesarean delivery, and she agrees. You perform a primary cesarean section and deliver a 3,050-g female infant through thick meconium with Apgar score of 6/7 at 1 and 5 minutes. The infant is initially taken to the neonatal intensive care unit for observation due to some respiratory grunting. By the second day of life, the baby is at the bedside, and on the fourth postpartum day you discharge the mother and the baby home together.

SUGGESTED READINGS

ACOG Practice Bulletin No. 9: antepartum fetal surveillance, October 1999. Int J Gynaecol Obstet. 2000;68(2):175–85. Reaffirmed 2009.

American College of Obstetricians and Gynecologists. ACOG Practice Bulletin No. 97: fetal lung maturity. Obstet Gynecol. 2008;112(3):717–26.

American College of Obstetricians and Gynecologists. ACOG Practice Bulletin No. 55: management of postterm pregnancy. Obstet Gynecol 2004;104:639. Reaffirmed 2009.

Caughey AB, Stotland NE, Washington AE, Escobar GJ. Maternal and obstetric complications of pregnancy are associated with increasing gestational age at term. Am J Obstet Gynecol. 2007; 196(2):155.e1–6.

Degani S. Fetal biometry: clinical, pathological, and technical considerations. Obstet Gynecol Surv. 2001;56(3):159–67. Review.

Hilder L, Costeloe K, Thilaganathan B. Prolonged pregnancy: evaluating gestation-specific risks of fetal and infant mortality. Br J Obstet Gynaecol. 1998;105(2):169–73.

Laursen M, Bille C, Olesen AW, Hjelmborg J, Skytthe A, Christensen K. Genetic influence on prolonged gestation: a population-based Danish twin study. Am J Obstet Gynecol. 2004;190(2):489–94.

Olesen AW, Westergaard JG, Olsen J. Prenatal risk indicators of a prolonged pregnancy. The Danish Birth Cohort 1998–2001. Acta Obstet Gynecol Scand. 2006;85(11):1338–41.

Abnormal Labor

34

Robert Eden

 CASE PRESENTATION

You arrive on labor and delivery at 8:30 following morning rounds to learn that last night at midnight, your colleague admitted Mrs. Olulu, a 30-year-old G1 P0 female at 41½ weeks, in the latent phase of labor with irregular contractions every 3 to 6 minutes. History reveals that uterine contractions had began 14 hours prior to admission. The patient states that fetal movements have been normal and that a nonstress test performed yesterday was normal. Her medical record reveals that her gestational dating is based on a first trimester ultrasound and that her pregnancy has been complicated only by maternal smoking. Her prenatal labs were within normal limits. The physical examination on admission reveals normal vital signs, fundal height of 40 cm, and an estimated fetal weight (EFW) of 3,500 g. A pelvic examination 6 hours ago revealed a 1 cm dilated cervix that was 50% effaced with the head at −2 station in the left occiput transverse (LOT) position; the cervix was moderately soft and in mid-position. Per your colleague's orders, the night duty nurse had placed misoprostol (Cytotec) 25 μg in the posterior fornix at 5:00 AM to initiate cervical ripening, with the plan to repeat the dose every 4 hours. Following a brief discussion with the patient, you perform a bedside ultrasound and confirm the vertex presentation and EFW (3,575 g) while revealing an anterior fundal placenta and normal amniotic fluid volume. The fetal heart rate (FHR) recording over 30 minutes is consistent with the 12-minute segment as shown in Figure 34.1.

On review of the FHR, you determine that the uterine activity is consistent with tachysystole, with contractions every 1 to 2 minutes, the heart rate is 150 bpm, it is reactive, with average variability and decelerations are absent. At 9:00 AM, you perform a bimanual examination of Mrs. Olulu, and find the cervix to be 2 to 3 cm dilated, 80% effaced, −1 station with a soft, anterior cervix and the fetus in the LOT position.

 Decision 1: Management

What should be your immediate management of this patient?

A. Permit the nurse to place a repeat dose of 50 μg misoprostol in the posterior fornix.
B. Cancel the misoprostol order and begin low-infusion rate oxytocin (2 mU/min) augmentation in 4 hours if the uterine activity subsides.
C. Cancel the misoprostol order and begin intrauterine resuscitation measures with intravenous (IV) fluids, positional change, and oxygen via mask.
D. Personally disconnect the monitor from the patient and take her to the operating room for emergency cesarean section.

The correct answer is B: Cancel the misoprostol order and begin low-infusion rate oxytocin (2 mU/min) augmentation in 4 hours if the uterine activity subsides. The information presented suggests that this patient now has a cervix that is favorable for labor induction, and that the fetus is tolerating the uterine contractions. Cervical ripening agents like misoprostol are used when the cervix is unfavorable for labor induction (when the cervix is relatively closed, thick and firm). The cervical examination of this patient at 8:00 AM is favorable, indicating no need for additional cervical ripening (Answer A). In addition, in the presence of tachysystole, cervical ripening agents are contraindicated and generally should not be readminstered. Tachysystole is defined as more than five contractions per 10 minutes, averaged over a 30-minute period. It may be associated with FHR changes suggestive of fetal compromise, but in the absence of these changes fetal resuscitation (Answer C) or emergent cesarean section (Answer D) is not appropriate.

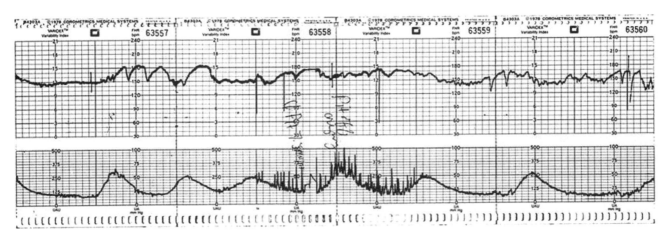

Figure 34.1 7:30 AM FHR TRACING (Bates 20860). UC: q1 to 2 minutes, tachysystole (6/10 minutes). FHR: Baseline 150 bpm, average FHR variability, No FHR decelerations, FHR accelerations (reactive). (Adapted from Cabaniss ML, Ross MG. Fetal Monitoring Interpretation, 2nd edition. Lippincott Williams & Wilkins. 2010.)

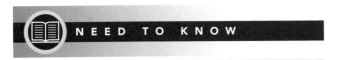

NEED TO KNOW

Labor Induction/Augmentation

Labor induction is the induction of uterine contractions artificially to promote delivery. Indications for labor induction include any condition that makes delivery of the pregnancy desirable. Common indications include postdate pregnancy, maternal medical illnesses such as preeclampsia, and fetal growth failure. No indication is absolute, and inductions may be performed for indications as serious as fetal demise and as trivial as a maternal desire to be delivered before a specific event.

In performing a labor induction, the cervix is commonly evaluated to estimate the likelihood of successful vaginal delivery. The most common method of evaluation involves a physical examination, and evaluation of the dilatation, effacement, position (anterior, posterior, or mid-position) and consistency (firm, soft, or mid-consistency) of the cervix and the station of the presenting part of the fetus. This evaluation is expressed as a number, called a Bishop score shown in Table 34.1. A Bishop score above 5 predicts successful labor induction, and is generally called a "favorable" score seen in Table 34.2. A lower Bishop score is usually addressed by attempts to "ripen" the cervix by increasing the Bishop score. Many studies indicate that, when cervical ripening is successful, the incidence of vaginal delivery is improved.

When cervical ripening is indicated, it may be affected by mechanical or pharmacologic means. Mechanical methods may include hygroscopic cervical dilators, or various balloon catheters that may be placed within the cervix. Mechanical methods may increase the risk for infection and are not used in a trial of labor induction (when the patient may be discharged undelivered) or when the amnion is ruptured. Pharmacologic methods generally include prostaglandins (dinoprostone) and prostaglandin analogues (misoprostol). Pharmacologic agents generally have the potential to induce uterine contractions and are contraindicated in a patient with a prior uterine scar or with preexisting uterine contractions. Most prostaglandins are administered vaginally, and are relatively contraindicated in the

TABLE 34.1
BISHOP SCORE

Dilation (cm)	Effacement (%)	Station	Consistency	Position	
0	Closed	0–30	−3	Firm	Posterior
1	1–2	40–50	−2	Medium	Midposition
2	3–4	60–70	−1/0	Soft	Anterior
3	≥5	≥80	+1, +2	—	—

TABLE 34.2

PREDICTION OF MODE OF DELIVERY USING THE BISHOP SCORE (NULLIPAROUS WOMEN, BISHOP SCORE ON ADMISSION FOR DELIVERY. IN THIS STUDY, SPONTANEOUS VS. INDUCED LABOR HAD NO EFFECT BEYOND THAT OF THE BISHOP SCORE)

Bishop Score	Cesarean Delivery (%)
≤5	25
6–8	13.60
≥9	6.20

TABLE 34.3

CARDINAL MOVEMENTS OF LABOR (VERTEX PRESENTATION)

1. Engagement	The biparietal diameter of the fetal head enters the true pelvis
2. Flexion	The fetal neck flexes, making the occiput the presenting part
3. Descent	The fetal head descends into the true pelvis, propelled by uterine contractions
4. Internal rotation	The fetal head rotates from occiput transverse to occiput anterior (or posterior) position to pass the ischial spines
5. Extension	The head delivers through the maternal perineum by extension around the symphysis pubis
6. External rotation	Following delivery, the fetal head returns to the original transverse position it occupied entering the pelvis
7. Expulsion	Delivery of the fetal body

context of ruptured membranes. Misoprostol, which may be administered orally, may be used with caution with ruptured fetal membranes. Protocols for cervical ripening usually involve the use of a ripening agent for 12 to 24 hours, followed by induction of labor with oxytocin. In some cases, if delivery is not urgent, failure of the cervix to ripen will lead to the patient being discharged with the plan to reinitiate induction some days later.

With a favorable cervix, or after a cervical ripening protocol, uterine contractions are induced. Although some patients may be induced simply by rupturing the amniotic membrane (amniotomy), most patients will be treated with oxytocin to provoke uterine contractions. Oxytocin is favored over prostaglandins for this indication as it can more easily be titrated to achieve the desired number of uterine contractions.

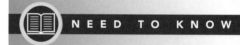

NEED TO KNOW

Latent Phase of Labor

Labor is characterized by a predictable pattern of cervical dilatation. This was originally described by Friedman in the 1950s, although recent reports suggest that the normal pattern may have changed over time as shown in Figure 34.2. Labor is traditionally divided into three stages: the first stage of labor begins with the onset of uterine contractions and ends with full cervical dilation. The first stage of labor is also divided into the latent phase and active phase of labor; the active phase begins when the cervical dilatation begins to change rapidly, usually between 4 and 6 cm. The second stage of labor begins with complete cervical dilation and ends with delivery of the fetus. The third stage of labor begins with the delivery of the fetus and ends with the delivery of the placenta. During labor, the fetus must perform the seven cardinal movements of labor as it passes through the birth canal seen in Table 34.3, and these movements correspond to the various stages of labor.

During the latent phase of labor, the cervix slowly dilates and the fetus generally performs the first two cardinal movements, if not completed prior to the onset of labor. The latent phase is extremely variable in duration, although many authors have found the latent phase to be shorter in multiparas than in nulliparas and a prolonged latent phase is generally described as a latent phase that exceeds 20 hours in a nullipara or 14 hours in a multipara. Because of difficulties in establishing the time of onset of contractions, and difficulties in

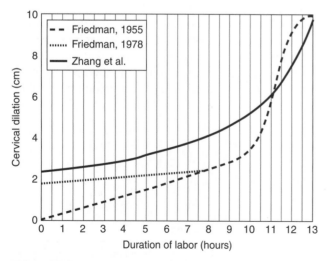

Figure 34.2 Progress of cervical dilatation over time (12388957). Friedman found that the active phase of labor began by 4 cm of dilatation, whereas Zhang, in 2002, found that cervical dilatation did not accelerate until 6 cm in their patients.

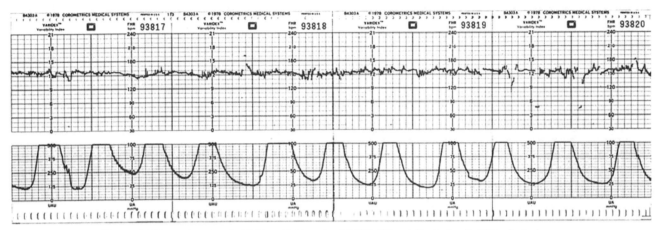

Figure 34.3 FHR tracing 2: 19:10 PM FHR tracing (20895). UC: q1–2 minutes (6–7/10 minutes), coupling (Tachysystole). FHR: 145 bpm, average variability, no FHR decelerations, no FHR accelerations. (Adapted from Cabaniss ML, Ross MG. Fetal Monitoring Interpretation, 2nd edition. Lippincott Williams & Wilkins. 2010.)

distinguishing latent phase labor from "false" labor, or Braxton–Hicks contractions the assessment of latent phase duration is quite inaccurate.

Prolongation of the latent phase of labor has often been attributed to the early use of narcotics or epidural anesthesia, although this has not been borne out in controlled trials. Retrospective data suggest that pregnancies with a prolonged latent phase of labor are characterized by an increase in cesarean delivery rates and in poor perinatal outcomes such as fetal meconium passage and the need for newborn intubation. These studies are compromised by the lack of a consistent definition of the latent phase. In a normal pregnancy, latent phase labor is generally not an indication for hospital admission or treatment. Treatment may become desirable when a gravida is so uncomfortable with contractions as to be unable to be rest, when the amnion is ruptured or when the maternal or fetal medical status is not reassuring. When treatment of the prolonged latent phase is indicated, it may consist of oxytocin stimulation of uterine activity or maternal sedation ("therapeutic rest"). Augmentation with oxytocin accelerates the progress of the latent phase of labor in many patients, especially those with favorable cervices. The alternate approach of "therapeutic rest" (maternal sedation) may allow the mother to be better prepared to cope with the physical and emotional demands of active labor and may allow identification of those who are not in true labor. The choice between uterine stimulation and therapeutic rest depends on the clinical situation. Either intervention has been reported to have an 85% success rate in terms of advancement to active labor.

 SUBSEQUENT CLINICAL COURSE

Thirty minutes after your initial examination, the patient grossly ruptures her membranes and contractions became more regular. At 11:00, the patient is 6 cm/100%/−1 station (LOT). Several hours later, at 14:00, the patient requests an epidural; you perform a pelvic examination, and her cervix is 8/100%/0 station (LOT). The FHR tracing is presented as shown in Figure 34.3, tachysystole is again present.

The oxytocin infusion is decreased while the patient is prepared for an epidural. Following the epidural, the oxytocin is restarted and increased per protocol to 16 mU/min. At 16:00, you are called to the bedside as the nurse is having difficulty in monitoring the contractions. You check the patient's cervix; the examination is anterior lip/100% effaced, 0 to +1 station (LOT). You attach a fetal scalp electrode and insert an intrauterine pressure catheter (IUPC) to evaluate uterine contractions. The FHR at this time is presented shown in Figure 34.4.

 Decision 2: Management

What is your management of the patient at this time?

A. Continue the oxytocin infusion rate at 16 mU/hr. Increase the oxytocin infusion rate to 18 mU/hr.
B. Stop the infusion of oxytocin and begin intrauterine resuscitation by maternal position.
C. Change, increased IV fluids, and oxygen by mask while observing the FHR.
D. Transfer to operating room for immediate cesarean section.

The correct answer is B: Stop the infusion of oxytocin and begin intrauterine resuscitation by maternal position. The presence of uterine tachysystole in the presence of repetitive FHR decelerations with slow return to FHR baseline requires a response on the part of the physician. The FHR pattern is classed as type II, meaning that the fetal acid–base status is uncertain due to the presence of repetitive decelerations with

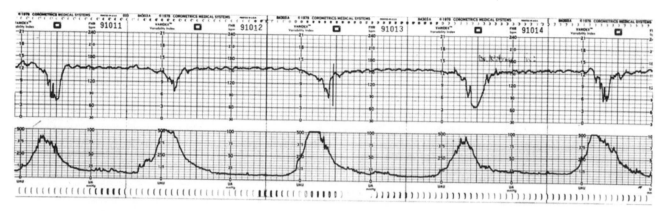

Figure 34.4 FHR tracing 3: 16:00 (Bates 20815). UC: 6/10 minutes. FHR: 150 bpm, average FHR variability, variable FHR decelerations with slow return to baseline, no FHR accelerations. (Adapted from Cabaniss ML, Ross MG. Fetal Monitoring Interpretation, 2nd edition. Lippincott Williams & Wilkins. 2010.)

average variability. In the face of this uncertainty and the presence of greater than normal uterine activity, prudent care might include the discontinuation of oxytocin and the institution of intrauterine resuscitation including maternal position change, IV fluids, and oxygen by mask. Persistence of uterine tachysystole may contribute to the likelihood of developing fetal metabolic acidosis and asphyxia because there is inadequate time for uterine–placental perfusion between contractions. When clinically indicated, uterine tachysystole in the active phase of labor can be treated with removal or reduction in uterotonic agents, or with the use of tocolytics such as magnesium sulfate or terbutaline.

Continuing or increasing the oxytocin infusion (Answers A and C) is inappropriate in this case as the patient already has an excessive number of uterine contractions, in addition to a poor fetal response to contractions. Immediate cesarean delivery (Answer D) is not appropriate with this presentation, especially prior to an attempt of intrauterine resuscitation.

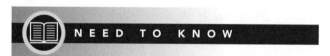

Active Phase of Labor/Second Stage of Labor

The active phase of labor begins when the cervix begins to rapidly dilate, usually between 4 and 6 cm of dilatation, and ends with complete cervical dilation. The second stage extends from complete dilatation to expulsion of the fetus. During the active phase, the fetus performs the third and fourth cardinal movements of labor, namely descent and internal rotation; the remainder of the cardinal movements is performed in the second stage. The expected minimum rate of cervical dilation for nulliparas in the active phase of labor is 1.0 cm/hr; for multiparas, it is 1.2 cm/hr. For descent of the fetal head in the second stage, the minimum rate for nulliparas is 1.0 cm/hr; for multiparas it is 2.0 cm/hr or more. These

criteria for minimal rates of cervical change and descent represent the 95th percentiles, based on Friedman's data, although several recent studies indicate that slower rates of cervical dilation and head descent are generally well tolerated in the presence of normal fetal heart tracings.

Prolongation of the active phase of labor may be due to slow progress (a protraction disorder) or to a lack of progress (an arrest disorder). Protraction disorders of the active phase of labor are usually associated with cephalopelvic disproportion (CPD), use of conduction anesthesia (epidural), and fetal malposition (asynclitism). Oxytocin augmentation may or may not improve the rate of cervical change. Recent evidence suggests that there are significant differences in collagen content and collagen remodeling of the cervix and lower uterine segment in patients with protracted active phase of labor when compared with normal labors possibly explaining why there may be an inadequate response to oxytocin augmentation. With continued progress in labor and acceptable fetal condition, protraction disorders can be managed expectantly.

Arrest disorders of the active phase of labor are characterized by the cessation of either cervical dilation or descent of the fetal head for longer than 2 hours. Before the arrest of progress the rate of cervical dilation or descent of the fetal head is normal. Arrest of progress can also complicate a protraction disorder. Approximately half of the cases are associated with CPD and may ultimately require cesarean section. Recent studies demonstrate that lack of progress up to 6 hours is not associated with fetal or neonatal morbidity and mortality provided the fetus is carefully monitored. Protocols for treating arrest disorders often include achieving a uterine contraction pattern of >200 Montevideo units measured by IUPC. Montevideo units are calculated as the increase in uterine pressure over baseline for each contraction, summed over a 10-minute period. Usually, a minimum of 2 to 4 hours of labor with a contraction pattern of

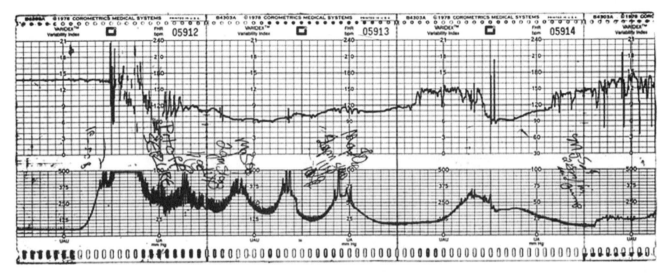

Figure 34.5 FHR tracing (20842) 3:50 AM. UC: Before dislodging of intrauterine pressure catheter (IUPC), pushing efforts q 1–2 minutes, then IUP dislodged. FHR: Salutatory FHR variability, prolonged FHR deceleration. (Adapted from Cabaniss ML, Ross MG. Fetal Monitoring Interpretation, 2nd edition. Lippincott Williams & Wilkins. 2010.)

>200 Montevideo units is observed before proceeding to cesarean delivery for active phase arrest in the presence of normal FHR. For patients who cannot achieve a sustained uterine contraction pattern of >200 Montevideo units, a minimum of 6 hours of oxytocin augmentation is observed before proceeding to cesarean delivery.

 SUBSEQUENT CLINICAL COURSE

At 17:00, you recheck the cervix and found that Mrs. Olulu fully dilated, 100% effaced, and LOA (left occiput anterior) at +1 station. The FHR baseline is 150 bpm, the tracing is devoid of FHR decelerations, FHR variability is normal, and FHR accelerations are present. Uterine contractions are occurring every 5 minutes. Mrs. Olulu has no urge to push since the epidural is providing effective pain relief.

By 19:00, the epidural has worn off and the patient begins pushing. At 21:00, you are called to the bedside to review the FHR tracing shown in Figure 34.5. As you examine the patient, the IUPC becomes dislodged. The cervix is C/100%/+1–2 with caput, LOA, and no descent with maternal pushing efforts. The labor curve is depicted in Figure 34.6.

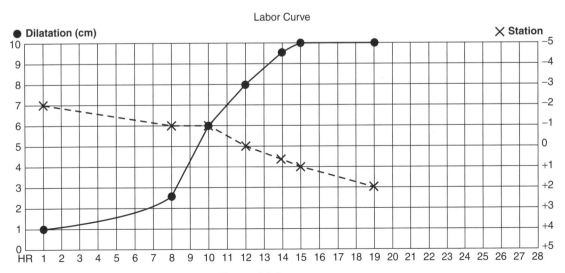

Figure 34.6 Labor curve.

Decision 3: Management

The management of this patient at this time should be?

A. Immediate discontinuation of the oxytocin induction and 0.25 mg subcutaneous terbutaline injection
B. Stop all maternal pushing efforts
C. Intrauterine resuscitation including positional change, IV fluids and oxygen by mask
D. All of the above

The answer is D: All of the above. In the presence of repetitive prolonged decelerations, the goal is to allow intrauterine resuscitation by removing the stressors on the fetus. To this end, all maternal pushing efforts are stopped, uterine contractions are abated by discontinuing the oxytocin infusion and injecting terbutaline, and intrauterine resuscitation is begun with fluids and oxygen. When there are no serious FHR abnormalities, if the mother is stable and there is some progress in descent or rotation of the fetal head, there is no need to hasten delivery. However, following the initiation of intrauterine resuscitation, if the FHR baseline rate and variability do not return to normal, operative intervention should be strongly considered.

CASE CONCLUSION

Despite your attempts at intrauterine resuscitation, the FHR abnormalities continue. You elect to proceed with cesarean delivery, as you do not believe that the head is low enough for forceps delivery. At cesarean, you deliver a 3,580-g female infant with Apgar score of 7/9 at 1 and 5 minutes. Mrs. Olulu does well postoperatively, and you discharge her home on postoperative day 4 with her baby.

SUGGESTED READINGS

Arthur P, Taggart MJ, Mitchell BF. Oxytocin and parturition: a role for increased myometrial calcium and calcium sensitization? Front Biosci. 2007;12:619–33.

Baacke KA, Edwards RK, Preinduction cervical assessment. Clin Obstet Gynecol. 2006;49(3):564–72.

Cardozo LD, Gibb DM, Studd JW, Vasant RV, Cooper DJ. Predictive value of cervimetric labour patterns in primigravidae. Br J Obstet Gynaecol. 1982;89(1):33–8.

Chelmow D, Kilpatrick SJ, Laros RK Jr. Maternal and neonatal outcomes after prolonged latent phase. Obstet Gynecol. 1993;81(4):486–91.

Gharoro EP, Enabudoso EJ. Labour management: an appraisal of the role of false labour and latent phase on the delivery mode. Obstet Gynecol Clin North Am. 2005;32(2):145–64, vii.

Liao JB, Buhimschi CS, Norwitz ER. Normal labor: mechanism and duration. J Obstet Gynaecol. 2006;26(6):534–7.

Ness A, Goldberg J, Berghella V. Abnormalities of the first and second stages of labor. Obstet Gynecol Clin North Am. 2005;32(2):201–20, viii.

Wang F, Shen X, Guo X, Peng Y, Gu X; The Labor Analgesia Examining Group (LAEG). Epidural analgesia in the latent phase of labor and the risk of cesarean delivery: a five-year randomized controlled trial. Anesthesiology. 2009. [Epub ahead of print].

Wong CA, McCarthy RJ, Sullivan JT, Scavone BM, Gerber SE, Yaghmour EA. Early compared with late neuraxial analgesia in nulliparous labor induction: a randomized controlled trial. Obstet Gynecol. 2009;113(5):1066–74.

Shoulder Dystocia

35

Sherri Jackson   Siegfried Rotmensch

CASE PRESENTATION

While taking in-house call at a busy Women and Children's Hospital, you are informed by a labor and delivery nurse that Mrs. Jackson, one of your private patients, is being admitted in active labor. You recall her pregnancy course thus far: She is a 35-year-old African-American woman G3 P2002 (gravid three, with two preterm deliveries and two living children), who is 1 week past her due date. She has had a relatively uncomplicated prenatal course except for an abnormal 1-hour glucose challenge test of 167 mg/dL, followed by a normal 3-hour glucose tolerance test (80, 195, 130, and 95 mg/dL for fasting, 1-hour, 2-hour, and 3-hour values, respectively) with one abnormal value out of four. She is 5 foot 5 inches tall and weighs 192 lbs.

Her prenatal chart is reviewed and reveals that you have attended her previous two deliveries. Her first son weighed 3,900 g and was delivered vaginally without complications. Her second son delivered vaginally with a birth weight of 4,200 g. Neither delivery was accompanied by shoulder dystocia nor fetal bone fractures. In the last interpregnancy interval, she has gained 30 lb but has had no other health problems.

On physical examination her cervix is 5 cm dilated and 75% effaced, and the fetal vertex is at 0 station. During this examination, you find her pubic arch to be wide with nonprominent and widely spaced ischial spines, and you cannot reach the sacral promontory with your fingertips. Your clinical estimate of fetal weight by manual palpation of the uterus is approximately 4,300 g. You share this finding with the patient, who also believes that this baby will be bigger than her last two. Fetal heart rate monitoring shows a baseline of 135 bpm, moderate variability, multiple accelerations, and no decelerations. Spontaneous uterine contractions are occurring every 3 minutes and lasting around 1 minute. The remainder of Mrs. Jackson's physical examination and her vital signs are within normal limits. She is then moved to a labor room for expectant labor management.

Decision 1: Diagnosis

What is the most widely accepted definition of macrosomia?

- **A.** Birth weight of 4,000 g
- **B.** Birth weight of 4,250 g
- **C.** Birth weight of 4,500 g
- **D.** Birth weight of 5,000 g

The correct answer is C: 4,500 g. Although macrosomia is not formally defined, the American Congress of Obstetricians and Gynecologists (ACOG) guidelines support a weight of 4,500 g in a nondiabetic pregnancy as macrosomia, since fetal and maternal morbidity increase sharply at this fetal weight. However, ACOG does not recommend changing pregnancy management due to the diagnosis of macrosomia. The point at which the fetal weight estimate should alter clinical management is controversial, especially as fetal weight estimates may be unreliable in this weight range and there is little evidence to suggest that management alterations improve outcomes.

NEED TO KNOW

Fetal Weight Estimation

There are multiple modalities to estimate fetal weight. Surprisingly, manual assessment of fetal weight by abdominal palpation was shown to be as least as accurate as ultrasound in the term fetus, although sonographic fetal biometry is also a useful method for fetal weight estimation. Ultrasound fetal weight estimation may be especially helpful in the patient with obesity in whom manual palpation is more difficult, although ultrasound measurements also may be limited under these conditions. It should be remembered that ultrasound weight estimation is calculated from the two-dimensional fetal biometry. A variety of protocols have been proposed, although methods that use three or four fetal measurements have been shown to have lower random and systematic error compared with methods using two measurements. The error of ultrasound measurement is a percentage of the total estimated weight. Generally speaking, the error in sonographic estimation of fetal weight is <10% in 80% of the cases, up to 20% in 90% of the cases, and it exceeds 20% of the actual birth weight in 10% of cases. Therefore, as the birth weight exceeds 4,000 g the estimation error may exceed a pound or more. Practitioners may use a combination of sonographic and clinical weight estimates for clinical decisions. Finally, as demonstrated by simple clinical studies, expectant mothers who have delivered previously have a fairly accurate sense of whether the current fetus is larger or smaller than their previous one. Therefore, an astute clinician may take into account all relevant information in estimating the fetal weight, including the mother's assessment.

Decision 2: Management

Your management plan at this point may include all of the following, except:

A. Close monitoring of labor progress
B. Discussion with nursing staff about the possibility of a shoulder dystocia
C. Discussion with pediatric staff about the possibility of a shoulder dystocia
D. Immediate cesarean delivery

The correct answer is D: Immediate cesarean section. Since your examination revealed a normal gynecoid pelvis, and the estimated weight is 4,300 g, there is no clear-cut indication for an abdominal delivery. ACOG guidelines recommend that elective cesarean delivery be offered only for an estimated fetal weight above 5,000 g (in a nondiabetic pregnancy), although many physicians would consider offering a nondiabetic patient with an estimated fetal weight above 4,500 g, an elective cesarean section due to the potential risk of shoulder dystocia.

Shoulder dystocia is the impaction of the bisacromial diameter (shoulders) of the fetus against the symphysis pubis anteriorly and the sacral promontory posteriorly after delivery of the fetal head. Shoulder dystocia occurs in 0.24% to 2% of deliveries, although the precise percentage is considerably in doubt. The diagnosis of "shoulder dystocia" is made when there is difficulty in delivering the fetal shoulders. Since the degree of difficulty is subjective, some investigators have attempted to objectify the diagnosis, by providing clinically relevant and measurable criteria. One common diagnostic criterion is a head-to-body delivery time of >60 seconds, or the use of additional maneuvers to effect delivery of the fetal body.

You consider that Mrs. Jackson may be at increased risk for shoulder dystocia due to her estimated fetal weight of 4,300 g, her borderline glucose tolerance, her obesity and weight gain, and her ethnicity. Since you and your patient have decided to proceed with a vaginal delivery, it is important to be prepared for the risk of a shoulder dystocia. A multidisciplinary team should be available, so that if action is required, it may be initiated without delay. At the time of delivery, it would be desirable to have the following team available, if not in the room: nurses to help with maneuvers and keep time, an anesthesiologist, a pediatric resuscitation team, and, if available, a second obstetrician.

NEED TO KNOW

Risk Factors for Birth Injury and Shoulder Dystocia

Many risk factors have been statistically linked with the occurrence of birth trauma and shoulder dystocia including macrosomia, diabetes, operative vaginal delivery (particularly mid-pelvic instrumentation), protracted labor, postterm pregnancy, male fetal gender, maternal obesity, increased maternal weight gain, advanced maternal age, prolonged second stage of labor, and African-American ethnicity. The dilemma for the clinician, however, is that accurate prediction of shoulder dystocia is not possible. More than 50% of pregnancies complicated by shoulder dystocia have no identifiable antepartum risk factor, making the predictive value of the above-mentioned factors quite low. The single most predictive risk factor is a history of a prior shoulder dystocia, although maternal diabetes and presumed fetal macrosomia also have relatively high predictive value. Maternal hyperglycemia has been shown to cause fetal hyperglycemia, which, in turn, leads to fetal hyperinsulinemia. As insulin is a growth hormone, excessive fetal growth may result. However, since brain size is only minimally affected by insulin, infants of diabetic mothers have larger than usual chest-to-head and shoulder-to-head ratios, which predispose them to shoulder dystocia, even at lower birth weights.

CASE CONTINUES

You are called for the delivery 6 hours after admission, and 1 hour after the second stage of labor began. You gown and glove and take your place at the perineum. Palpation of the fetal vertex reveals a right occiput anterior (ROA) position. Your team is in the room, as planned. After a few more minutes of pushing, the fetal head delivers slowly and is then "drawn back" tightly against the maternal perineal body. This has been described as the "turtle sign." You suspect shoulder dystocia. Indeed, the usual downward traction on the fetal head fails to deliver the anterior shoulder.

 Decision 3: Management

Which action should be initiated first in attempting to deliver a shoulder dystocia?

A. Apply additional traction, since the shoulder might dislodge with somewhat increased traction force.
B. Wood's screw maneuver
C. Perform the McRoberts maneuver, and apply suprapubic pressure.
D. Apply suprapubic pressure.

The correct answer is C: Perform the McRoberts maneuver, and apply suprapubic pressure. Shoulder dystocia is a true obstetric emergency. At this point, your manual skills and ability to function under stress will be tested. In most fetuses, delivery of the fetal head implies that the fetal abdomen and umbilical cord have entered the pelvic canal, and fetal circulation to the placenta has stopped. The fetus will get no additional oxygen until the chest is delivered, allowing expansion of the lungs.

Answer A describes additional traction. Exaggerated traction forces can injure the brachial plexus and cause Erb's palsy (affecting spinal roots C_5 through C_7) or Klumpke's palsy (affecting spinal nerves C_8 through T_1). Increased traction, however, is not helpful in dislodging the impacted anterior shoulder. Answer B, the Wood's screw maneuver, will be discussed shortly, but is generally not considered the first measure to be used, although there is no strong evidence to guide the sequence of measures to be taken in this obstetric emergency. Answer D, suprapubic pressure may be attempted alone, but most often is used in conjunction with the McRoberts maneuver.

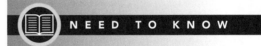 **NEED TO KNOW**

Maneuvers for Shoulder Dystocia

In managing a shoulder dystocia, clinicians usually begin with the least invasive maneuvers, with the lowest rate of complications. The McRoberts' maneuver refers to hyperflexing the maternal thighs against the maternal abdomen (Fig. 35.1) and is intended to straighten the sacrum relative to the lumbar spine (Fig. 35.2). This

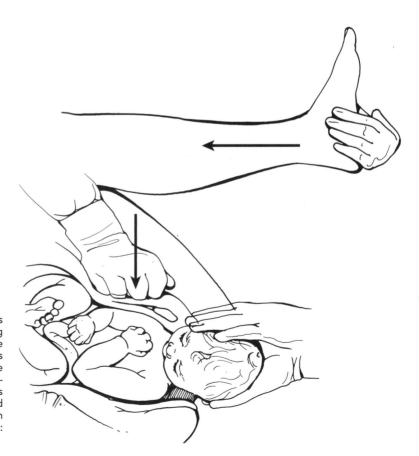

Figure 35.1 McRoberts' maneuver. The mother's thighs are flexed onto her abdomen, straightening her sacrum, and increasing the pelvic diameter for the fetal shoulder. In the illustration, the assistant is also providing suprapubic pressure to dislodge the fetal shoulder from behind the pubic symphysis. Approximately 50% of shoulder dystocias are relieved by these two maneuvers. (Adapted from Baxley EG, Gobbo RW. Shoulder dystocia. Am Fam Physician. 2004;69(7):1707–14. PubMed PMID: 15086043.)

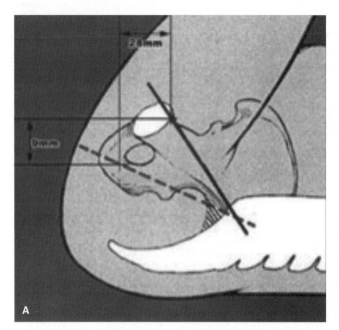
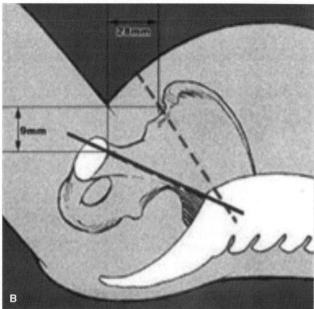

Figure 35.2 Change of the pelvic geometry with McRoberts maneuver. **A:** Maternal pelvis after McRoberts maneuver **B:** Maternal pelvis in standard lithotomy position. (Adapted from Poggi SH, Spong CY, Allen RH. Prioritizing posterior arm delivery during severe shoulder dystocia. Obstet Gynecol. 2003;101(5 Part 2):1068–72.)

position may allow the pubic bone to rotate cephalad and thereby slip over the fetal shoulder. The maneuver is often combined with suprapubic pressure, (Rubin I maneuver, shown in Figure 35.1), exerted by an assistant, attempting to enhance the downward movement of the anterior shoulder. If possible, suprapubic pressure should be exerted from a location slightly lateral to the midline, to facilitate the adduction of the shoulders and rotation of the shoulder from its impacted position behind the pubic bone. Therefore, in the present case, suprapubic pressure should be applied from the maternal right to adduct the infant's shoulders, since the fetal head is in the ROA position.

If the McRoberts maneuver is unsuccessful in relieving the shoulder dystocia, cutting a wide episiotomy may be somewhat helpful in creating more room posteriorly; however, it is unlikely that an episiotomy will extend far enough up the vagina to allow the anterior shoulder to "drop" below the pubic arch. An episiotomy also may be needed to place a hand in the vagina and to perform any of the following maneuvers. At the same time, consideration should be given to anesthesia. In the patient without a regional anesthetic, general anesthesia may be required for some of the internal maneuvers. In addition, in some cases, maternal muscle relaxation is the key to releasing the fetal shoulder.

After the McRoberts maneuver has been tried, maneuvers to relieve shoulder dystocia involve direct manipulation of the fetus. In fact, some have argued that these maneuvers should be the primary means of approaching shoulder dystocia. The two types of fetal rotational maneuvers and the delivery of the posterior arm are all known by their eponyms. The Wood's screw maneuver involves applying pressure with the fingers to the anterior surface (or clavicular surface) of the posterior shoulder, attempting to turn the fetus until the anterior shoulder is displaced from beneath the pubic bone. Rotational pressure can be simultaneously applied with the second hand to the posterior aspect of the anterior shoulder. This maneuver uses the relatively fixed dimensions of the bisacromial diameter as a lever to turn the entire fetus like a screw. The Rubin II maneuver consists of applying pressure with your hand to the posterior surface of the most accessible part of the fetal shoulder (anterior or posterior) to cause shoulder adduction, thus decreasing the bisacromial diameter and turning the shoulders into the oblique position as shown in Figure 35.3. Another maneuver to use either before or after the rotational maneuvers is the delivery of the posterior arm shown in Figure 35.4. This is best accomplished with adequate analgesia and involves insertion of the attendants' hand into the posterior vagina, reaching

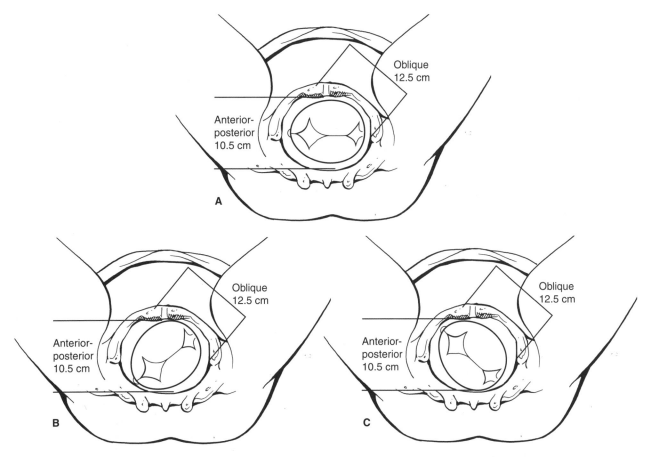

Figure 35.3 Rubin maneuver. Panel **A** shows the fetal shoulders in the direct AP, with shoulder dystocia in a gynecoid pelvis. After an anterior (panel **B**) or posterior (panel **C**) Rubin maneuver, the shoulders have been rotated into the larger oblique diameter of the pelvis and can be delivered. (Adapted from Gurewitsch ED, Kim EJ, Yang JH, Outland KE, McDonald MK, Allen RH. Comparing McRoberts' and Rubin's maneuvers for initial management of shoulder dystocia: an objective evaluation. Am J Obstet Gynecol. 2005;192(1):153–60.)

for the fetal humerus. Pressure is then applied to the antecubital fossa to flex the fetal forearm. The flexed forearm is then swept over the fetal chest and delivered. In some cases, it is necessary to turn the fetus over and repeat the delivery of the posterior arm on the second arm. It is usual to attempt all of these maneuvers more than once before going on to the more aggressive maneuvers below. In particular, previously unsuccessful maneuvers may become successful after maternal anesthesia and muscle relaxation.

The three preceding maneuvers may involve some risk of fetal injury, but they are typically expected to result in delivery of an uninjured fetus if used with caution. If delivery of the fetal shoulders still cannot be achieved, it may become necessary to use techniques with a higher risk of fetal injury. First, an attempt can be made to deliver the posterior shoulder by pulling the shoulder out of the birth canal with two fingers placed

in the fetal axilla (Fig. 35.5). This is associated with an increased chance of injuring the brachial plexus. However, in an emergent situation, the risk may be justified.

Intentional fetal clavicular fracture may be attempted by hooking the index finger beneath the clavicle and pushing the bone upwards away from the fetal chest (toward the operator). This is technically difficult to perform.

Although rarely performed in modern medicine, symphysiotomy should be mentioned for the sake of completeness. This refers to intentional splitting of the symphysis pubis with a scalpel.

Truly a measure of last resort is the Zavanelli maneuver. This requires flexing the fetal head and pushing it back into the uterine cavity for delivery by cesarean section. An attempt should be made to reverse the cardinal movements of the fetal head during delivery. This maneuver is difficult to perform, and tocolysis will be

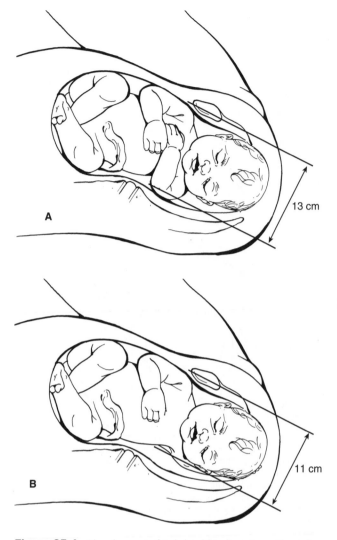

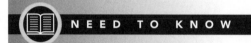

Figure 35.4 The change in fetal shoulder diameter with performance of the Barnum maneuver (delivery of the posterior arm). In panel **A,** the bisacromial diameter is 13 cm. In panel **B,** after delivery of the posterior arm the remaining diameter is 11 cm. (Adapted from Poggi SH, Spong CY, Allen RH. Prioritizing posterior arm delivery during severe shoulder dystocia. Obstet Gynecol 2003; 101(5 Part 2):1068–72.)

required since the uterus is firmly contracted behind the partially delivered fetus. The maneuver may cause fetal injury, including spinal cord transection, and may cause fetal death or uterine rupture. There are many reports of fetal harm caused by this maneuver, and the chance of harm may exceed the chance of a successful outcome.

Finally, there are some maneuvers that should never be attempted. Fundal pressure generally should not be applied, as it may further impact the fetal shoulder and may cause uterine rupture. An exception to this policy would be in circumstances in which maternal pushing is ineffective. Nuchal cords should not be clamped and cut as they may provide some blood circulation during the dystocia or if the Zavanelli maneuver must be performed.

NEED TO KNOW

Risks of Fetal Injury During Shoulder Dystocia

As previously described, the most frequent injuries during shoulder dystocia are brachial plexus injuries. Others include clavicular or humeral fractures, and rarely, hypoxic injury and fetal death. Most brachial plexus injuries are due to damage to spinal nerve roots C_5 through C_7 leading to Erb's palsy, in which the affected arm is pronated, internally rotated, and extended, known classically as the "waiter's tip" position. The majority of brachial plexus injuries resolve with conservative therapy, but up to 20% may have some residual deficit. It is also important to note that brachial plexus injuries have occurred in normal vaginal deliveries without dystocia and even in cesarean sections. Clavicular and humeral fractures usually resolve spontaneously with conservative management.

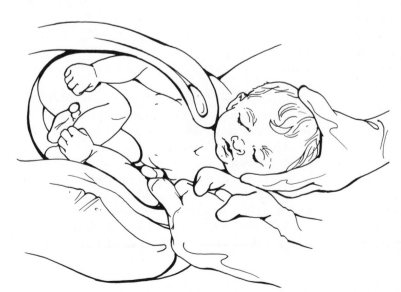

Figure 35.5 Delivery of the posterior shoulder (modified Barnum procedure). The operator's finger is used to hook the fetal axilla and pull the shoulder out of the birth canal. This procedure has a high likelihood of causing injury and should be used only when other measures have been unsuccessful. (Adapted from Menticoglou SM. A modified technique to deliver the posterior arm in severe shoulder dystocia. Obstet Gynecol. 2006; 108(3 Part 2):755–7.)

Maternal risks with shoulder dystocia include hemorrhage and third- or fourth-degree lacerations in addition to minor trauma. Less common complications include symphyseal separation and femoral neuropathy often due to prolonged adoption of McRoberts' position.

 CASE CONTINUES

Upon recognition of the "turtle sign" you call for help from pediatrics, anesthesia, and the obstetrics team. You instruct Mrs. Jackson to stop pushing until you tell her to do so. The nurses immediately put her in the McRoberts position and begin suprapubic pressure. Continued traction is unsuccessful in delivery of the infant. You attempt a Rubin II maneuver to adduct the shoulders, followed by a Wood's screw without success. At this point, a nurse in the room tells you that it has been 3 minutes since head delivery. After an episiotomy is cut, you are able to reach in, flex the infant's posterior right arm, and deliver it. Immediately after delivery of the posterior arm, the infant delivers and is pale and limp in your arms. You clamp and cut the cord and hand the infant off to the waiting pediatrics team. While delivering the placenta you can hear crying from the infant warmer. Apgar score given to the infant are 2 at 1 minute and 6 at 5 minutes.

 Decision 4: Counseling

What is this mother's risk of a shoulder dystocia in the next delivery?

A. <25%
B. 25% to 50%
C. 50% to 75%
D. 75% to 100%

The correct answer is A: <25%. The recurrence risk for shoulder dystocia ranges from 1% to 16.7%. The risk of a repeat shoulder dystocia has been reported to be 10 times that in the general population. Although cesarean delivery in a subsequent pregnancy is not mandatory, any decision on the route of delivery in a future pregnancy should take into account the fetal estimated weight relative to weight of the "index" fetus, presence or absence of maternal diabetes, gestational age, maternal anxiety, and the extent of previous fetal injuries. The patient should be involved in the decision regarding route of delivery, and should make an informed choice regarding delivery, once these topics are addressed.

 CASE CONCLUSION

On postpartum day 2 you stop in to say goodbye before Mrs. Jackson is discharged home. You hold her newest son who is crying and moving all extremities, and she thanks you for delivering him to her safely.

SUGGESTED READINGS

ACOG Practice Bulletin No 22, November 2000, Reaffirmed 2008. Fetal Macrosomia.
ACOG Practice Bulletin No 40, November 2002, Reaffirmed 2008. Shoulder Dystocia.
Beall MH, Spong C, McKay J, Ross M. Objective definition of shoulder dystocia: a prospective evaluation. Am J Obstet Gynecol. 1998; 179(4):934–7.
Chauhan SP, Luttone PM, Bailey KJ, Guerieri JP, Morrison JC. Intrapartum clinical, sonographic, and parous patients' estimates of newborn birth weight. Obstet Gynecol. 1992;79(6):956–8.
Dildy GA, Clark SL. Shoulder dystocia: risk identification. Clin Obstet Gynecol. 2000;43(2):265–82.
Gottlieb AG, Galan HL. Shoulder dystocia: an update. Obstet Gynecol Clin N Am. 2007;34(3):501–31, xii.
Gurewitsch ED, Kim EJ, Yang JH, Outland KE, McDonald MK, Allen RH. Comparing McRoberts' and Rubin's maneuvers for initial management of shoulder dystocia: an objective evaluation. Am J Obstet Gynecol. 2005;192(1):153–60.
Hendrix NW, Grady CS, Chauhan SP. Clinical vs. sonographic estimate of birth weight in term parturients. A randomized clinical trial. J Reprod Med. 2000;45(4):317–22.
Irion O, Boulvain M. Induction of labour for suspected fetal macrosomia. Cochrane Database Syst Rev. 2000;(2):CD000938.
McFarland MB, Trylovich CG, Langer O. Anthropometric differences in macrosomic infants of diabetic and nondiabetic mothers. J Matern Fetal Med. 1998;7(6):292–5.
Ouzounian JG, Gherman RB. Shoulder dystocia: are historic risk factors reliable predictors? Am J Obstet Gynecol. 2005;192(6):1933–8.

Postpartum Hemorrhage

36

Diana S. Wolfe

 CASE PRESENTATION

Ms. Kent, a 34-year-old G8 P6026 with an intrauterine pregnancy at 39 weeks of gestation arrives to labor and delivery in active labor. Her prenatal records are available, and you ascertain that she has had no complications in the present pregnancy. She has a history of asthma, but no other significant medical problems. Her previous pregnancies included six vaginal deliveries and two first trimester spontaneous abortions that required dilation and curettage. She reports that she had to be given a blood transfusion after two of her deliveries because she bled more than normal; the records in her chart report that she had a postpartum hemorrhage (PPH). Her largest baby weighed 4,600 g, but she reports that this baby does not feel as large. Her hemoglobin is 12 g/dL and blood type is O positive. Her sterile vaginal examination is reported as 4 cm dilated/80% effaced/fetal head at −2 station.

 NEED TO KNOW

What is a Postpartum Hemorrhage?

A PPH is defined (in the United States) as a blood loss of ≥500 mL after a vaginal delivery and ≥1,000 mL after a cesarean delivery. This definition is problematic for a number of reasons: In the absence of special techniques, the estimation of blood loss at delivery is inaccurate, and when these techniques are used, the normal blood loss at delivery is close to the values proposed to define hemorrhage (Table 36.1). In the United States, about 3% of deliveries are complicated by PPH as reported by diagnosis coding (Fig. 36.1), suggesting that a more stringent criterion is used in clinical practice; however, this criterion has not been codified.

PPH can be either immediate or delayed; the American Congress of Obstetricians and Gynecologists (ACOG) categorizes an immediate PPH as "primary," and defines it as a hemorrhage occurring in the first 24 hours after delivery. A "secondary" or delayed PPH occurs more than 24 hours after delivery. The major source of bleeding in PPH is the uterus, with uterine atony the most common etiology. During pregnancy, the placenta is perfused via spiral arteries that penetrate the myometrium. After delivery of the placenta, uterine contraction normally constricts these arteries and limits blood loss. If the uterus fails to contract, blood loss may be profuse. Other uterine etiologies for primary PPH include a partial placental separation, especially with a placenta previa, a uterine rupture or inversion, placenta accrete, or a coagulopathy. Following cesarean section, uterine lacerations or inadequate hemostasis at the incision site may contribute. Although less common, cervical or vaginal lacerations may be etiologic. Secondary PPH is more likely to be due to uterine infection or retained products of conception. Secondary PPH may also be the first indication of maternal Von Willibrand's disease or other maternal coagulopathies.

PPH is the leading cause of maternal death in developing countries, where women may deliver without access to medications and banked blood. PPH remains an important cause of preventable maternal mortality in developed countries, often associated with delays in treatment. Fatal PPH is most likely to be due to uterine bleeding, as opposed to genital lacerations, a result of the amount of blood flow to the term pregnant uterus (~600 mL/min).

? **Decision 1:** Risk assessment

What risk factors does this patient have for a PPH?

- **A.** Maternal asthma history
- **B.** History of prior PPH
- **C.** History of prior macrosomic fetus
- **D.** History of prior spontaneous abortions

The correct answer is B: a history of a prior PPH. Women with a prior PPH have an increased risk of PPH in a subsequent pregnancy, even if they have had other pregnancies without PPH. In one study, the risk of PPH after two prior episodes was about 20%. In contrast, maternal asthma (Answer A) has not been reported as a risk factor for PPH. A prior macrosomic fetus (Answer B) is not a risk factor for PPH in the present pregnancy, unless the current

TABLE 36.1

AVERAGE BLOOD LOSS AT DELIVERY[a]

Method	RBC Loss	Hematocrit	Blood Loss
Vaginal delivery			
Single fetus	190	37.5	505
Twins	320	35.5	905
Repeat cesarean section	340	36.5	930
Repeat cesarean section hyst.	425	36.5	1,435

[a]Note that the average blood loss for a singleton delivery was 505 cc, and the average for a repeat cesarean section was 930 cc, both very similar to the cutoffs recommended for the diagnosis of postpartum hemorrhage. Pritchard JA. Changes in the blood volume during pregnancy and delivery. Anesthesiology. 1965;26:393–9, used with permission.

fetus is also macrosomic. Although some authors have associated prior abortions (Answer D) with PPH, the association is not strong and the finding is not consistent. A list of factors known to confer risk for PPH is found in Table 36.2. In many women, the risk for PPH can be assessed in advance of delivery due to the presence of risk factors. To

reduce the occurrence of PPH, a program of active management of the third stage of labor has been proposed; this includes early use of uterotonics (immediately after delivery of the baby or even after delivery of the anterior shoulder), and uterine massage and gentle traction on the umbilical cord to deliver the placenta as expeditiously as possible. Active management of the third stage has been shown to result in less PPH and less need for blood transfusion when compared with awaiting spontaneous delivery of the placenta.

 CASE CONTINUES

Ms. Kent progresses to 8 cm of cervical dilatation after 2 hours of spontaneous labor. Thirty minutes later, she delivers a female fetus weighing 4,100 g with Apgar score of 8/9 at 1 and 5 minutes. After handing the newborn off to the nurse, you turn back to the patient. On inspection of the vagina, a bleeding laceration is noted in the right sulcus, and you quickly repair it with 2–0 chromic suture. As you are repairing the laceration, the

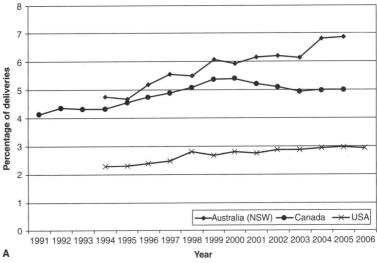

A

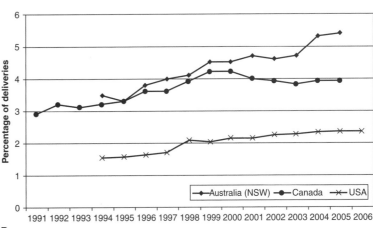

B

Figure 36.1 Diagnosis of postpartum hemorrhage in the United States, Australia, and Canada, based on medical record diagnosis coding. In all three countries, there was an increase in postpartum hemorrhage from 1991 to 2006, attributable to an increase in the incidence of uterine atony. Difference between countries may represent real difference, or may be due to differences in coding or case definition practices. **A:** All cases of postpartum hemorrhage. **B:** Postpartum hemorrhage attributed to uterine atony. (From Knight M, Callaghan WM, Berg C, et al. Trends in postpartum hemorrhage in high resource countries: a review and recommendations from the International Postpartum Hemorrhage Collaborative Group. BMC Pregnancy Childbirth. 2009;9:55.)

TABLE 36.2

RISK FACTORS FOR POSTPARTUM HEMORRHAGE (MODIFIED FROM ACOG PRACTICE BULLETIN NO. 76).

Prolonged labor
Augmented labor
Rapid labor
History of postpartum hemorrhage
Episiotomy, especially mediolateral
Preeclampsia
Overdistended uterus (macrosomia, twins, hydramnios)
Operative delivery
Asian or Hispanic ethnicity
Chorioamnionitis
Grand multiparity (five or more prior deliveries)
Placental anomalies (placenta accreta)

vaginal bleeding becomes heavier, and you note a continuous flow of bright red blood from the vagina. You place a speculum in the vagina. However, the quantity of bleeding is too great to allow you to visualize the source.

Decision 2: Management

What is the most appropriate immediate management of this patient's bleeding?

A. Resuture the vaginal tear
B. Administer oxytocin
C. Order two units of packed red blood cells (PRBCs)
D. Perform a manual examination of the uterus

The best answer is D: Perform a manual examination of the uterus. In the case described, the placenta has not yet delivered. Among the leading causes of primary PPH is uterine atony and retained placenta. A vaginal examination will allow you to assess the location of the placenta, to remove it if possible, and to perform manual compression to reduce uterine bleeding. Given the history above, with worsening bleeding after suturing the laceration, the laceration is less likely to be the source of the bleeding, and time spent in resuturing the laceration (Answer A) will be time lost in gaining control of the patient's hemorrhage. Administering oxytocin (Answer B) is a part of the prophylactic procedures for PPH. It may help to control uterine hemorrhage, but it will not assess placental separation, and it is not as prompt as uterine compression. Although this patient may require a blood transfusion (Answer C), ordering blood products will not stop the acute bleeding.

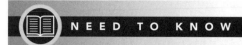

Evaluation of Postpartum Hemorrhage

The first step in assessing the patient with PPH is physical examination: To assist in the examination and to allow for uterine contraction, the bladder is typically emptied using a urinary catheter. The uterine fundus should be palpated, to ascertain whether it is well-contracted and the placenta evaluated for completeness. An atonic uterus will feel soft, and may appear to be larger than normal. Failure to palpate a uterine fundus may indicate a uterine inversion. If a portion of the placenta is missing (following inspection), the attendant can rapidly explore the uterine cavity for retained placental fragments. In the patient with a prior cesarean delivery, the uterine scar can be palpated for intactness. If the uterus is firm, the vagina and cervix are explored for lacerations; this can also be done before delivery of the placenta. This examination can rapidly be performed at the bedside, and fundal palpation and inspection of the placenta and vagina/cervix are a usual part of the delivery routine for all patients.

With excessive bleeding, additional studies may be indicated: Clotting studies may be of help, especially in the patient with a history of bleeding diathesis or with obstetrical complications such as severe preeclampsia. In an emergent situation, 5 mL of blood may be placed in a plain tube (a red-topped tube in the United States). Normal blood will clot within 8 to 10 minutes, and the clot will remain intact. Failure to clot, or rapid clot dissolution may indicate an underlying coagulopathy. Imaging studies are seldom required for primary PPH, but ultrasound of the uterus may be of benefit in the diagnosis of retained products of conception with secondary PPH, and pelvic imaging by ultrasound or computed tomography scanner may help to establish a diagnosis of intraabdominal processes such as a broad ligament hematoma. Genital tract lacerations can cause an extensive amount of bleeding in rare cases. Cervical tears can extend into the lower uterine segment, involving the uterine artery and its major branches. Extensive vaginal tears must be carefully inspected. If a peritoneal perforation or retroperitoneal hemorrhage is suspected, an exploratory laparotomy may be necessary to identify the source and stop the bleeding.

CASE CONTINUES

On manual examination, Ms. Kent's fundus is soft and boggy. It does not respond to uterine massage and there is no further contraction after 300 mL of urine are drained with a bladder catheter. Her vagina is reinspected and the area you repaired continues to ooze bright red blood. In addition, bright red blood continues to flow from the uterus. You order stat labs, including a complete blood cell count, prothrombin time, partial thromboplastin time, and a clot tube. You request an additional large bore IV to be placed in the patient's opposite arm and order 4 units of PRBC to be crossmatched.

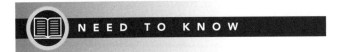

Management of Atony

PPH due to uterine atony is a medical emergency. As with other emergent situations, results are optimized when there is a clear protocol for patient management (Table 36.3 presents one protocol). In general, bladder drainage and uterine massage (Fig. 36.2) are followed by uterotonic use (Table 36.4). Uterine packing, either with sponges or a balloon catheter may be considered. In the face of ongoing bleeding, surgical treatment must be considered (see below).

 CASE CONTINUES

Ms. Kent has no retained placenta after manual exploration of the uterus. A total of 40 units of oxytocin is added to her intravenous fluid followed by Methergine

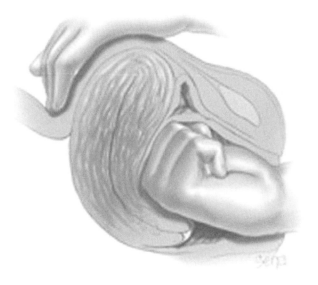

Figure 36.2 Bimanual compression of uterus: first step in management of uterine atony. This technique consists of massage of the posterior aspect of the uterus with a hand on the abdomen and massage through the vagina of the anterior uterine wall with the other hand made into a fist. (From Anderson JM, Etches D. Prevention and management of postpartum hemorrhage. Am Fam Physician. 2007;75(6):875–82, used with permission.)

0.2 mg IM. The uterus continues atonic. Cytotec 1,000 μg is given per rectum and the second unit of PRBCs is started. An attempt is made to pack the uterus, but the packing is not retained. You are informed that the hemoglobin level is 6.5 g/dL. You elect to take Ms. Kent to the operating room with a blood transfusion ongoing. At laparotomy, a retroperitoneal hematoma is revealed.

TABLE 36.3
PROTOCOL FOR MANAGEMENT OF POSTPARTUM HEMORRHAGE

Action	
Initial Evaluation	Catheterize bladder Bimanual exam (to identify uterine tone) Blood for crossmatch and clotting studies as appropriate. This may include a tube for bedside observation of clotting. Visual assessment of cervix, vagina and preineum
If atony suspected: evaluate for retained products of conception	Examine placenta for defects Consider uterine curettage
Treat for atony	Utertonics 　Oxytocin 　Methylergonivine 　15-methyl prostaglandin (PG) F2α 　Misoprostol Bimanual uterine compression
If ongoing bleeding: Consider uterine tamponade	Intrauterine balloon for tamponade
If ongoing bleeding: Consider laparotomy	Uterine devascularization Uterine compression stitch (B-Lynch suture) Hysterectomy

TABLE 36.4

UTEROTONIC USE IN POSTPARTUM HEMORRHAGE

Drug[a]	Dose/Route	Frequency	Comment
Oxytocin (Pitocin)	IV: 10–40 units in 1 L normal saline or lactated Ringer's solution IM: 10 units	Continuous	Avoid undiluted rapid IV infusion, which causes hypotension.
Methylergonovine (Methergine)	IM: 0.2 mg	Every 2–4 hr	Avoid if patient is hypertensive.
15-Methyl $PGF_{2\alpha}$ (carboprost) (Hemabate)	IM: 0.25 mg	Every 15–90 min, eight doses maximum	Avoid in asthmatic patients; relative contraindication if hepatic, renal, and cardiac disease. Diarrhea, fever, and tachycardia can occur.
Dinoprostone (Prostin E_2)	Suppository: vaginal or rectal 20 mg	Every 2 hr	Avoid if patient is hypotensive. Fever is common. Stored frozen, it must be thawed to room temperature.
Misoprostol (Cytotec, PGE_1)	800–1,000 μg rectally		

[a]All agents can cause nausea and vomiting.
IM, intramuscularly; IV, intravenously; PG, prostaglandin.
From American College of Obstetricians and Gynecologists. ACOG practice bulletin: clinical management guidelines for obstetrician-gynecologists Number 76, October 2006: postpartum hemorrhage. Obstet Gynecol. 2006;108(4):1039–47, used with permission.

 Decision 3: Management

What are the surgical options for this patient?

A. Ligate the uterine arteries
B. Perform a B-Lynch suture
C. Explore the retroperitoneum
D. Ligate the ovarian arteries

Surgical approaches to the patient with uterine atony include the B-Lynch suture (Fig. 36.3) and ligation of the vessels supplying the uterus. The B-Lynch suture (Answer B) compresses the fundus of the uterus and may control

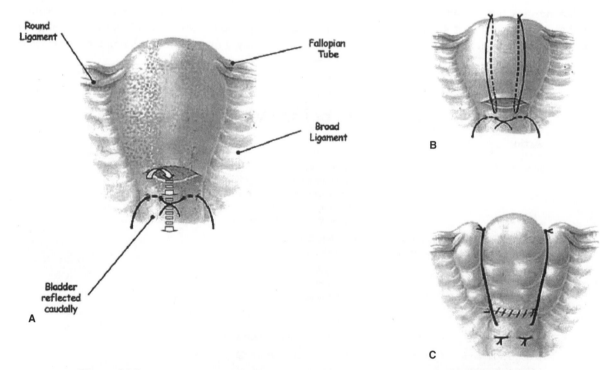

Figure 36.3 B-Lynch suture: A surgical option in postpartum hemorrhage. The suture is shown on a uterus postcesarean section. The B-Lynch suture is anchored in the lower uterine segment (**A**) and passes over the fundus (like a pair of suspenders) (**B**). When the suture is tightened, the uterus is compressed (**C**). From: Hayman RG, Arulkumaran S, Steer PJ. Uterine compression sutures: surgical management of postpartum hemorrhage. Obstet Gynecol. 2002 Mar;99(3):502–6, used with permission.

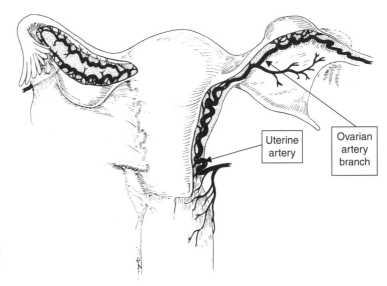

Figure 36.4 Sites of ligation of the uterine artery and ovarian artery branch in post partum hemorrhage. (image copyright fotosearch)

the bleeding of uterine atony. Ligation of the uterine arteries at the level of the internal os (O'Leary suture, Answer A) is often combined with ligation of the uterine branch of the ovarian arteries (Fig. 36.4). However, ligation of the main ovarian artery (Answer D) is not usually performed. None of these treatments would, however, address the patient's retroperitoneal bleeding. Therefore, the best of the answers above is C: explore the retroperitoneum to identify and repair the site of bleeding.

 CASE CONCLUSION

You open the retroperitoneum and identify rapid bleeding from a branch of the uterine artery. The vessel is ligated securely and hemostasis achieved. The patient is given a total of 10 units of PRBCs, 6 units of fresh frozen plasma, and 3 units of platelets. She is transferred to the intensive care unit where she is hemodynamically stable. She is extubated on postoperative day 2 and resumes routine postoperative care. She is discharged home with her baby on postoperative day 8.

SUGGESTED READINGS

Akwuruoha E, Kamanu C, Onwere S, Chigbu B, Aluka C, Umezuruike C. Grand multiparity and pregnancy outcome in Aba, Nigeria: a case-control study. Arch Gynecol Obstet. 2009. [Epub ahead of print]

American College of Obstetricians and Gynecologists. ACOG practice bulletin: clinical management guidelines for obstetrician-gynecologists Number 76, October 2006: postpartum hemorrhage. Obstet Gynecol. 2006;108(4):1039–47.

Audureau E, Deneux-Tharaux C, Lefèvre P, et al. Practices for prevention, diagnosis and management of postpartum haemorrhage: impact of a regional multifaceted intervention. BJOG. 2009;116(10): 1325–33. Epub 2009 Jun 17.

Ford JB, Roberts CL, Bell JC, Algert CS, Morris JM. Postpartum haemorrhage occurrence and recurrence: a population-based study. Med J Aust. 2007;187(7):391–3.

Knight M, Callaghan WM, Berg C, et al. Trends in postpartum hemorrhage in high resource countries: a review and recommendations from the International Postpartum Hemorrhage Collaborative Group. BMC Pregnancy Childbirth. 2009;9:55. Review.

Pritchard JA. Changes in the blood volume during pregnancy and delivery. Anesthesiology. 1965;26:393–9. Review.

Rajan PV, Wing DA. Postpartum hemorrhage: evidence-based medical interventions for prevention and treatment. Clin Obstet Gynecol. 2010;53(1):165–81.

Uterine Rupture

John D. Richard

 CASE PRESENTATION

Your patient, Ms. Jordan presents to labor and delivery with a complaint of a large gush of fluid approximately 1 hour ago. She is a 39-year-old G3 P2 who is presently at 39 weeks of gestation by last menstrual period, confirmed by a first-trimester ultrasound. Ms. Jordan has been receiving care in your office since 10 weeks of gestation. Her pregnancy course has been unremarkable, and her prenatal screening predicted a low risk of fetal Down syndrome. Her past obstetrical history is significant for a spontaneous vaginal delivery of her first child, and a cesarean delivery of her second due to nonreassuring fetal heart tracing. These children both weighed about 7.5 lb and are now doing well. She has no other significant past medical or surgical history, takes no medication and uses no tobacco or alcohol. Her prepregnant BMI was 29. During the course of her prenatal care, Ms. Jordan had inquired about the possibility of a vaginal delivery in this pregnancy. The patient had been counseled regarding the risks of a vaginal birth after cesarean (VBAC), and she has indicated that she would like a trial of labor, which is her current delivery plan. At present, Ms. Jordan denies contractions, but states that at her last delivery the contractions started shortly after her "water broke."

On physical examination, this is a well-developed Caucasian female. Her blood pressure is 130/75 mm Hg, her pulse is 90 bpm, and she is afebrile. Her abdomen is nontender, and there is a well-healed lower abdominal transverse scar. Evaluation reveals gross rupture of membranes with copious fluid coming from the vagina. On the speculum examination, the cervical dilation appears to be about 4 cm. The fetal heart rate is 140 bpm and is category 1; there are irregular contractions seen on the monitor. The remainder of the physical examination is unremarkable. The patient is admitted for management of labor.

 Decision 1: Counseling

What are the important risks of VBAC?

A. Maternal infection
B. Uterine rupture
C. Maternal mortality
D. Fetal mortality

The correct answers are B and D: Uterine rupture and fetal mortality. Meta-analyses of the numerous studies in this area suggest that the risk of uterine rupture is significantly increased (from about 0.5% to about 1%) in patients undergoing VBAC compared with those having an elective repeat cesarean delivery. Those who fail to deliver vaginally after a trial of labor had a uterine rupture rate of 4% (Fig. 37.1). In addition, the risk of fetal or neonatal mortality nearly doubled (from about 0.3% to 0.6%) in those undergoing VBAC. By contrast, maternal mortality (Answer C) is not significantly increased by VBAC, and maternal febrile morbidity (Answer A) is decreased in those undergoing VBAC. Significant risks of VBAC are listed in Table 37.1.

 N E E D   T O   K N O W

Selection of the Patient for a VBAC

When a patient with a prior cesarean delivery becomes pregnant again, consideration may be given to a trial of labor. If a VBAC is to be considered, the patient must not have an absolute contraindications to the procedure. One group of contraindications involves the uterine incision made at the prior cesarean. There is a large degree of variation in the subsequent risk of uterine rupture based on the type of surgery performed on the uterus. A standard low-transverse uterine incision carries approximately a 1% chance of rupture during labor. In contrast, a classical cesarean incision, which extends vertically up above the level of the round ligaments, carries a 7% to 8% risk. In current practice in the United States, a prior classical uterine scar is a contraindication to an attempted VBAC. Other contraindications to VBAC are any contraindication to vaginal delivery (such as fetal malpresentation), and maternal refusal. Many practices will not allow a VBAC if the patient has had more than one prior cesarean delivery as the uterine rupture rate increases with the number of prior uterine incisions. Given that the rupture rate is about

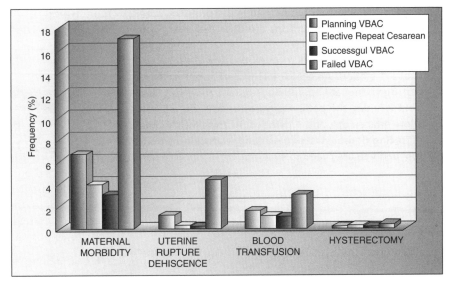

Figure 37.1 Maternal morbidity related to vaginal birth after cesarean (VBAC). Rates of uterine rupture, blood transfusion, and hysterectomy were increased in patients undergoing VBAC compared with those having an elective repeat cesarean delivery. The risk in patients undergoing VBAC was greatly increased in those failing to deliver vaginally; successful VBAC had the lowest risk of any group. (From Rossi AC, D'Addario V. Maternal morbidity following a trial of labor after cesarean section vs elective repeat cesarean delivery: a systematic review with metaanalysis. Am J Obstet Gynecol. 2008;199(3):224–31. Used with permission.)

VBAC: vaginal birth after caution
ERCS: elective regulate caution section
F-TOL: failer trial of labor

1.5% after two prior cesareans, some practitioners will allow a VBAC with up to two prior low transverse cesarean deliveries. Although the data are not as good, practitioners may also regard other uterine incisions in the same light as cesarean sections. The most common such incision is made for a myomectomy; if the incision is made through the uterine wall most practitioners would perform a cesarean delivery in a subsequent pregnancy. Importantly, if the practitioner performing the prior surgery indicates in the medical record that future deliveries should be by cesarean section, this advice is generally complied with. Finally, VBAC is contraindicated in the absence of suitable facilities. There must be anesthesia and an operating room available, and a physician able to perform an emergency cesarean.

When planning a delivery after a previous cesarean, the group at highest risk are those mothers who attempt to deliver vaginally and fail. For this reason, it is also desirable to attempt VBAC in patients with a high likelihood of success. Factors predicting a successful VBAC include a history of a prior vaginal delivery, maternal age <40 years, spontaneous initiation of labor, cervical examination on admission of >4 cm, and fetal weight

<4,000 g. Women whose prior cesarean was for a malpresentation are also more likely to successfully deliver vaginally (Table 37.2).

The patient contemplating a VBAC is informed of these risks, and is asked to indicate her consent to the trial of labor, usually by signing a formal informed consent form.

 CASE CONTINUES

Ms. Jordan is observed for 2 hours in labor and delivery. During this time, no increase in uterine activity is observed, and the patient reports no increase in discomfort. You

TABLE 37.1

SIGNIFICANT RISKS OF AN ATTEMPTED VAGINAL DELIVERY AFTER CESAREAN

	Odds Ratio (vs. planned cesarean delivery)
Uterine rupture	2.1
Fetal/neonatal mortality	1.7
5-minute Apgar <7	2.24

TABLE 37.2

SUCCESS RATES FOR TRIAL OF LABOR

	VBAC Success (%)
Prior Indication	
CPD/FTP	63.5
NRFWB	72.6
Malpresentation	83.8
Prior Vaginal Delivery	
Yes	86.6
No	60.9
Labor Type	
Induction	67.4
Augmented	73.9
Spontaneous	80.6

CPD, cephalopelvic disproportion; FTP, failure to progress; NRFWB, nonreassuring fetal well-being; VBAC, vaginal birth after cesarean. (From: Landon MB. Vaginal birth after cesarean delivery. Clin Perinatol. 2008 Sep;35(3):491–504, ix–x, used with permission.)

decide to begin oxytocin augmentation per protocol. After 30 minutes, uterine contractions are observed every 3 to 4 minutes; the fetal heart rate tracing remains category 1. After 3 hours, the patient is 6 cm dilated and the fetal vertex is at −1 station. An epidural is placed at the patient's request, and adequate pain management is achieved. Over the next 2 hours, the patient progresses to 9 cm dilation, complete effacement, and +1 station. At this time the fetal heart tracing demonstrates a prolonged deceleration to 60 bpm and you are called to evaluate.

Decision 2: Diagnosis

What additional finding would be likely in a uterine rupture?

A. Blood in the bladder catheter
B. High baseline uterine tone with rapid uterine contractions
C. Maternal loss of consciousness
D. Loss of fetal station

Although all of the above situations can occur in uterine rupture, the most typical is **D:** Loss of fetal station. The typical presentation of uterine rupture is a maternal complaint of tearing, constant abdominal pain, accompanied by a fetal heart rate deceleration. On physical examination, the fetal head is found to have lost station, and, if an intrauterine pressure catheter is used, there may be a loss of intrauterine pressure. Sometimes, fetal small parts may be palpable through the maternal abdomen. In some cases, the uterine scar separation may be nearly bloodless (usually called a dehiscence). In other cases, there may be profuse maternal bleeding leading to maternal shock (Answer C). Bladder injury (Answer A) is possible if the uterine tear extends into the bladder. A high baseline tone with rapid contractions (Answer B) is more typical of a placental abruption, but a high baseline tone may also be seen in a uterine rupture.

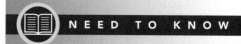

Outcome of Uterine Rupture

The reported outcome of uterine rupture includes serious or terminal events in both mother and infant. The likelihood of these events varies widely in different reported series (Table 37.3). The difference in reported outcomes appears to be related to three factors:

- The definition of uterine rupture. Most authors exclude cases of uterine scar separation not requiring treatment; however, there is a difference in reports with respect to the proportion of patients with full-thickness uterine separations and uterine bleeding. Ruptures associated with significant maternal hemorrhage would be expected to involve more morbidity.
- The proportion of ruptures in unscarred uteri. Many reports of uterine rupture originate from developing countries, where the primary risk factor for uterine rupture is obstructed labor. Uterine ruptures in unscarred uteri may have a more morbid course.
- The availability of facilities to rapidly address fetal or maternal distress.

Recent reports from the United States would suggest that the most significant maternal risk is for blood loss with blood transfusion and the need for additional surgery. Long-term risks include loss of fertility, surgical complications (such as ureteral injury) and blood-borne infections.

TABLE 37.3
OUTCOME OF UTERINE RUPTURE IN THE UNITED STATES AND INDIA

Outcome	United States (Yap et al., 2001) N = 21 Patients	India (Gupta and Nanda, 2009) N = 57 Patients
Maternal Complications		
Rupture of unscarred uterus	3/21 (14%)	37/57 (65%)
Blood transfusion	4/21 (19%)	N/A
Hysterectomy	2/21 (10%)	17/57 (30%)
Maternal mortality	0	0
Fetal Complications		
Acidemia (cord blood pH <7)	4/17 (24%)[a]	N/A
Perinatal mortality	(Corrected) 0[b]	54/57 (95%)

[a]Decreasing fetal pH below 7 may be associated with neurologic damage; however, most such fetuses will have a normal outcome. Damaged fetuses are found in the group with a metabolic component to the acidosis (data not reported in this study).
[b]Two perinatal deaths occurred, neither due to uterine rupture. One fetus died prior to labor and one newborn with a lethal congenital anomaly.

Although the risk of fetal death due to uterine rupture in labor is relatively low when the patient is labored in a controlled setting, the risk of fetal acidemia appears to be elevated. There are no studies on this population to indicate the long-term outcome of these infants, although studies in other populations suggest an increase in hypoxic-ischemic encephalopathy in acidemic fetuses with a pH below 7.0 and a metabolic component to the acidosis (suggesting more severe or prolonged oxygen deficit). It should be emphasized that, even in the group with pH below 7.0, most newborn outcomes were normal.

 CASE CONTINUES

When you arrive on labor and delivery, Ms. Jordan appears appropriately anxious. Her blood pressure is 100/60 mm Hg, and her pulse is 110 bpm. Palpation of the uterus reveals apparent increased resting tone, and a bulge in the lower segment that was not previously appreciated. On vaginal examination, the cervix is 9 cm dilated with the presenting part at −2 station. The fetal heart rate is 60 bpm and has been 60 for 4.5 minutes.

 Decision 3: Management

What is the best treatment at this point?

A. Increase oxytocin and await vaginal delivery
B. Maternal fluid resuscitation
C. Cesarean delivery
D. Operative vaginal delivery

The correct answer is C: Cesarean delivery. The fetal heart rate tracing has evolved to category 3, indicating a need for emergent delivery. Operative vaginal delivery (Answer D) would only be appropriate when the cervix is completely dilated and when the fetus is at +2 station or below. If the uterine scar has ruptured, increasing the oxytocin (Answer A) is contraindicated, because delivery uterine contraction may worsen the rupture. Maternal fluid resuscitation (Answer B) will not be harmful, but surgery should not be delayed to administer maternal fluids; the treatment of this condition is to remove the fetus from an environment where it is being insufficiently oxygenated and to control any maternal hemorrhage.

 CASE CONTINUES

You diagnose a uterine rupture, and preparations are made for an immediate cesarean delivery. The epidural dose is increased on the way to the operating room, and a uterine incision is made 11 minutes after your arrival at the delivery room. On opening the abdomen, you find that the prior uterine incision is completely separated. There is a 1 L hemoperitoneum, and the fetal arm and umbilical cord protrude into the maternal abdomen. The male infant weighs 3,260 g and the Apgar scores are 1 and 9 at 1 and 5 minutes. Umbilical cord gases are obtained and show an arterial pH of 7.10, and a base excess of −11 mmol/L. You repair the uterine incision with good hemostasis, and you decide against further surgical intervention. The infant is taken to the neonatal intensive care unit for observation. Ms. Jordan's vital signs remain stable, and the remainder of her surgery is without incident. In the recovery room, she asks you whether she made a foolish decision to try to deliver vaginally. She is concerned that she should have known that she would rupture.

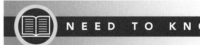

Risk Factors for Uterine Rupture

In the United States, the single greatest risk factor for uterine rupture is the presence of a uterine scar. As stated previously, rupture the uterus in labor occurs in 1% of patients after a prior low transverse uterine incision, and in 1/10,000 patients without a prior uterine surgery. A variety of factors have been described that are associated with uterine rupture in scarred and unscarred uteri (Table 37.4); however, the predictive value of these is minimal, and it is not possible to predict with confidence whether a particular individual will experience a uterine rupture in labor.

TABLE 37.4

FACTORS ASSOCIATED WITH AN INCREASED RISK OF UTERINE RUPTURE. NOTE THAT NOT ALL FACTORS ARE CONFIRMED IN ALL STUDIES

Unscarred uterus	Uterine anomalies
	Connective tissue disease (Ehlers–Danlos syndrome)
	Trauma
	Abnormal placentation (placenta accreta)
	Labor induction/augmentation
	Obstructed labor
Prior uterine incision	Prior classical incision
	Prior single-layer closure
	More than one prior uterine incision
	No prior vaginal delivery
	Interdelivery interval <2 yr
	Obesity
	Term (as opposed to preterm) delivery
	Use of medications for cervical ripening
	Labor induction

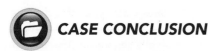

CASE CONCLUSION

You inform Ms. Jordan that based upon risk assessment, she had a high likelihood of a successful delivery and low risk of uterine rupture. She feels reassured regarding her original decision. She experiences postpartum endometritis that responds to antibiotic treatment. Her postoperative course is otherwise uneventful. Her baby does well and is ready to be discharged with her on postoperative day number 5.

SUGGESTED READINGS

Gupta A, Nanda S. Uterine rupture in pregnancy: a five-year study. Arch Gynecol Obstet. 2010 Jan 28. [Epub ahead of print].

Landon MB. Vaginal birth after cesarean delivery. Clin Perinatol. 2008;35(3):491–504.

Mukhopadhaya N, De Silva C, Manyonda IT. Conventional myomectomy. Best Pract Res Clin Obstet Gynaecol. 2008;22(4): 677–705.

Mozurkewich EL, Hutton EK. Elective repeat cesarean delivery versus trial of labor: a meta-analysis of the literature from 1989 to 1999. Am J Obstet Gynecol. 2000;183(5):1187–97.

Rossi AC, D'Addario V. Maternal morbidity following a trial of labor after cesarean section vs elective repeat cesarean delivery: a systematic review with metaanalysis. Am J Obstet Gynecol. 2008; 199(3): 224–31.

Smith JG, Mertz HL, Merrill DC. Identifying risk factors for uterine rupture. Clin Perinatol. 2008;35(1):85–99.

Yap OW, Kim ES, Laros RK Jr. Maternal and neonatal outcomes after uterine rupture in labor. Am J Obstet Gynecol. 2001;184(7): 1576–81.

Amniotic Fluid Embolism

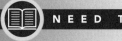

Robert Eden

 CASE PRESENTATION

You are called to labor and delivery to admit Ms. Ruiz, a 37-year-old G4 P3003 female at 39½ weeks in the latent phase of labor, with irregular contractions every 3 to 5 minutes. Her contractions began 3 hours prior to admission, and she denies rupture of membranes. Review of her prenatal chart reveals that dating criteria are based on a first trimester ultrasound, and her obstetrical history is significant for three uneventful spontaneous vaginal deliveries. Her prenatal labs are within normal limits. Your physical examination reveals normal vital signs, a fundal height of 40 cm, and clinical estimated fetal weight of 3,600 g. The pelvic examination reveals a cervix that is 1 cm dilated and 60% effaced with a vertex presentation, left occiput transverse at −2 station (1/60%/−2). The cervix is soft and anterior giving a Bishop score of 8. The admission fetal heart rate (FHR) tracing is unremarkable.

Eight hours later, the cervix is unchanged at 2 cm/60%/−2 with contractions every 4 to 5 minutes, and oxytocin is started. Three hours after initiation, the oxytocin infusion is at 6 mU/min. The patient spontaneously ruptures membranes and 1+ meconium is noted by the nurse. You arrive to find the FHR tracing following membrane rupture depicted in Figure 38.1.

You perform a pelvic examination finding the cervix to be 4 cm/80%/−2 without a prolapsed cord, and you place a fetal scalp electrode. After stopping the oxytocin infusion, turning the patient on her side, increasing IV fluids, and placing an oxygen mask on her face, you assist the nursing staff in moving the patient to the operating room and placing her on the operating table. While the FHR monitor is being reattached, the anesthesiologist and neonatal intensive care unit (NICU) team arrive and you describe the clinical situation. Shortly thereafter, the patient becomes agitated and complains of difficulty breathing. The maternal oxygen saturation is reported to be 75%. The following FHR monitor strip appears as seen below (Fig. 38.2):

 Decision 1: Management

What is your management of the FHR bradycardia at this time?

A. Immediate IV injection of 0.25 mg terbutaline and continued observation with initiation of regional anesthesia for delivery
B. Continue to perform intrauterine resuscitation by maternal position change, increased IV fluids, O₂ by mask while observing the FHR
C. Fetal scalp stimulation to provoke an FHR acceleration and return to baseline FHR
D. Immediate maternal intubation and cesarean delivery

The correct answer is D: Since the patient has begun to demonstrate signs of respiratory compromise, maternal intubation must be initiated as soon as possible so you can perform a cesarean section delivery on the patient. Answers A and B are not indicated for this patient because of the need to perform an immediate delivery. Answer C is not correct due to the fact that a fetal bradycardia induced by intense vagal or hypoxic stimulation will not be relieved by scalp stimulation. Vagal tone actually may be increased by aggressive scalp stimulation.

NEED TO KNOW

Prolonged Fetal Heart Rate Decelerations

Prolonged FHR decelerations are characterized by an abrupt onset of the deceleration (decrease of at least 15 bpm) for at least 2 minutes, but <10 minutes. The FHR pattern may be associated with normal or abnormal baseline heart rate, variability, and the presence or absence of FHR accelerations. The ability of the fetus to

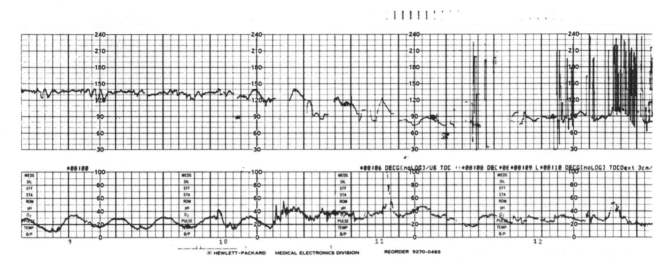

Figure 38.1 Fetal heart rate (FHR) tracing immediately after SROM. From Cabaniss ML and Ross MG. Fetal Monitoring Interpretation 2nd edition. Philadelphia, PA: Lippincott Williams & Wilkins; 2010 p. 329, used with permission.

tolerate prolonged decelerations is directly related to the fetal status prior to the onset of the deceleration: the presence of a normal baseline rate, with normal FHR variability and accelerations is associated with the absence of preexisting fetal hypoxia and acidosis while fetal tachycardia, decreased or absent FHR variability, and loss of accelerations may indicate the presence of fetal hypoxia.

Since prolonged FHR deceleration carries an associated risk of cessation of blood and oxygen flow to the fetus, the initial management may include (1) reducing uterine contractions by stopping oxytocin adminis-

tration or by the use of a tocolytic; (2) maximizing uterine blood flow by turning the patient on her left side to increase venous return to the maternal heart, and by increasing IV fluid infusion; and (3) enhancing maternal oxygenation by placing an O_2 mask on the mother's face.

Depending upon the degree of bradycardia, one should perform a vaginal examination (to diagnose a prolapsed umbilical cord) while observing the FHR response. Normal FHR variability prior to the deceleration, or an FHR acceleration in response to vaginal examination are predictive of good fetal condition,

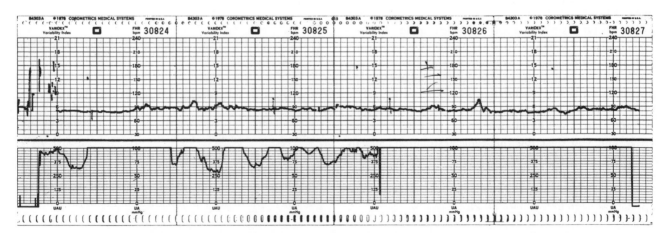

Figure 38.2 Fetal heart rate (FHR) monitor strip in the operating room at 19:25. From Cabaniss ML and Ross MG. Fetal Monitoring Interpretation 2nd edition. Philadelphia, PA: Lippincott Williams & Wilkins; 2010 p. 328, used with permission.

while reduced FHR variability prior to the deceleration is a predictor of fetal acidemia in response to the deceleration.

The mechanism of FHR decelerations is most often vagal or hypoxia mediated. The etiology of the prolonged deceleration includes uterine hypertonus (from abruption, excessive use of oxytocin or prostaglandins, eclampsia, or amniotic fluid embolism [AFE]), or from fetal manipulation, including vaginal examination or scalp sampling, maternal position change, or acute fetal hemorrhage. Prolonged FHR decelerations most often occur in the second stage of labor. In this case, the etiology of the prolonged FHR deceleration was the increase in contraction frequency and intensity associated with rupture of membranes. This may be associated with placental abruption or AFE, conditions that are unlikely to respond to intrauterine resuscitation. The most prudent course of action to take is to immediately begin intrauterine resuscitation, alert the OR team (anesthesia, NICU), and transfer the patient to the operating room for immediate operative delivery. Since the cervix was noted to be 4 cm on pelvic examination, operative vaginal delivery is not possible, and you must anticipate the need for emergent cesarean section if the fetus does not recover from the prolonged deceleration.

 CASE CONTINUES

After 8 minutes in the OR, the maternal airway is secured by the anesthesiologist; Ms. Ruiz is intubated and sedated. Once under general anesthesia, you operatively deliver the fetus. You hand the male infant weighing 3,905 g to the NICU team and immediately the neonate is intubated and resuscitation begun. The Apgar scores are 2, 4, and 5 at 1, 5, and 10 minutes, respectively. The umbilical arterial cord gas reveals a pH of 6.86, PO_2 17 mm Hg, PCO_2 95 mm Hg, and base excess −13.6 mmol/L consistent with a combined respiratory and metabolic acidosis. The interval of time from the onset of the FHR deceleration to delivery of the fetus is 17 minutes.

While you are closing the uterus, you note that the mother's blood has become dark, purplish red. You alert the anesthesiologist who reports that her blood pressure is not detectable despite a faint carotid pulse of 122 bpm. Immediately, the anesthesiologist injects 15 mg of ephedrine and 200 μg phenylephrine (Neo-Synephrine); the maternal pulse immediately increases to 140 bpm, but the blood pressure is still not obtainable. The cardiac rhythm further deteriorates to ventricular fibrillation. You instruct the head nurse to call the Code team stat.

 Decision 2: Diagnosis

Which of the following four choices would you consider your primary etiology for the onset of the acute cardiovascular collapse?

A. Cardiac arrest
B. AFE
C. Pulmonary embolism
D. Eclamptic seizures

The answer is B: AFE. Answer A: Cardiac arrest is not correct as this patient has not experienced cardiac arrest. Answer D is unlikely as the patient was able to communicate until anesthetized and showed no evidence of either seizure activity or a postictal state. Although answer C is a possibility that must be excluded, an acute event following uterine tachysystole and hypertonus with spontaneous rupture of membranes and associated with FHR deceleration is a typical presentation for AFE.

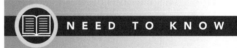 **NEED TO KNOW**

Management of Amniotic Fluid Embolism

This case presentation of AFE is a very typical, though unfortunate scenario with maternal collapse following rupture of membranes and the onset of uterine tachysystole and hypertonus. However, not all cases of AFE present in such a classical fashion.

AFE has an incidence ranging from 1 in 8,000 to 1 in 80,000 pregnancies. Overall mortality is 50%, with half of the deaths occurring within the first hour. Among survivors, 75% to 85% may be expected to have long-term neurologic deficits due to the initial profound hypoxemia. Maternal survival is dependent upon rapidly reestablishing adequate oxygenation and cardiovascular circulation to the mother. As exemplified by this case, nearly all cases are accompanied by evidence of fetal compromise. Depending upon the surgical management, up to 70% of fetuses will survive, though nearly 50% of survivors have neurologic damage. Risk factors for AFE are multiple, although few have a definitive etiologic mechanism shown in Table 38.1.

Since maternal survival is improved with early diagnosis, AFE should be considered whenever there is a sudden onset of signs and symptoms. About 27% to 51% of patients with AFE present with acute respiratory distress (tachypnea and shortness of breath) followed by maternal cyanosis and sudden cardiovascular collapse. Alternatively, 13% to 27% present

TABLE 38.1

RISK FACTORS FOR AMNIOTIC FLUID EMBOLISM

Advanced maternal age	Placenta accrete
Multiparity	Polyhydramnios
Meconium	Uterine rupture
Cervical laceration	Maternal history of atopy
Intrauterine fetal death	Chorioamnionitis
Uterine tachysystole or hypertonus	Macrosomia
Rapid labor	Oxytocin (controversial)

with acute hypotension, whereas approximately 30% demonstrate convulsions prior to other signs or symptoms. Respiratory distress is often followed by hemorrhage, maternal coma, seizures, and nearly always fetal distress.

There is no specific laboratory testing available for AFE. On autopsy, patients dying with an AFE have classically demonstrated fetal squamous cells, as well as lanugo hairs, vernix, and meconium in the maternal pulmonary circulation. The diagnosis of AFE in a living patient is confirmed by the clinical presentation; the finding of squamous cells in blood obtained from the pulmonary circulation via a pulmonary artery catheter is not exclusive to patients with AFE. Serum tryptase (a measure of mast cell degranulation) as well as sialyl Tn (a fetal antigen) has been found to be elevated in some women with AFE. Neither of these tests is in widespread clinical use for the diagnosis of AFE. Nonspecific laboratory assessments that are of value in concurrent management of the patient include complete blood cell count, coagulation parameters including fibrin degradation products and fibrinogen, arterial blood gases, chest x-ray, EKG, VQ scan, and echocardiogram as shown in Table 38.2.

TABLE 38.2

LABORATORY INVESTIGATION IN SUSPECTED AMNIOTIC FLUID EMBOLISM

Nonspecific	Specific
CBC	Serum tryptase
Coagulation parameters including fibrin degradation products (FDP) Fibrinogen	Serum sialyl Tn antigen
Arterial blood gas	
Chest x-ray	
Electrocardiogram	
V/Q scan or spiral CT	

CBC, complete blood cell count.

There is no specific intervention for AFE; treatment is supportive. Clinical management of AFE includes maintenance of oxygenation, maternal circulatory support, and correction of coagulopathy (disseminated intravascular coagulopathy [DIC]). Cesarean section should be instituted as soon as possible, despite maternal cardiopulmonary compromise. The immediate measures include establishment of multiple large-bore IV sites, maternal oxygen administration, airway control, including endotracheal intubation with maximal ventilation. Initial therapy when hypotension occurs is to rapidly expand the maternal blood volume and to administer direct-acting vasopressors such as phenylephrine to maintain perfusion pressure and dopamine to improve myocardial function. Coagulopathy may be treated rapidly with cryoprecipitate as well as fresh frozen plasma. Platelets should be transfused if the platelet count is <20,000/mm^3 and O-negative blood may be used for rapid transfusion if crossmatched blood is unavailable. Experimental approaches include the use of high-dose corticosteroids, cardiopulmonary bypass for persistent respiratory distress, nitric oxide, and inhaled prostacyclin.

NEED TO KNOW

Pathophysiology of Amniotic Fluid Embolism

The pathophysiology of AFE is thought to involve amniotic fluid and fetal cells entering the maternal circulation via open uterine venous sinusoids and being deposited in the lung shown in Figure 38.3. Amniotic fluid and fetal cells induce inflammatory biochemical mediators leading to pulmonary artery vasospasm, pulmonary hypertension, and elevated right ventricular pressure. This effect may be similar to an anaphylactic reaction, and AFE has been called anaphylactoid syndrome of pregnancy. The resulting hypoxia leads to myocardial and pulmonary capillary damage, left heart failure, and acute respiratory distress syndrome. In support of this hypothesis, animal models demonstrate the initial cardiovascular event to be pulmonary hypertension. In humans, pulmonary artery pressures have not been measured in the acute phase; the later evolution of AFE may involve severe systemic hypotension due to left ventricular dysfunction. During the evolution of AFE, biochemical mediators may also be responsible for a maternal coagulopathic phase characterized by massive hemorrhage and uterine atony. Maternal coagulopathy (DIC) typically occurs 30 minutes to 4 hours after the initial phase (Fig. 38.4).

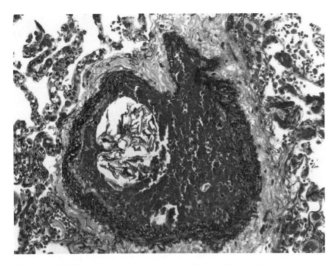

Figure 38.3 Pulmonary artery capillary filled with fetal squamous cells. From Marcus BJ, Collins KA, Harley RA. Ancillary studies in amniotic fluid embolism: a case report and review of the literature. Am J Forensic Med Pathol. 2005;26(1):92–5, used with permission.

 CASE CONTINUES

Following the Code team arrival, you quickly pack the maternal wound to allow resuscitation. One ampule of epinephrine (1 mg) and one ampule of atropine (1 mg) are given without effect and chest compressions and immediate electrocardioversion is performed. The patient converts to sinus tachycardia then progresses to a wide complex tachycardia. Amiodarone 150 mg and sodium bicarbonate (total 50 mL of 8.4% solution) are then administered resulting in a ventricular tachycardia.

A second cardioversion results in a sinus tachycardia. A right groin central line is then placed and the blood pressure noted to be 128/88 mm Hg, pulse 156 bpm, and O_2 saturation 94%. The patient begins to stabilize. Her arterial gas reveals: pH 7.02, PCO_2: 85 mm Hg, PO_2: 67 mm Hg, HCO_3: 22 mmol/L, and base excess of −10 mmol/L. The patient is transferred to the intensive care unit (ICU). Echocardiography is performed by the cardiologist and a small ventricular septal defect is noted without evidence of a pulmonary embolus. During the next few hours, the patient receives 3 units of packed red blood cells, 12 units of fresh frozen plasma, 1 unit of platelets, and 10 units of cryoprecipitate. On the third postoperative day, you discharge her from the ICU to the postpartum ward, and the patient then experiences a relatively normal postpartum course. On the ward, her husband asks if she should attempt to have other children.

 Decision 3: Counseling

How should an AFE survivor be counseled about future pregnancy?

A. The condition is likely to recur if she attempts another pregnancy.
B. The condition is unlikely to recur if she attempts another pregnancy.
C. There is limited information, but recurrence appears likely.
D. There is limited information, but recurrence appears unlikely.

Mediators of Anaphylactoid Syndrome of Pregnancy

Amniotic Fluid Components

In Solution (biochemical mediators)

Surfactant
Endothelin
Leukotrienes
IL-1 and TNFα
Thromboxane A2
Prostaglandins
Arachidonic acid
Thromboplastin
Collagen and tissue factor III
Phospholipase A2
PF III

In Suspension (mechanical mediators)

Lanugo hair
Vernix
Fetal cells
Meconium
Fetal mucin
Trophoblasts

Figure 38.4 Presumed mediators of the anaphylactoid syndrome of pregnancy. Adapted from theories of Clark, SL.

The correct answer is D: There are fewer than 10 cases of pregnancy after AFE in the literature, with no clear cases of recurrence. Although encouraging, this data is insufficient to support a conclusion that pregnancy is safe after AFE. Many AFE survivors also have significant neurologic and psychological sequelae of the event, and these may impact on the advisability of future pregnancy.

 CASE CONCLUSION

On postpartum day 5, both Ms. Ruiz and her infant are discharged home. You arrange with your office a follow-up for Ms. Ruiz in 1 week to check her surgical wound and to assess her coping. In addition, she is given a follow-up appointment with a psychotherapist, at her request, to help her to deal with depression and anxiety following the event. Finally, she is to be followed by the neurologist to assess her cognitive functioning.

SUGGESTED READINGS

Clark J, But M. Maternal collapse. Curr Opin Obstet Gynecol. 2006; 17:157–60.

Clark SL. New concepts of amniotic fluid embolism: a review. Obstet Gynecol Surv. 1990;45:360–8.

Clark SL, Hankins GD, Dudley DA, Dildy GA, Porter TF. Amniotic fluid embolism: analysis of the national registry. Am J Obstet Gynecol. 1995;172:1159–69.

Davies S. Amniotic fluid embolus: a review of literature. Can J Anaesth. 2001;48:88–98.

Electronic fetal heart rate monitoring: research guidelines for interpretation. National Institute of Child Health and Human Development Research Planning Workshop. Am J Obstet Gynecol. 1997;177(6): 1385–90.

Meyer JR. Embolus pulmonar-caseosa. Braz J Med Bio Res. 1926;2: 301–3.

Moore J, Baldisseri MR. Amniotic fluid embolism. Crit Care Med. 2005;33:S279–85.

Perozzi KJ, Englert NC. Amniotic fluid embolism: an obstetric emergency. Crit Care Nurse. 2004;4:54–61.

Westgate JA, Wibbens B, Bennet L, Wassink G, Parer JT, Gunn AJ. The intrapartum deceleration in center stage: a physiologic approach to the interpretation of fetal heart rate changes in labor. Am J Obstet Gynecol. 2007;197(3):236.e1–11.

Operative Delivery

John Richard

39

CASE PRESENTATION

Ms. Johnson, a 32-year-old G1 P0 woman at 38 weeks of estimated gestational age presents to labor and delivery with chief complaint of regular uterine contractions every 5 to 6 minutes. She reports that contractions began approximately 6 hours ago and have become increasingly painful over the past hour. She states that the fetus has been moving well and denies fluid loss. She reports no significant past medical history and no problems during this pregnancy. Your evaluation reveals that the cervix is dilated to 5 cm, is 75% effaced, and the fetal vertex is at 0 station. The estimated fetal weight by Leopold's maneuvers (manual palpation) is 3,600 g. You elect to admit Ms. Johnson, believing that she is in active labor.

After 6 hours of active labor, Ms. Johnson is found to be fully dilated. The fetal vertex is now at +1−2 station (of 5) and is noted to be in the left occiput anterior position. The head descends well with each maternal contraction, and you have Ms. Johnson begin to push. At this point (the commencement of the second stage of labor) the fetal heart tracing shows a baseline of 140 bpm, normal variability, and occasional accelerations. Contractions are every 2 minutes. The patient has an epidural that provides adequate pain relief, but the patient is still aware of her contractions.

After approximately 30 minutes of effective pushing, the fetal heart tracing demonstrates a deceleration to 60 bpm, continuing now for 2 minutes. You are called urgently to evaluate. The fetal vertex is +1 to +2 station, and still left occiput anterior. The maternal pelvis is gynecoid.

Decision 1: Management

What immediate **delivery** options are available at this time?

A. Cesarean delivery
B. Vacuum delivery
C. Midpelvic forceps
D. Low forceps

The correct answer is C: Midpelvic forceps and **A:** Cesarean section. The fetus is experiencing a severe deceleration, which will ultimately result in fetal acidemia if not

corrected. In this situation, steps should be undertaken to attempt to resolve the deceleration. These steps could include repositioning the patient, administration of oxygen by nasal cannula, or possibly administration of a quick-acting tocolytic agent such as terbutaline. Should these interventions not be effective, consideration should be taken for immediate delivery. Because the fetus has achieved a positive station, delivery could be facilitated via forceps in skilled hands. Fetuses at this high station are frequently in a mal-rotated state, as internal rotation has not been completed by this time, especially in multiparous patients. For such cases, a rotational maneuver with forceps may be required before delivery can be safely accomplished. When this level of expertise is not available, or if the patient is not a candidate for forceps delivery for other reasons, a cesarean delivery is appropriate if the fetal heart rate deceleration cannot be resolved.

In the present case, answer D is not correct, as the fetus has not descended far enough in the pelvis for a low forceps delivery, and answer B is less correct, as the vacuum extractor is unlikely to effect delivery rapidly from this station in a primigravida.

NEED TO KNOW

Types of Instrumental Deliveries

Instrumental (or operative vaginal) deliveries require that the cervix be fully dilated, the fetal vertex engaged, and the position known, that the mother consent to the procedure and have anesthesia adequate for the procedure to be performed. Operative vaginal deliveries are categorized both by the station and position of the fetal head and by the instrument used. The categories used are "outlet," "low," or "mid" pelvic, depending on the station of the fetal head at the time of application of the instrument and on the degree of rotation of the fetal head necessary to effect delivery (Table 39.1). Indications for instrumental delivery include (1) prolonged second stage of labor, (2) suspicion of fetal compromise, and (3) shortening the second stage for maternal benefit.

CLASSIFICATION OF FORCEPS DELIVERY (AMERICAN COLLEGE OF OB/GYN)[a]

Criteria for Types of Forceps Deliveries

Outlet Forceps
1. Scalp is visible at the introitus without separating labia.
2. Fetal skull has reached pelvic floor.
3. Sagittal suture is in anteroposterior diameter or right or left occiput anterior or posterior position.
4. Fetal head is at or on perineum.
5. Rotation does not exceed 45°.

Low Forceps
1. Leading point of fetal skull is at station $\geq$+2 cm and not on the pelvic floor.
2. Rotation is 45° or less (left or right occiput anterior to occiput anterior, or left or right occiput posterior to occiput posterior).
3. Rotation is greater than 45°.

Midforceps
Station is above +2 cm but head is engaged.

[a]High forceps refer to procedures performed when the fetal vertex is above 0 station; these are associated with an unacceptable degree of risk to the fetus and are not considered a part of current practice.

The risk of an instrumental delivery to both mother and fetus increases with higher station and greater degree of rotation, therefore the expected benefit must be greater to justify instrumental delivery at a higher station.

CASE CONTINUES

Ms. Johnson is instructed to stop pushing with each contraction. She complies and completes a rest period of 15 minutes, during which time the monitoring demonstrates good return to baseline with intermittent accelerations, a reassuring pattern. Pushing resumes, and the patient pushes for an additional 45 minutes. The vertex is now at +3 station, position confirmed to be direct occiput anterior. At this time the fetal heart rate again demonstrates another severe deceleration to 60 bpm, lasting 2 minutes.

Decision 2: Treatment

What delivery options are available from +3 station?

A. Mid forceps rotation
B. Vacuum delivery
C. Low forceps
D. Cesarean section

Both B: Vacuum delivery **and C:** Low forceps are viable options. In the current case the patient has achieved a deep positive station and requires no rotation to achieve delivery. Either instrument will suffice, with the choice being left to operator preference. It is important to note the differences in complications for each instrument. For the vacuum, complications include cephalohematoma, subgaleal hemorrhage, retinal hemorrhage, and intracranial hemorrhage. Forceps also increase maternal pelvic trauma, and carry additional risks for facial lacerations and bruising, facial nerve palsies, and, rarely, skull fracture. It is believed that with the vacuum it is easier to place the instrument, and that the patient may require less anesthesia for a successful delivery. The relative severity and frequency of each complication balances equally between the two, and, as stated previously, the instrument used is largely a choice based on operator preference and experience.

N E E D   T O   K N O W

Indications/Contraindications for Instrumental Delivery

As described above, indications for instrumental delivery include (1) prolonged second stage of labor, (2) suspicion of fetal compromise, and (3) shortening the second stage for maternal benefit. Therefore, instrumental delivery may be indicated under circumstances of nonreassuring fetal status remote from delivery, maternal exhaustion, arrest of descent in certain circumstances, or any condition in the mother that precludes Valsalva maneuver. In the current example, the use of forceps would be indicated because of the fetal deceleration with accompanying concern for fetal compromise.

Maternal exhaustion is another common indication for forceps or vacuum, and this condition is typically described as the mother's inability to continue pushing efforts. Care must be taken in this circumstance that the maternal pelvis and fetal size are evaluated to assess if vaginal delivery is likely, as maternal exhaustion can be an indicator of cephalopelvic disproportion. Evaluation of the progress of labor can also be helpful with this assessment.

Arrest of descent may be the result of many factors, either in isolation or in combination. These include cephalopelvic disproportion or maternal exhaustion. However, a common cause of arrest of descent involves malposition of the fetal head such as occiput transverse or posterior position, or asynclitism of the fetal head. Asynclitism is a common condition, especially in rapid deliveries, in which the planes of the fetal head are not parallel to the planes of the maternal pelvis. This results in a presenting diameter of the fetal head, which is larger than it would be if the fetal head was aligned correctly. Malposition of the fetal head represents a correctable cause of arrest of descent, as the use of forceps allows correction of the malposition prior to delivery.

Contraindications to operative vaginal deliveries include any contraindication to vaginal delivery. In addition, a fetal bleeding diathesis or bone mineralization defect is a contraindication. Vacuum extraction is considered inappropriate for a fetus at <34 weeks of gestation. Although special forceps are designed for preterm babies, they typically are not appropriate for gestations <32 weeks. Operative vaginal delivery is also contraindicated with an unengaged fetal head or when the cervix is not completely dilated.

CASE CONTINUES

The fetal heart pattern again recovers after a brief rest period and the patient resumes pushing. After approximately 1 hour of continuous pushing effort the patient becomes visibly exhausted, and descent with each push is noticeably less. At this time, the fetal vertex is visible at the introitus, but the patient states that she cannot continue pushing any longer.

Decision 3: Options

What are delivery options at this point?

A. Mid forceps rotation
B. Vacuum delivery
C. Outlet forceps
D. Cesarean section

Both B: Vacuum delivery *and C:* Outlet forceps are viable options. As with decision 2, either vacuum or forceps would be appropriate in this case, with choice left to operator preference. In this case, maternal exhaustion would be the indication for the operative delivery with a proposed outlet procedure. Because of the ready availability of the vacuum in most delivery suites, it would be the most likely choice. However, the above situation can also be resolved with the use of forceps. In either case,

instrumental delivery from the outlet station is associated with a similar risk compared with spontaneous vaginal delivery.

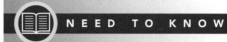

Instruments Available for Operative Delivery

The instruments available for instrumental delivery include the vacuum and forceps, both of which include several types. Vacuum cups may include rigid or flexible cups in a variety of shapes and sizes. Suction is provided either by an external vacuum pump attached by a hose or a smaller, hand-held device connected to the cup (Fig. 39.1). Both devices are still in common use, with the hand-held devices becoming increasingly more common. In use, the vacuum is applied to the fetal vertex at the median flexion point (in the midline about 2 cm anterior to the posterior fontanelle. Suction is applied with a pump, and traction is applied during maternal pushing (Fig. 39.2).

Forceps can generally be classified as either being "classic" or special purpose (Fig. 39.3). Those types in the classic group are designed to deliver only a fetus in the vertex position, and for which no rotation is required. The classic group includes such forceps as Simpson, McLane-Tucker, and others. Special purpose forceps, as the name implies, are designed for a specific task. For example, Keilland forceps are used in rotational maneuvers for fetuses with a malrotation of the fetal vertex. Piper forceps are only designed to deliver the after-following head in a breech delivery. In use, the two halves of the forceps are placed in the posterior vagina and advanced to the side of the fetal head. After the forceps are adjusted to be symmetrical on the fetal head, traction is applied to the fetal head (Fig. 39.4).

Forceps are divided into three parts: the blades, the shanks, and the handles (Fig. 39.5). The blades will generally have a similar shape, but a great deal of variation occurs with the curvature, fenestration, and size. Fenestrated blades may give a better grip on the fetal head, allowing for more traction. Variation also exists in the shanks of the instruments, where the locking device for the blades is found. Simpson forceps have overlapping shanks with considerable space between to allow for fetal caput, whereas McLane forceps have little room for caput, but distend the vaginal opening much less. Locks can be either rigid, sometimes describes as an "English" lock, or sliding, which allow for correction of asynclitism, as in the Keilland forceps. Handles can also vary widely in shape.

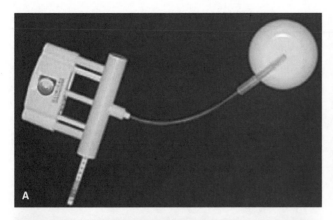

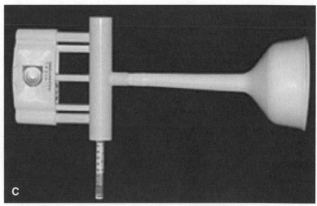

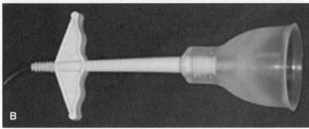

Figure 39.1 Vacuum extraction. Different cup shapes have been developed. The flat cup **(A)** has been developed to allow for placement of the vacuum on a part of the fetal head not directly presenting. **B** and **C** represent two types of soft cups; **B** is designed to be used with a separate suction pump, **C** has a hand-held pump attached. From Hook CD, Damos JR. Vacuum-assisted vaginal delivery. Am Fam Physician. 2008;78(8):953–60.

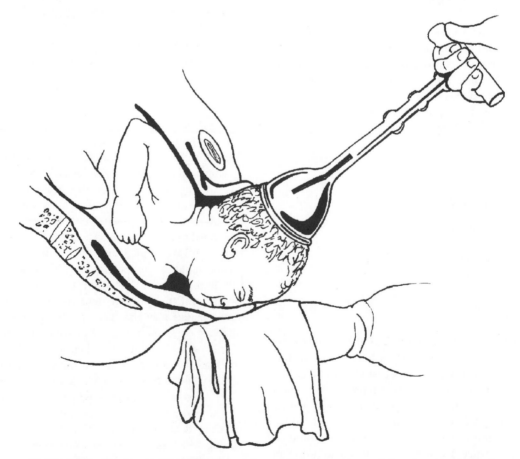

Figure 39.2 The vacuum in use. The device is inserted into the vagina and placed against the fetal head. Suction is applied. With maternal pushing, traction is applied to the cup and fetal head. The cup is removed after delivery of the fetal head. (copyright fotosearch).

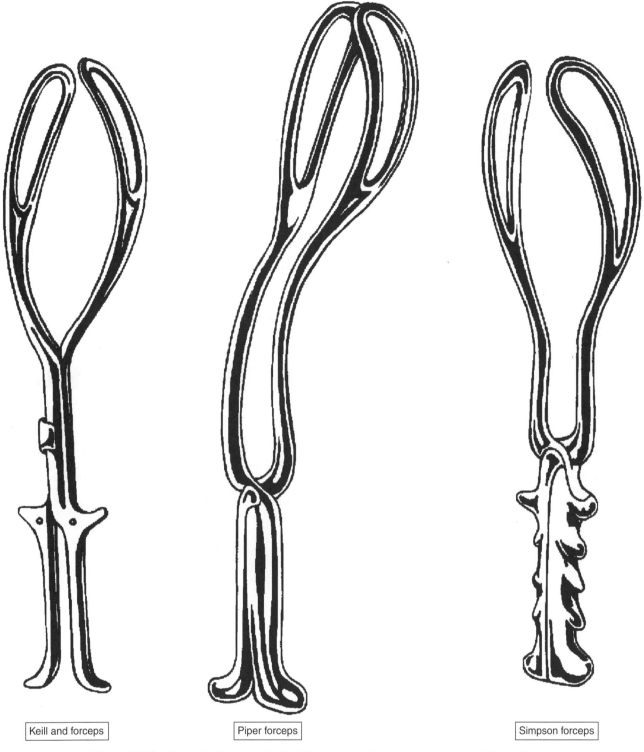

Keill and forceps

Piper forceps

Simpson forceps

Figure 39.3 Obstetrical forceps. Keilland forceps are designed for rotation of the fetal head within the maternal pelvis. Piper forceps are for the after-coming head of a breech birth. Simpson forceps have an elongated cephalic curve for delivery of a molded head, whereas other types, such as McLean forceps are designed for the rounded head of the fetus of a multigravida. Any of the fenestrated forceps (with a hole in the blade) may be made in the Luikart variation, with a ridge inside the bladeand no fenestration. (copyright fotosearch).

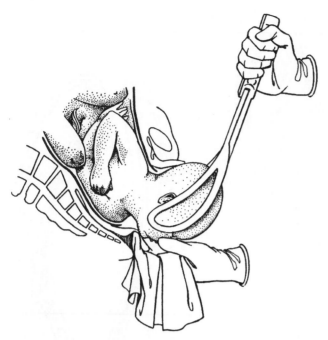

Figure 39.4 Obstetrical forceps in use. The instrument is placed into the vagina, one blade at a time, and adjusted until the blades are symmetrically placed on the fetal head. Traction is then applied to the fetal head to effect delivery. (copyright fotosearch)

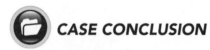 **CASE CONCLUSION**

Simpson forceps were applied and an outlet forceps delivery was completed. Traction was applied with maternal expulsive effort, and the fetal head delivered

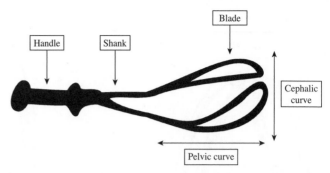

Figure 39.5 Parts of Simpson forceps (labeled). The cephalic curve fits the fetal head. The pelvic curve follows the maternal pelvis in this instrument not intended for rotational maneuvers. (copyright fotosearch)

on the third attempt. Forceps were disengaged, and the remainder of the fetus delivered without difficulty over a second-degree perineal laceration. Examination of the fetus demonstrated superficial indentations over the bilateral malar eminences, indicting appropriate placement.

SUGGESTED READINGS

ACOG Practice Bulletin No. 17: June 2000. Operative Vaginal Delivery.

Dennen PC. Dennen's Forceps Deliveries. Philadelphia, PA: F.A. Days Co; 1989.

Goetzinger KR, Macones GA. Operative vaginal delivery: current trends in obstetrics. Women's Health. 2008;4(3):281–90.

Laufe L, Berkus B. Assisted Vaginal Delivery: Obstetric forceps and Vacuum Extraction Techniques. Columbus, OH, McGraw-Hill; 1992.

Towner DR, Ciotti MC. Operative vaginal delivery: a cause of birth injury or is it? Clin Obstet Gynecol. 2007;50(3):563–8.

Breastfeeding

Jennifer Benedict

40

CASE PRESENTATION

You are at the bedside of Ms. DiGregorio, a 32-year-old G1 P1 who had a primary cesarean delivery for arrest of dilation yesterday. She delivered a healthy baby girl weighing 3,600 g with Apgar scores of 9 and 9 at one and five minutes. Ms. DiGregorio considered breastfeeding while she was pregnant, but is now ambivalent. Her mother did not breastfeed, but one of her sisters successfully breastfed two children. She is concerned about the antibiotics and pain medication she is currently taking and worries that she will be too uncomfortable with a recent abdominal incision. She wants to know if it is really important to breastfeed her infant. How would you counsel her?

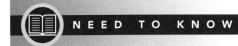

NEED TO KNOW

Advantages of Breastfeeding

The advantages of breastfeeding can be broken up into two categories; benefits to the mother and benefits to the newborn. Benefits to the mother include enhanced bonding, decreased postpartum blood loss, and more rapid uterine involution. As the baby feeds, he or she stimulates the release of prolactin (milk production hormone) and oxytocin (milk ejection hormone). Oxytocin stimulates the myoepithelial cells to contract around the alveoli, pushing the milk down through the ducts to the lactiferous sinuses, and it also stimulates the uterus to contract.

In addition, women who breastfeed may have a decreased risk of developing ovarian and premenopausal breast cancers. Mothers can also use breastfeeding as a natural means of family spacing, although not as effective as other methods. Mothers who breastfeed exclusively during the first 6 months with no signs of menstruation reduce the likelihood of pregnancy to <2%. Finally, breastfeeding is the least expensive and one of the safest sources of nutrition for the infant.

Women who breastfeed do not have to spend additional time or money preparing formula and cleaning bottles, and they do not have to worry about formula becoming contaminated through poor storage.

The newborn who breastfeeds benefits from a myriad of improved health outcomes. Colostrum, the first product of the breast after parturition, is a rich source of antibodies for the newborn. There is strong evidence that breastfeeding decreases the incidence and/or severity of diarrhea, lower respiratory tract infection, otitis media, bacteremia, bacterial meningitis, botulism, urinary tract infection, and necrotizing enterocolitis. Many studies show a possible protective effect against sudden infant death syndrome, insulin-dependent diabetes mellitus, Crohn's disease, ulcerative colitis, and allergic diseases. Breastfeeding has also been related to possible enhancement of cognitive development.

Every patient should be counseled about all of these benefits both to her and her newborn. The very best time to discuss the mother's breastfeeding plans is during routine prenatal care visits. By discussing breastfeeding prior to the birth of the baby the mother has the opportunity to ask questions and the provider can address any concerns she may have. The provider should also identify additional resources to support her decision to breastfeed; in this case the patient's sister would be an excellent resource.

CASE CONTINUES

During the first postoperative days, Ms. DiGregorio takes hydrocodone bitartrate and acetaminophen (Vicodin) two tablets as needed every 6 hours for pain and ibuprofen (Motrin) 600 mg three times a day. One of the nurses told her that the baby may become sleepy if she breastfeeds while she is taking so much pain medication. She usually needs at least five tablets of Vicodin a day and she is very concerned about how this might affect her baby.

❓ Decision 1: Counseling

How would you advise your patient about breastfeeding while on pain medication?

A. Withhold breastfeeding if breastfeeding is painful
B. Refuse narcotics
C. Supplement the infant with formula while she is on narcotics
D. Withhold breastfeeding if infant is lethargic

The correct answer is D: The patient should not refuse narcotics if they are needed for postoperative pain control. Oral narcotics (fentanyl, codeine, propoxyphene, methadone, morphine) are excreted into breast milk, but at low concentrations and have short half-lives. They are compatible with breastfeeding. Meperidine may accumulate in breast milk with repetitive use and should be avoided in breastfeeding mothers. Nonsteroidal anti-inflammatory drugs have short half-lives and primarily inert metabolites. They are excreted into breast milk in low or undetectable amounts and are compatible with breastfeeding. A few general guidelines for breastfeeding and medication use are as follows:

1. Avoid drugs with long half-lives or sustained-release preparations.
2. Take the lowest dose possible for the shortest period of time necessary.
3. Take the medication just after breastfeeding so that the lowest concentration is transferred into the milk.

The mother should be educated about potential side effects in the infant as a result of drugs that have been prescribed for her. Many women are anxious about breastfeeding while taking medications but may not express this and may not ask about potential side effects to the baby. It is important to address the topic before the medication is initiated to minimize any disruption in breastfeeding. The mother should be advised that narcotics may cause lethargy in the infant, and if this is noted breastfeeding may be held until the infant is alert.

If the patient is complaining of pain with breastfeeding, observe her during a feeding to ensure that the baby is correctly latching on. The infant obtains milk during breastfeeding by compressing the breast between the palate and the tongue, which is forcefully stroked down the areola. A common problem is the baby latching onto only the tip of the nipple, which can cause pain. If the baby is latched on correctly, then the baby's nose just touches the breast, the lips are flanged out like "fish lips," the chin is against the breast and more areola is visible above the upper lip than below the lower lip as seen in Figure 40.1.

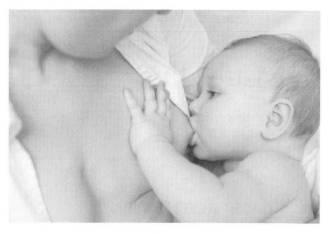

Figure 40.1 Breastfeeding infant. Note that nearly the entire areola of the breast is in the infant's mouth. (Shutterstock Image ID 55166842)

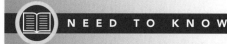

NEED TO KNOW

Drugs Contraindicated in Lactation

Very few drugs are strictly contraindicated during lactation. As a general rule, if a drug is prescribed for infants then it is not contraindicated during breastfeeding. The American Academy of Pediatrics Committee on Drugs publishes a list of drugs and chemicals that are transferred into human milk. The list is divided into those that are contraindicated, drugs of abuse, those that require temporary cessation of breastfeeding, drugs with unknown effects that may be of concern, and drugs that should be given with caution. Many antianxiety, antidepressant, and antipsychotic medications are classified as drugs of concern. Of the antidepressants, many have been associated with birth defects when used during pregnancy, but their long-term effects are not known. Fluoxetine has been reported to be associated with colic, irritability, feeding, sleep disorders, and slow weight gain. Table 40.1 is an abbreviated summary of commonly used drugs that are contraindicated or should be used with caution. (For the full list please see: American Academy of Pediatrics. The transfer of drugs and other chemicals into human milk.)

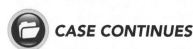

🗂 CASE CONTINUES

Ms. DiGregorio has an uneventful postoperative course and is ready for discharge on postoperative day 4. During her hospital stay, she has received assistance from the

TABLE 40.1

EXAMPLES OF THE CATEGORIES OF DRUGS IN BREASTFEEDING

Drug	Effect on Infant
Drugs that require temporary or total cessation of breastfeeding	
Cyclophosphamide	Possible immune suppression; unknown effect on growth or association with carcinogenesis; neutropenia
Doxorubicin	Possible immune suppression; unknown effect on growth or association with carcinogenesis
Iodine 123	Radioactivity in milk present up to 36 hr
Radioactive sodium	Radioactivity in milk present 96 hr
Technetium 99 m	Radioactivity in milk present 15 hr to 3 d
Drugs of abuse with reported adverse effects on the infant	
Amphetamine	Irritability, poor sleeping pattern
Cocaine	Cocaine intoxication
Heroin	Tremors, restlessness, vomiting, poor feeding
Marijuana	Only one report in the literature; no effect mentioned; very long half-life for some components
Phencyclidine	Potent hallucinogen
Drugs associated with significant effects on infants and should be given with caution	
Aspirin	Metabolic acidosis (one case)
Atenolol	Cyanosis; bradycardia
Bromocriptine	Suppresses lactation
Ergotamine	Vomiting, diarrhea, convulsions (doses used in migraine medications)
Lithium	One third to one half of therapeutic blood concentrations in infants
Phenobarbital	Sedation; infantile spasms after weaning from milk
Primidone	Sedation, feeding problems
Sulfasalazine	Bloody diarrhea (one case)
Drugs for which the effect on nursing infants is unknown but may be of concern	
Diazepam	None
Fluoxetine	Colic, irritability, feeding and sleep disorders, slow weight gain
Imipramine	None
Paroxetine	None
Amiodarone	Possible hypothyroidism

Adapted from American Academy of Pediatrics Committee on Drugs. Transfer of drugs and other chemicals into human milk. Pediatrics. 2001;108(3):776–89.

nurses several times a day to help her with breastfeeding the baby. Her sister visited her in the hospital and has stated that she will be available to help continue breastfeeding at home. You also give her information on community resources, including a referral to the lactation consultant.

Ms. DiGregorio remains a little anxious about having to breastfeed the baby on her own. You want to ease her anxiety by explaining what problems are concerning and reviewing some things that she might notice but are actually normal.

Decision 2: Abnormalities

What should the patient call about after she goes home?

A. Breasts different sizes
B. Infant not sleeping more than 4 hours
C. Milk leaking from breasts
D. Infant eating every hour

The correct answer is D: From 4 hours after birth through day 4 of life it is expected that the baby will breastfeed every 1.5 to 3 hours (8–12 times in 24 hours). On day 5 of life the baby may have one longer interval of up to 5 hours, but this may not happen before 2 to 3 months for some infants. A baby who is feeding every hour may be feeding too frequently, indicating that the infant is not getting sufficiently full at each feeding. This may be due to the infant not fully emptying the breast or the infant not latching on appropriately. Patients should also be instructed to report increasing breast tenderness and redness or fever, which may indicate mastitis.

With initiation of lactation, there is normally an increase in the size of the breasts, and this may be asymmetrical. In the absence of signs of infection, this is not of concern. Similarly, leakage of milk from the breasts is common, and is not of concern, although it may be helpful to use absorbent pads so as to keep the breasts dry. Other common discomforts include uterine contractions, which are a consequence of the oxytocin released with breastfeeding, and nipple soreness. Many patients complain of sore nipples after several days of breastfeeding.

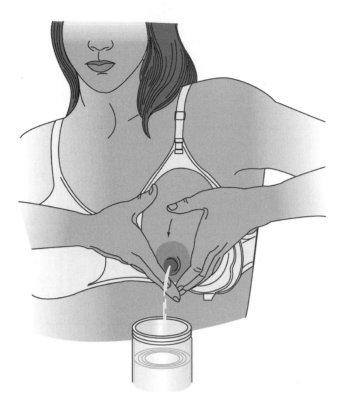

Figure 40.2 Manual expression of breast milk. The left hand supports the breast, while the fingers of the right hand compress the areola, expressing milk. In practice, the milk is collected in a clean bottle or storage container. (fotosearch.com/LIF139/nu118002/)

Improper latching on, with direct contact of the infant's tongue to the nipple may be contribute to this, but many patients experience sore nipples even with proper latching. Sore nipples may be helped by keeping the nipples dry, and with the use of lanolin cream. The patient should be cautioned against using other preparations, as anything put on the nipples will go into the infant's mouth. Except in very unusual circumstances, it's better not to feed the infant with a bottle, even with bottled breast milk, as exposure to artificial nipples has been shown to reduce the duration of breastfeeding.

NEED TO KNOW

Collection and Storage of Breast Milk (Breast Pumping)

Breast milk can be collected in several ways. First, it can be expressed by hand and the technique can be mastered with only a little practice. When using hand expression, the mother should be instructed to apply warm compresses to the breast then massage each quadrant of the breast. Then, the thumb and forefingers of one hand are placed in opposition (e.g., one at 12 and one at 6 o'clock) about 1 to 1.5 inches behind the nipple and the other hand is used to push straight against the chest wall. The mother leans over and directs sprays of milk into a container (Fig. 40.2).

Breast milk can also be collected with a manual pump shown in Figure 40.3. Manual pumps are usually less expensive than electric pumps and are lightweight and easily portable. They may require significant energy to use. Mothers who only occasionally need to pump are good candidates for a hand pump.

There are also battery-operated and electric pumps. Hospital-grade electric pumps are the gold standard for pumps and may be easier for the mother because they require less mechanical effort on her part. One disadvantage is the cost; however, insurance or social programs will sometimes cover the cost of a breast pump rental.

Breast milk can be stored at room temperature for up to 4 hours in sealed, sterile containers, stored in the refrigerator for 48 hours or in the freezer for 3 months. Milk should be thawed rapidly by placing the container under running tepid water. Milk should not be thawed in a microwave. After milk has been thawed it can be stored for up to 24 hours in a refrigerator.

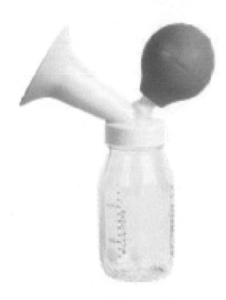

Example of a bicycle horn pump

Figure 40.3 Manual breast pump (there are a number of different designs). (www.fda.gov/MedicalDevices/ProductsandMedicalProcedures/HomeHealthandConsumer/ConsumerProducts/BreastPumps/ucm061584.htm (public domain)).

CASE CONTINUES

Ms. DiGregorio decides to resume work after 6 weeks. She had asked her employer about breastfeeding facilities and was informed that her company provides a lactation room that she could use to express her milk as needed. She purchases an electric pump and uses it to express her breast milk when she is away from home. She went back to work requesting that the first few days of work be half-days so that the transition would be gradual. The baby did well with the transition and successfully bottle feeds while the patient is at work and breastfeeds when she is at home. However, she reports that the infant is fussy and wants to feed much more often.

 ## Decision 3: Problems

What is your response to an increase in newborn hunger?

A. This is unexpected, probably due to maternal work schedule.

B. This is unexpected, probably due to reduced maternal milk supply.

C. This is expected, probably due to separation from infant.

D. This is expected, probably due to newborn growth spurt.

The answer is D: There are transient periods of time when the baby demands to feed more often. This will happen several times in the first 3 months (typically at 2–3 weeks, 6 weeks, and 3 months). The mother may feel that she has lost her milk supply because the baby has become fussy and suddenly wants to feed more often, and this may lead to her abandoning breastfeeding, or supplementing with formula. Although maternal work per se will have no effect on milk supply, return to work is a time at which cessation of breastfeeding may occur, due both to the fetal growth spurt described, and to a reduction in maternal breast stimulation. Milk should be expressed at least once every 4 hours when the mother and infant are separated (the same frequency that the infant would be expected to feed). More frequent emptying of the breast will stimulate a larger milk supply. The infant should be allowed to breastfeed as often as desired in the evening and overnight to encourage continued milk supply. Having the baby close by at night may help to facilitate frequent feedings. Anticipatory guidance regarding normal infant feeding patterns often helps mothers avoid unnecessary supplementation and premature weaning. If the problem persists for more than 3 or 4 days, then the mother and infant should be evaluated to determine the adequacy of the mother's milk supply and the infant's weight gain.

 ## CASE CONCLUSION

The patient continues to successfully breastfeed her infant and at 6 months of age begins introducing complementary foods rich in iron. When she saw you for her 6 week postpartum visit she inquired about the recommended length of time for breastfeeding. You counseled her that the American Academy of Pediatrics recommends breastfeeding for at least the first year of life and beyond for as long as mutually desired. She continues to breastfeed and decides to wean her infant at 1 year of age.

SUGGESTED READINGS

American Academy of Pediatrics. Breastfeeding and the use of human milk. Pediatrics. 2005;115:496–506.

American Academy of Pediatrics. The transfer of drugs and other chemicals into human milk. Pediatrics. 2001;108:776–89.

Biancuzzo M. Breastfeeding the Newborn. St. Louis: Mosby Inc.; 1999.

Collaborative Group on Hormonal Factors in Breast Cancer. Breast cancer and breastfeeding: collaborative reanalysis of individual data from 47 epidemiological studies in 30 countries, including 50302 women with breast cancer and 96973 women without the disease. Lancet. 2002;360(9328):187–95.

Danforth KN, Tworoger SS, Hecht JL, Rosner BA, Colditz GA, Hankinson SE. Breastfeeding and risk of ovarian cancer in two prospective cohorts. Cancer Causes Control. 2007;18:517–23.

Goldfarb J, Tibbetts E. Breastfeeding Handbook. Berkeley Heights, NJ: Enslow Publishers; 1980.

Lawrence RA, Lawrence RM. Breastfeeding A Guide for the Medical Profession. 6th ed. Philadelphia, PA: Mosby, Inc.: 2005.

LaCerva V, Breastfeeding A Manual for Health Professionals. New York, NY: Medical Examination Publishing Co., Inc.; 1981.

Riordan J, Auerbach K. Breastfeeding and Human Lactation. 2nd ed. Boston: Jones and Bartlett Publishers; 1999.

Schanler R, ed. Breastfeeding Handbook for Physicians. Washington, DC: American Academy of Pediatrics and The American College of Obstetricians and Gynecologists; 2006.

Wellstart International. Lactation Management Self-Study Modules, Level I. 2nd ed. San Diego, CA: Wellstart International; 2004.

Index

Note: Page locators followed by f and t indicate figures and tables respectively.

A

Abacavir, 84
Abdominal cerclage, 140
Abdominal pain, diagnosis of, 51
Abdominal surgery, maternal, 50
Abnormal labor
 active phase of labor, 192
 Bishop score, 189t, 190t
 case presentation, 188, 191, 193, 194
 labor induction/augmentation, 189–190
 latent phase of labor, 190–191
 patient management, 188, 191–192, 194
 second stage of labor, 192–193
Access express HIV-1 test system, 83
Acetylcholinesterase, 92
ACLS. See Advanced cardiac life support
ACOG. See American College of Obstetricians and Gynecologists
Active preterm labor, 139
Acute abdominal pain
 anesthesia in pregnancy, 90
 case presentation, 87, 89, 91
 differential diagnosis of, 87, 88f
 patient management, 88–89
 during delivery, 90–91
 during surgery, 89–90
Acute appendicitis, 87
Acute respiratory distress syndrome (ARDS), 15
Acute severe hypertension, treatment for, 21t
Adnexal masses in pregnancy, 49, 49t, 50f
Advanced cardiac life support (ACLS), 64
AFE. See Amniotic fluid embolism
Agenerase (amprenavir), 84
Agranulocytosis, 77
Albuterol, inhaled, 7, 8
Algorithms, fetal weight calculation for, 110t
American Academy of Pediatrics Committee on Drugs, 226
American College of Obstetricians and Gynecologists (ACOG), 12, 56, 63, 114, 146, 156, 157t, 195
 guidelines for perinatal care of, 154
American Heart Association, 64, 65t
American Red Cross criteria, the, 82
American Society for Reproductive Medicine, the, 150
Amniocentesis, 43, 94, 122
Amnioinfusion, 124
Amnioreduction, 128, 139
Amniotic fluid bilirubin, 43, 44

Amniotic fluid dynamics, 126–128
Amniotic fluid embolism (AFE), 64
 about future pregnancy, 217–218
 case presentation, 213, 214f, 215, 217
 diagnosis of, 215
 FHR bradycardia, management of, 213
 laboratory investigation in, 216t
 management of, 215–216, 216t
 pathophysiology of, 216
 prolonged FHR decelerations, 213–215
 risk factors for, 216t
Amniotic fluid index (AFI), 27, 119, 120f, 125
 over gestation, 126f
 single deepest pocket of, 125
Amniotic fluid volume, 119, 125, 126f
 normal in human pregnancy, 120f
 perinatal mortality related to, 123t
 ultrasound examination of, 154
Ampicillin, 14
Anaphylactoid syndrome of pregnancy, 216, 217f
Anemia, 15
 fetal, 128
Anencephaly, 160
Anesthesia, 29, 50
 in pregnancy, 90
Aneuploidy, 133
Angiotens-in-converting enzyme inhibitors, 121
Antenatal corticosteroids, 158
Antenatal fetal surveillance, 83
Antenatal testing. See under Postdated pregnancy
Antepartum surveillance, 77
Antibiotic prophylaxis, 5
Antibiotics, 141, 148, 158
Antibodies, atypical, 42t
Anticoagulation therapy, 56
Antidepressants, 226
Antihuman immunoglobulin, 81
Apgar scores, 114
Appendicitis, acute, 87
ARDS. See Acute respiratory distress syndrome
Arms of breech, delivery of, 163f
ASB. See Asymptomatic bacteriuria1
Aspirin, 57
Asthma
 management of, 8
 maternal obesity in, 10
 prognosis of, 10–11
 stages, definition of, 9t
 step therapy of, 9t
 triggers, category of, 8t

 See also Pulmonary disease
Asymptomatic bacteriuria (ASB), 12–13
Azithromycin, 68

B

Back-down transverse lie, 163, 164f
Bacterial vaginosis (BV), 143
Barnum maneuver, 200
Beckwith–Weidemann syndrome (BWS), 114
Benzathine penicillin, 72t
Beta–blockers, 77
Betamethasone, 146
Bicornuate uterus, 151
Bimanual compression of uterus, 205f
Bilirubin, 43
Biophysical profile (BPP), 184t, 185, 186f
Birth injury rate, 115t
Bisacromial diameter (shoulders) of fetus, 196
Bishop score, 189, 189t, 190t
Bladder injury, 210
Blood
 replacement in DIC, 180, 180t
 transfusion, 172
Blood loss at delivery, average, 203t
Blood sugar management, 36
Blood urea nitrogen (BUN), 12
Blunt force trauma, 61
B-Lynch suture, 206
BMI. See Body mass index
Body mass index (BMI), 32, 115
BPP. See Biophysical profile
Bradycardia, 213
Breastfeeding, 39
 abnormalities, 227–228
 advantages of, 225
 case presentation, 225, 226, 229
 collection and storage of breast milk, 228, 228f
 drugs contraindicated in lactation, 226, 227t
 as mother on pain medication, 226, 226f
 in newborn hunger, 229
Breast milk, collection and storage of, 228, 228f
Breech presentation
back-down transverse lie, 163, 164f
 case presentation, 160, 161, 163, 164
 definition of, 160
 diagnosis of, 160
 facts regarding
 breech delivery technique, 162, 163f
 external cephalic version, 162, 162f

Breech presentation (*Continued*)
  patient advice with breech, 161
  patient management, 161
  premature fetuses, 161t
  types of, 160, 161f
Bronchoconstrictor, 11
BWS. *See* Beckwith-Weidemann
    syndrome

C

Calcium channel blocker, 147
Carboprost tromethamine (hemabate), 11
Cardiac arrest, 215
Cardiac disease
  case presentation, 1, 2, 3, 4
  evaluation, 1
  facts regarding
    cardiac physiology in pregnancy, 1–2
    counseling for patient, 2–3
    inheritance of heart disease, 4, 4t
    optimum delivery plan, 5
    risk assessment, 2
Cardiac output, 1, 2, 2f
Cardiopulmonary resuscitation (CPR), 64,
    65t, 66
Caudal regression syndrome, 38
Ceftriaxone, 69
Centers for disease control and prevention
    (CDC), 67, 72t
Centric fusion, 97
Cephalopelvic disproportion (CPD),
    192, 220
Cerclage, 138–140. *See also under* Cervical
    incompetence
Cervical dilatation over time, 190f
Cervical incompetence
  case presentation, 137, 138, 140, 141
  cerclage
    based on indication class, 139t
    preparation for, 138–139
    technique, 139–140
  characteristics of, 137, 138t
  patient management, 141
  risk factors, 137–138
Cervical insufficiency. *See* Cervical
    incompetence
Cervical length measurements,
    distribution of, 138f
Cervical ripening, 189
Cesarean delivery, 30, 64, 85, 116, 161,
    211, 219
Cesarean hysterectomy, 169
Chest x-ray, 83
Chlamydia trachomatis, 68
Chorioamniotics. *See* Rupture of
    membranes
Chromosomal trisomies, 97
Chronic hypertension (CHTN)
  blood pressure changes, 26f
  categorization of, 23
  definition of, 23
  case presentation, 23, 24–25, 26, 27
  essential hypertension
    nontreatable risks for, 24
    treatable risks for, 24
  etiology of, 24
  evaluation, 23–24

fetal evaluation, 27
  risk assessment, 25
  secondary hypertension, 25t
  second-trimester drop in BP, 26
  treatment of, 25–26
CHTN. *See* Chronic hypertension
Clark's mortality index, 3t
Cleft lip diagnosis, 134f
Clotting studies, 204
Coagulopathy, 55, 63, 179, 180, 180t, 204
Coarctation of aorta, 25t
Color Doppler sonography, 50f
Colostrum, 225
Complete breech, 161f
Complete placenta previa, 172, 172f
Compression ultrasound, 53
Computed tomography pulmonary
    angiography (CTPA), 54
Congenital syphilis. *See under* Sexually
    transmitted diseases
Contraction stress test (CST), 184, 184t
Contrecoup effect, 62
Cord occlusion, 107
Corticosteroids, 148
Couvelaire uterus, 178
CPD. *See* Cephalopelvic disproportion
CPR. *See* Cardiopulmonary resuscitation
Cromolyn sodium, 7
Crystalloid infusion, 21
CST. *See* Contraction stress test
CTPA. *See* Computed tomography
    pulmonary angiography
Cushing Syndrome, 25t
Cyanotic congenital heart disease, 3
Cyclooxygenase inhibitors, 94
Cystitis, 12

D

D-dimer, 54
Deep venous thrombosis (DVT), 53
  algorithm for, 54f
Desmopressin, 124
Diabetes in pregnancy
  blood sugar management, 36
  case presentation, 36, 37, 39, 40
  classification of, 37
  on fetus and neonate, diabetes,
    38–39, 39t
  insulin dose calculation, 37, 37t
  intra and postpartum management, 39
  natural history of, 36–37, 37t
  patient management, 39
Diabetic ketoacidosis, 36
  fetal consequence, 37f
Diamniotic twins, 105, 106
DIC. *See* Disseminated intravascular
    coagulation
Didelphic uterus, 150–151
Disseminated intravascular coagulation
    (DIC), 61, 180t, 216
Diuretics, 26
Dizygotic twins, 103
DNA (genetic) testing, 96
Doppler of ductus venosus, 111
Down syndrome
  adults with, 100t
  child with, 98f, 99–100

karyotype of female with translocation,
    97, 98f
  newborn with, 101
  risk for, 97
  See also Fetal chromosomal anomaly
Duodenal atresia, double bubble sign of,
    129f
DVT. *See* Deep venous thrombosis

E

Early ultrasound, 96
Echocardiography, 217
Edwards syndrome, 100
EFW. *See* Estimated fetal weight
EIA. *See* Enzyme immunoassay
Eisenmenger's syndrome, 2
ELISA. *See* Enzyme-linked
    immunosorbent assay
Env (envelope glycoprotein), 81
Enzyme immunoassay (EIA), 81
Enzyme-linked immunosorbent assay
    (ELISA), 81
Episiotomy, 198
Erythromycin, 68
Escherichia coli, 14
Essential hypertension
  nontreatable risks for, 24
  treatable risks for, 24
  See also Chronic hypertension
Estimated fetal weight (EFW), 156
External cephalic version (ECV), 162, 162f
Extraamniotic coelom, 103
Extramedullary hematopoiesis, 41

F

Familial down syndrome, 97
FASD. *See* Fetal alcohol spectrum
    disorders
Fasting, 35
Female genital tract, 150
Ferning of amniotic fluid, 155f
Fetal alcohol spectrum disorders (FASD),
    135
Fetal anomaly, 128
Fetal chromosomal anomaly
  adults with down syndrome, 100t
  child with down syndrome, 98f, 99–100
  chromosomal abnormalities, prognosis
    of, 100
  chromosomal rearrangements, 97–99,
    98f, 99f
  clinical case, 97, 99, 101–102
  down syndrome risk for, 97
  fetal echocardiogram, 99
  newborn with down syndrome, 101
Fetal dose estimation (radiation), 131t
Fetal echocardiogram, 39, 99, 135
Fetal fibronectin, 144
Fetal gestational ages, 157t
Fetal goiter, 77
Fetal growth, 9
  evaluation, 27
  monitoring, 116
Fetal head delivery, 163
Fetal heart rate (FHR), 214t
  acceleration, 185f
  management of, 213

prolonged decelerations, 213–215
    tracing, 88f, 170, 189f, 191f, 192f, 193f
Fetal hyperinsulinemia, 196
Fetal intraperitoneal transfusion, 46
Fetal macrosomia, 114–115, 115t
Fetal renal agenesis, 125
Fetal renal arteries, 123f
Fetal renal function, 121
Fetal station, loss of, 210
Fetal surveillance, 38
Fetal swallowing, 127
Fetal testing, 111, 112t
Fetal trauma, 61
Fetal urine flow, 127
Fetal weight estimation , 195–196
    in large fetus, 117, 117t
    by ultrasound, 110–111, 110t
Fetocide, 107
Fetomaternal hemorrhage, 62
Fetus, normal, 128
FHR. *See* Fetal heart rate
Fibrin split products (FSP), 61
First trimester screening, 96
First trimester twin pregnancy, 104f
Fluorescent treponemal antibody
        absorption test (FTA-ABS), 68
Follow-up ultrasound, 48
Footling breech, 161f
Forceps delivery, classification of, 220t
Four-quadrant AFI, 120f
Frank breech, 161f
Frank coagulopathy, 20
Fundal pressure, 200

G
Gadolinium, 131
Gallbladder disease, 87
Gastroparesis, 36
Gastroschisis
    fetus with, prognosis of, 93–94
    perinatal/neonatal management
        immediate postnatal management, 95
        long-term management, 95
        mode of delivery, 95
        surgical closure, 95
        timing of delivery, 95
    risk factors for, 94–95
GBS. *See* Group B streptococcus
Genetic syndromes, 121
    as cystic kidneys, 122t
    with unilateral/bilateral renal agenesis,
        121t
Genital tract lacerations, 204
Gestational diabetes mellitus (GDM), 115
    case presentation, 32, 34, 35
    definition of, 32
    detection of, 33t
    diagnosis of, 33, 33t
    glucose control in, 34t
    patient management, 35
    predictors of diabetes, 32
    risks of GDM, 34
    shoulder dystocia by birth weight, 35t
    White's classification of, 34t
Gestational thrombocytopenia, 28
Gestational transient thyrotoxicosis, 76
GFR. *See* Glomerular filtration rate

Glomerular filtration rate (GFR), 12
Glucose tolerance, 196
Glucose tolerance test (GTT), 32
Gonorrhea, 68–69
Graves' disease, 75
Group B streptococcus (GBS), 158
    infection, 148
GTT. *See* Glucose tolerance test

H
HAART (highly active antiretroviral
        therapy) treatment, 84
Hashimoto's disease, 76
Heart rate, increase in, 1
HELLP syndrome
    case presentation, 28, 29, 30, 31
    classification system, 29
    complications of, 30, 31t
    definition of, 28
    diagnosis of, 28
    mode of delivery in, 30
    patient management, 29–30
    treatments of, 30
Hematocrit, 15
Hemoconcentration, 20
Hemodynamics during parturition, 2f
Heparin, 56, 58t
Hepatitis B, 69
    vaccination, 83
Hepatitis B immune globulin (HBIG), 69
Hepatitis B surface antigen (HBsAg), 69
Highly active antiretroviral therapy
        (HAART), 84
HIV, 67
    case presentation, 80, 83, 85, 86
    delivery
        cesarean, 85
        with HIV infection, 85
    counseling for patient, 84
    HAART treatment, 84
    HIV-infected women, 83
    patient management, 80, 81t
    testing modalities, 80–83
        confirmatory test, 81
        ELISA, 81
        enzyme immunoassay, 81
        Western blot test, 81, 82
Home test kits, 82
Hospital-grade electric pumps, 228
Human chorionic gonadotropin (hCG),
        74
Human fetal urine flow, 127
Human papillomavirus (HPV) testing, 83
Human teratogens, 133t
Hydralazine, 21, 21t
Hydration, 88
Hydrops
    fetal, 42, 42t
    nonanemic, 128
Hydroureter, 12
Hyperglycemia
    fetal, 38
    maternal, 38
Hyperinsulinism, 38
Hyperlipidemia, 24
Hyperosmolarity, maternal, 129
Hyperparathyroidism, 25t

Hypertension
    chronic, 18t
    definition of, 17
    gestational, 18t
    secondary, 25t
    treatment for, 21t
    See also Chronic hypertension; Essential
        hypertension
Hypertensive disorders, 17, 18t, 19f, 21t
Hypertrophic congestive cardiomyopathy,
        38
Hyperventilation of pregnancy, 7
Hypoglycemia, 36
Hyperthyroidism, 75, 76
    treatment of, 77
Hypovolemic shock, 62
Hypoxia, 130
Hysterectomy, 168, 169
Hysterosalpingogram (HSG), 149
Hysteroscopy, 149
    with septoplasty, 152

I
Immunofluorescence assay (IFA), 82
Incomplete breech, 161f
Indomethacin, 139, 147
Indomethacin tocolysis, 51
Inhaled albuterol, 7, 8
Inherited down syndrome, 97
Insulin, 35, 114
    dose calculation, 37, 37t
    therapy, 36
Insulin-like growth factor (IGF), 115
Intentional fetal clavicular fracture, 199
Intraabdominal processes, 204
Intraamniotic infection, 139
Intramembranous flow, 127
Intrapartum therapy, 84
Intrauterine fetal death, 70
Intrauterine growth restriction (IUGR)
    case presentation, 109, 111, 113
    etiologies of, 110t
    fetal testing, 111, 112t
    fetal weight estimation, 110–111, 110t
    management of, 109–110, 113
    risk factors for, 109, 110t
Intrauterine transfusion, 46
Intravenous antibiotics, 13–14, 14t
Intravenous (IV) fluid, 5, 176
Intravenous immunoglobulin (IVIG), 47
Intravenous terbutaline, 147
Iodine, 131
Ionizing radiation, 130
Islet cell hypertrophy, 38
IUGR. *See* Intrauterine growth restriction

J
Jarisch–Herxheimer reaction, 70

K
Kaletra, 84
Keilland forceps, 221

L
Labetalol, 21, 21t, 26
Labor
    cardinal movements of, 190t

Labor (*Continued*)
  induction/augmentation, 189–190
  latent phase of, 190–191
  second stage of , 192–193
Laceration, 204
Lactation, drugs contraindicated in, 226, 227t
Laparoscopy, 149
Laparotomy, 205
Latent syphilis, 68
Latent tuberculosis 83
Leopold's maneuvers, 117f
Leukemia, childhood, 131
Liley curve for ΔOD450, 43f
Low-lying placenta, 172, 172f
Lung maturity amniocentesis, 39

M
Macrosomia
  case presentation, 114, 115, 116, 118
  definition of, 195
  delivery planning, 116
  fetal growth monitoring, 116
  fetal macrosomia, 114–115, 115t
  fetal weight estimation, 117, 117t
  patient counseling, 115
  Magnesium sulfate (MgSO4), 18, 129, 146–147
Magnesium sulfate tocolysis, 146
Magnetic resonance imaging (MRI), 151, 166
Maintenance therapy, 56
Manual breast pump, 228, 228f
Marginal placenta previa, 172, 172f
Maternal blood work, 127–128
Maternal cardiac arrest, 64
Maternal coagulopathy, 216
Maternal diabetes, 125
Maternal ECHO, 2
Maternal exhaustion, 220
Maternal febrile morbidity, 208, 209f
Maternal fluid resuscitation, 211
Maternal glucocorticoid therapy, 113
Maternal hydration, 124
Maternal hyperglycemia, 196
Maternal hypertension, 24
Maternal laceration at delivery, 183
Maternal morbidity, 2, 3t
  Clark's mortality index, 3t
Maternal pyelonephritis 15, 15t
Maternal quadruple serum screen, 133
Maternal resuscitation, 64
Maternal serum alpha fetoprotein (MSAFP)
  elevated, differential diagnosis of, 92–93, 93t
  false-positive, eliminating, 92
Maternal survival, 215
Maternal trauma, 60–61
Mauriceau maneuver, 163f
McDonald cerclage, 140
McLean forceps, 221, 223f
McRoberts' maneuver, 197–200, 197f, 198f, 200f
Medical imaging, 88, 89t
Mendelian inheritance of heart disease, 4, 4t

Methimazole (MMU), 77
Methyldopa, 26
Methylergonovine, 11, 181
Methylmercury, 135
Microhemagglutination assay for treponema pallidum (MHA-TP), 68
Middle cerebral artery (MCA), 44–45, 46
  Doppler evaluation of, 44f
Midpelvic forceps, 219
Mild hypertension, 23
Milk ejection hormone, 225
Milk production hormone, 225
Misoprostol, 188
Monochorionic twins, 103, 105, 106
Monozygotic twins, 103
Montevideo units, 192
Motor vehicle accidents, 61
MSAFP. *See* Maternal serum alpha fetoprotein
Mullerian abnormalities, classification of, 151
Multifactorial inheritance of heart disease, 4, 4t
Multiple gestation
  case presentation, 103, 106, 107
  diagnosis of, 103
  management of, 106–107
  twin gestation
    fetal risks of, 103–106
    maternal risks of, 103–106
  twin pregnancy, maternal complications in, 104
  twin–twin transfusion system, 105f, 107t
  twinning, physiology of, 103

N
National High Blood Pressure Education Program Working Group, 21
Neisseria gonorrhoeae, 68
Neonatal intensive care unit (NICU), 213
Neural tube defects (NTDs), 92
Neuraxial (regional) anesthesia, 58t
Neuroprotective peptides, 101
New York Heart Association Functional Classification of heart disease, 2, 3t
Nifedipine, 147
Nitabuch's layer, 166
Nitrazine test, 155
Nitrofurantoin, 14
Nonanemic hydrops, 128
Nonnucleoside reverse transcriptase inhibitors (NNRTIs), 84
Nonselective cyclooxygenase (COX)-2 inhibitor, 147
Nonsteroidal anti-inflammatory drugs, 226
Nonstress test (NST), 27, 111, 184, 184t
Nonsyndromic congenital heart disease, risk for, 5t
Northern California Kaiser Permanente study, 32
NST. *See* Nonstress test
Nuchal cords, 200
Nuchal translucency screening, 133
Nuclear medicine studies, 131
Nucleic acid hybridization tests (NAATs), 68

Nucleoside reverse transcriptase inhibitors (NRTIs), 84

O
Obesity 24
Obstetric events, adverse, 4t
Obstetrical forceps, 223f, 224f
Obstetrical hemorrhage, approach to, 173t, 174, 174t
Oligohydramnios, 186
  case presentation, 119, 122, 123, 124
  definition of, 119, 120f
  diagnosis of, 119–120
  evaluation of, 123
  genetic syndromes, 121t, 122t
  pathophysiology of, 121–122, 121t, 122t, 123f
  prognosis of, 123, 123t
Oliguria, 20
Operative delivery
  case presentation, 219, 220, 221, 224
  instrumental deliveries
    indications/contraindications for, 220–221
    types of, 219–220, 220t
  instruments available for, 221
  management of, 219
Operative vaginal delivery, 211
Oral contraceptive pills (OCPs), 132
Oral desensitization protocol, 71t
Oral narcotics, 226
Ovarian malignancies, 49t
Ovarian neoplasms in young women, 48
Oxytocin, 85, 204, 211, 225
  augmentation, 192
  infusion, 191, 192

P
Pancreatitis, 87
Papanicolaou test, 83
Partial placenta previa, 172, 172f
Patau syndrome, 100
Paternal blood type evaluation, 42
Peak expiratory flow (PEF), 8, 10f
Peak expiratory flow rate (PEFR), 8
Pelvic inflammatory disease (PID), 68
Pelvic mass in pregnancy
  abdominal pain, diagnosis of, 51
  case presentation, 48–52
  decision making, 48
  facts regarding
    ovarian neoplasms in young women, 48
    predictors of malignancy, 49
    risks of surgery, 50–51
  patient management during surgery, 51
Penicillin, 148
  desensitization in STD, 69
  treatment, congenital syphilis and, 70, 70f
Percutaneous umbilical blood sampling (PUBS), 43, 46
Perinatal mortality and BPP score, 186f
Phenytoin (dilantin), 132
Pheochromocytoma, 25t
Placenta accrete
  case presentation, 165, 166, 168, 169
  diagnosis of, 165, 166, 168

incidence and types of, 165–166
management of, 169
pathophysiology of, 166, 168f
surgical options with, 168
ultrasound findings of, 167f
Placenta percreta, 165, 166f
Placenta previa, 178
case presentation, 170, 171, 174, 175
definition of, 172
evaluation, 171
management of, 172–173
obstetrical hemorrhage, approach to,
173t, 174, 174t
recurrent acute bleed management, 174
third trimester vaginal bleeding,
170–171, 171f
types of, 172, 172f
Placental abruption, 60, 63, 120, 170,
171t, 178–179, 179t
abruption classification, 179t
blood replacement in DIC, 180, 180t
case presentation, 176, 178, 179, 180,
181
diagnosis of, 178, 179–180, 180t
evaluation of, 176
vaginal bleeding
diagnosis, 177–178, 177t
resuscitation, 176–177
Placental perfusion, 20
Plasmapheresis, 30
Platelet transfusion, 29
Pneumococcal vaccine, 83
Pneumocystis jiroveci pneumonia
(PCP), 83
Pol, 81
Polycythemia, 38
Polyhydramnios, 37, 121
abnormalities associated with, 126f
amniotic fluid dynamics, 126–128
case presentation, 125, 127, 128, 129
definition of, 125
differential diagnosis of, 125, 127t
duodenal atresia, double bubble sign
of, 129f
patient evaluation
fetal anemia, 128
fetal anomaly, 128
maternal blood work, 127–128
nonanemic hydrops, 128
normal fetus, 128
targeted ultrasound, 127
patient management, 128–129
Polymerized chain reaction (PCR), 82
Postdated pregnancy
antenatal testing, 184t
biophysical profile, 185, 186f
contraction stress test, 184
nonstress test, 184
case presentation, 182, 183, 184
patient counseling, 183–184, 183f
patient management, 182
postterm pregnancy, 184
pregnancy dating, 182–183, 183t
Postmaturity syndrome, 186
Postpartum hemorrhage (PPH)
case presentation, 202, 203–204, 205,
206, 207f

cause of maternal death, 202
definition of, 202, 203f, 203t
evaluation of, 204–205
patient management, 204
risk assessment, 202–203, 204t
surgical options for, 206, 206f
uterine atony, management of, 205,
205f, 205t, 206t
Postpartum thyroiditis, 76
Postterm pregnancy, 184
Potassium iodide, 77
PPH. See Postpartum hemorrhage
Preeclampsia, 15, 37
case presentation, 17, 18, 20, 21, 22
diagnosis of, 17, 18t
facts regarding
hypertensive disorders in pregnancy,
17, 18t, 19f
recurrence of preeclampsia, 21–22
systemic effects of preeclampsia, 20
patient management, 18, 20, 21
medications for, 21t
severe, 19t, 28, 29t
Pregestational diabetes, 36
Pregnancy
associated thyroid disease, 76
dating, 182–183, 183t
loss rates, 183
outcomes
with Mullerian anomalies, 152t
with septate uterus, 152t
Pregnant trauma patient, acute
management of, 62f
Premature rupture of membranes
(PROM), 154
Preterm labor (PTL), 51
case presentation, 142, 143, 146,
148
definition of, 142
and delivery, 142, 143f
diagnosis of, 146
risk management for, 142–143, 144t
screening for, 144–145
treatment of
antibiotics, 148
corticosteroids, 148
indomethacin, 147
magnesium sulfate, 146–147
nifedipine, 147
Preterm premature rupture of membrane
(PPROM), 120, 154
Primary aldosteronism, 25t
Primary syphilis, 68
Prior cesarean section, 165
Prior uterine incision, 211
Progesterone, 143
Prolactin, 225
Propylthiouracil (PTU), 77
Protease inhibitors (PIs), 84
Proteinuria, 17, 18t
PTL. See Preterm labor
PUBS. See Percutaneous umbilical blood
sampling
Pulmonary artery capillary, 217f
Pulmonary disease
case presentation, 7, 9, 11
changes in pulmonary function, 8f

facts regarding
asthma management, 8, 8t, 9, 9t
prognosis of asthma, 10–11
respiratory physiology in pregnancy, 7
outpatient management algorithm
for, 10f
prenatal care, 9–10
treatment of, 7–8, 10
See also Asthma
Pyelonephritis, 36
case presentation, 12, 14, 16
facts regarding
asymptomatic bacteriuria, definitions
of, 12–13
maternal and fetal complications of,
15, 15t
physiologic changes in urinary tract,
12, 13f
intravenous antibiotics for, 13–14, 14t
failure of, 14
maternal risks of, 15, 15t
Pyrazinamide, 83

Q
Queenan curve for ?OD450, 44f
Quintero system, 106, 107t

R
Radiation
on fetus, 130–132, 131t
intrauterine exposure to, 130
Radioablation, thyroid, 78
Rales on lung examination, 1
Rapid HIV testing, 67, 82
Rapid plasma reagin (RPR) test, 68, 71,
72, 73
RBC alloimmunization. See Red Blood
Cell Alloimmunization
Recurrent acute bleed management, 174
Red Blood Cell Alloimmunization
case presentation, 41, 42–43, 45–46, 47
counseling for mother, 47
definition of, 41, 42t
evaluation, 41–42
fetal anemia, risk for, 43–45, 43f,
44f
management of, 46
pathophysiology of, 42f
Renal agenesis, 121, 121t
Renal insufficiency, 15
Renal parenchyma, 14
Renal parenchymal disease, 25t
Renal ultrasound, 14
Renal vascular disease, 25t
Resuscitation, 176–177
blood components in, 174t
Rh alloimmunization, 45f
RhD–immune globulin, 174
RNA viral load test, 82
Robertsonian translocation, 97
Rubin maneuver, 198, 199f
Rupture of membranes
case presentation, 154, 155–156, 158,
159
clinical decision making, 15
delivery planning, 156
delivery timing, 159

Rupture of membranes (*Continued*)
  interventions to prolong latent period
    antenatal corticosteroids, 158
    antibiotics, 158
    tocolytics, 158
  patient counseling, 156
  preterm premature rupture of
      membranes, 157t
    contraindications to, 158t
    definition of, 154
    diagnosis of, 154–155, 155t
  premature rupture of membranes, 154
  spontaneous rupture of membranes, 154

S
Second trimester loss, etiologies of, 149,
    150t
Second trimester serum screening, 96
Secondary hypertension, 24, 25t
Secondary syphilis, 68
Seizures, 20
Septate uterus, 151
Septostomy, 107
Serial amnioreduction, 106, 107
Seroconversion in pregnancy, 81, 81t
Serologic test for syphilis, 68
Serum tryptase, 216
Severe hypertension, 23, 26
Sexually transmitted diseases (STD)
  case presentation, 67, 69, 71, 72
  congenital syphilis
    CDC recommendations for
        treatment, 72t
    infants at risk, evaluation for, 72–73
    and penicillin treatment, 70, 70f
  patient management, 71–72
  penicillin desensitization in, 69
  screening and treatment
    chlamydia, 68
    gonorrhea, 68–69
    hepatitis B, 69
    HIV, 67,
    syphilis, 68
  testing, 67
Shirdokar cerclage, 140
Shoulder dystocia, 116
  case presentation, 195, 196, 201
  fetal weight estimation, 195–196
  macrosomia, definition of, 195
  management of, 196, 197
  maneuvers for, 197–200, 197f, 198f,
      200f
  risk factors for birth injury, 196
  risks
    of fetal injury during, 200–201
    for mothers, 201
Simpson forceps, 223f, 224f
Single deepest pocket (SDP) of amniotic
    fluid, 125
Sinus tachycardia, 217
Smoking, 142
Sonographic fetal biometry, 195
Sonohysterogram, 149
Spectinomycin, 69
Spontaneous Rupture of Membranes
    (SROM), 154
STD. *See* Sexually transmitted diseases

Step therapy of asthma, 9t
Sterile speculum examination, 178
Steroids, 141
  inhaled, 7
Stillbirth, 183
Stroke volume, increase in, 1
Subclinical hypothyroidism, 76
Symphysiotomy, 199
Syphilis, 68
Syphilis spirochetes, 70

T
TBII. *See* TSH binding inhibitory
    immunoglobulin
Tennessee classification (HELLP
    syndrome), 28
Terbutaline, 138
Term Breech Trial in 2000, 161
Tertiary syphilis, 68
Tetracycline, 69
Teratogens
  case presentation, 130, 132, 134, 136
  risk identification, 130
  facts regarding
    drug teratogen categorization, 132,
        132t, 133t
    fetal effects of exposure to radiation,
        130–132, 131t
    first trimester fetal anatomy survey,
        134
    neurobehavioral alterations, 135
  fetal diagnosis of, 133–134
  pregnancy management, 135
Theophylline, 7
Thioamides, 77
Third trimester vaginal bleeding, 170–171,
    171f
Thrombocytopenia, 20
Thrombophilia, testing for, 57t
Thrombosis, 51
Thyroid-binding globulin (TBG), 74
Thyroid disease, 25t
  case presentation, 74, 76, 77, 78, 79
  counseling, 78–79
  facts regarding
    hyperthyroidism, 75, 77
    hypothyroidism, 76
    pregnancy-associated thyroid disease,
        76
    thyroid physiology, 74
    thyroid storm, treatment of, 78, 78t
  pregnancy on thyroid hormones, 75f
  signs/symptoms of, 75t
  thyroid function tests, 74
Thyroid storm, treatment of, 78, 78t
Thyroidectomy, 77
Thyroid-stimulating hormone (TSH), 74
Thyrotoxicosis, 76, 77
Tocodynamometer, 61
Tocolysis, 20, 51, 89, 146, 158, 173
Total parenteral nutrition (TPN), 94
Toxoplasma gondii, 83
Transabdominal amnioinfusion, 124
Transvaginal placement, 140
Transvaginal sonography (TVS), 171
Trauma
  case presentation, 60, 63, 64, 66

diagnosis of, 63–64
facts regarding
    cardiopulmonary resuscitation, 64,
        65t, 66
    fetal trauma, 61
    maternal trauma, 60–61
    fetal and neonatal consequences, 61, 63
    guidelines for stable patient, 60
    management of patient, 61, 62f
    obstetric management, 64
Treponemal-specific antibody tests, 71
Trial labor, 209t
Triglyceride, 115
Trophoblast, 166
TSH binding inhibitory immunoglobulin
    (TBII), 75
TTTS. *See* Twin–twin transfusion
    syndrome
Twin gestation, 103–106
Twin pregnancy
  first trimester, 104f
  maternal complications in, 104
Twinning
  monochorionic, 103
  physiology of, 103
Twin–twin transfusion syndrome (TTTS),
    105f, 107t

U
Ultrasound, 39, 42, 195
  abdominal, 88
  for amniotic fluid volume assessment,
      154
  for cervical cerclage, 139
  fetal measurement, 183
  fetal weight estimation by, 110–111, 110t
  for macrosomia, 117
  for multiple gestation, 106
  for pelvic masses, 49, 50
  placenta previa, 171
  targeted, 127
  teratogens, 133
  in thyroid disease, 77
  for trauma patient, 60
  uterine anomalies, 149
  vaginal, 144
  venous thromboembolism, 53
Ultrasound diagnosis of congenital
    anomaly
  case presentation, 92, 93, 93t, 95, 96
  elevated MSAFP, differential diagnosis
      of, 92–93, 93t
  false-positive MSAFP, eliminating, 92
  gastroschisis
    fetus with, prognosis of, 93–94
    perinatal/neonatal management, 95
    risk factors for, 94–95
  patient counseling, 96
  umbilical artery Doppler assessment, 94
Ultrasound transvaginal examination of
    cervix, 145
Umbilical artery Doppler assessment, 94
Umbilical artery Doppler flow
    velocimetry, fetal, 135
Unicornuate uterus, 150
Unscarred uterus, 211
Ureteral stent, 14

Urinary obstructions, fetal, 122, 122t
Urinary tract, physiologic changes in, 12, 13f
Urothelium, 12
Uterine anomalies
    case presentation, 149, 151
    developmental abnormalities, types of
        bicornuate uterus, 151
        didelphic uterus, 150–151
        septate uterus, 151
        unicornuate uterus, 150
    diagnostic testing for, 151–152
    management options, 152–153
    Mullerian abnormalities, classification of, 151
    pregnancy outcomes with, 152, 152t
    screening for, 149–150
    second trimester loss, etiologies of, 149, 150t
Uterine artery branches, anatomy of, 207f
Uterine atony, management of, 205, 205f, 205t, 206t
Uterine packing, 205
Uterine reunification (Strassman), 153
Uterine rupture
    bladder injury, 210
    case presentation, 208, 209–210, 211, 212
    cesarean delivery, 211

loss of fetal station, 210
maternal bleeding, 210
outcome of (in USA and India), 210t, 21211
risk factors for, 211, 211t
VBAC
    patient selection for, 208–209, 209t
    risks of, 208, 209t
Uterine vasculature in pregnancy, 19f
Uterotonic use in PPH, 206t

V
Vacuum delivery, 220, 221
Vacuum extraction, 221, 222
Vagal tone, 213Vaginal birth after cesarean (VBAC)
    patient selection for, 208–209
    risks of, 208, 209f, 209t
Vaginal bleeding. *See under* Placental abruption
Vaginal delivery, 90–91, 162
    after cesarean, 209t
Vaginal ultrasound, 144
Valsalva maneuver, 220
Vasa previa, 171, 171t
Vascular resistance, 2
VBAC. *See* Vaginal birth after cesarean
VDRL test. *See* Venereal disease research laboratory

Venereal disease research laboratory (VDRL) test, 68, 71
Venous thromboembolism (VTE)
    case presentation, 53, 55–56, 57, 58
    diagnostic test, 53–55, 54f
        additional, 56–57, 57t
    facts regarding
        anticoagulated patient, delivery planning in, 58, 58t
        thromboembolic disease in pregnancy, 55
    management of, 57
    treatment of, 56
Ventilation perfusion (VQ) scanning, 54
Virchow's triad in pregnancy, 55f
VTE. *See* Venous thromboembolism

W
Warfarin, 3
Western blot test, 81, 82
White's classification of, 34t
Wood's screw maneuver, 198

Z
Zavanelli maneuver, 199, 200
Zidovudine (ZDV), 80, 84
Zygosity, 42, 103